Empowering Behavior Change in Patients

Empowering Behavior Change in Patients: Practical Strategies for the Healthcare Professional reviews medical research and pairs it with behavior change theories to create counseling strategies and tools that equip the reader to empower others to adopt and sustain change. With contributions by leading physicians, PhDs, Doctorates in Behavioral Health, health coaches, and other experts in behavior change, this book presents a variety of perspectives, backgrounds, and educational experiences encouraging readers to alter their counseling practices to include more behavior change and coaching strategies.

Features

- Gives guidance from renowned behavior change experts, as well as medical students and healthcare professional students in training, to create a unique mix of well-established theories and practices, review articles and research, and tools and strategies in addition to perspectives on change to use when counseling individuals with chronic conditions and those looking to prevent disease. It is written for people who are just starting their journey in behavior change counseling to those who have been practicing for years.
- Gives healthcare professionals tools to be empowering messengers by relaying this information to patients in relatable, inspiring ways.
- Features successful case studies throughout and provides examples of language to use when counseling individuals.
- Provides cutting-edge examples of the effectiveness of group visits to help create sustainable change which is a healthcare trend that is up and coming.
- Shares concrete strategies to help readers move forward in their own behavior change journeys as well as to help others, whether patients, colleagues, students, or loved ones, in making strides toward optimal health and well-being.
- Implements lifestyle medicine concepts and principles.
- Includes a summary and takeaway points for the reader in each chapter.

A volume in the *Lifestyle Medicine* series, this book is intended for healthcare professionals who want to empower people to adopt and sustain healthy lifestyles based on the six pillars of lifestyle medicine, which include routine physical activity, nutritious eating patterns, sound sleep, positive social connections, stress resilience, and avoidance of risky substances. This book is a solid resource for information on behavior change in healthcare benefiting not only the healthcare industry and students, but also parents, teachers, and anyone who cares for an individual with a chronic condition such as diabetes, heart disease, hypertension, or obesity, as well as those looking to prevent the onset of disease.

Lifestyle Medicine

Series Editor

James M. Rippe

Professor of Medicine,
University of Massachusetts Medical School

Led by James M. Rippe, MD, founder of the Rippe Lifestyle Institute, this series is directed to a broad range of researchers and professionals consisting of topical books with clinical applications in nutrition and health, physical activity, obesity management, and applicable subjects in lifestyle medicine.

Manual of Lifestyle Medicine

James M. Rippe

Obesity Prevention and Treatment

A Practical Guide

James M. Rippe and John P. Foreyt

Improving Women's Health Across the Lifespan

Michelle Tollefson, Nancy Eriksen, and Neha Pathak

Lifestyle Nursing

Gia Merlo and Kathy Berra

Integrating Lifestyle Medicine in Cardiovascular Health and Disease Prevention

James M. Rippe

Lifestyle Medicine for Prediabetes, Type 2 Diabetes, and Cardiometabolic Disease

Michael A. Via and Jeffrey Mechanick

Empowering Behavior Change in Patients

Practical Strategies for the Healthcare Professional

Beth Frates, MD and Mark D. Faries, PhD

For more information, please visit: www.routledge.com/Lifestyle-Medicine/book-series/CRCLM

Empowering Behavior Change in Patients
Practical Strategies for the Healthcare Professional

Edited by
Beth Frates, MD and
Mark D. Faries, PhD

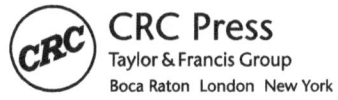

CRC Press
Taylor & Francis Group
Boca Raton London New York

CRC Press is an imprint of the
Taylor & Francis Group, an **informa** business

First edition published 2024
by CRC Press
6000 Broken Sound Parkway NW, Suite 300, Boca Raton, FL 33487-2742

and by CRC Press
4 Park Square, Milton Park, Abingdon, Oxon, OX14 4RN

CRC Press is an imprint of Taylor & Francis Group, LLC

© 2024 selection and editorial matter, Beth Frates and Mark D. Faries; individual chapters, the contributors

ISBN: 9780367751517 (hbk)
ISBN: 9780367751500 (pbk)
ISBN: 9781003161226 (ebk)

DOI: 10.1201/9781003161226

Typeset in Times
by codeMantra

Contents

Preface

In our earliest conversations about this book, we discussed how wonderful it would be to have a book that practitioners could pull off their bookshelves and directly apply the material in that book to their practice of helping others initiate, adopt, and maintain healthy lifestyles. From one aspect, it needed to be a practical resource–less like a sterile manual and more like a trusted, well-worn tool. Of course, behavior change is complex, so instructions were needed, but they are provided as more of a companion, mentor, and guide–directions, not dogma. Each chapter needed to be written by evidence-based experts, not only in knowledge, but also in experience– who not only have passion, but also compassion. It would help us meet others where they are while also reminding us that others meet us where we are. It would be the book that we desired for ourselves, the one we would pull off the bookshelves throughout our careers. We now hope it will be that book for you.

Series Preface

"How beautiful the river flows and the birds they sing. But you and I we're messier things."

Bruce Springstein
The Big Muddy

"They won't care about what you know until they know that you care."

Nick Saban
Six Time National Champion Alabama Football Coach

It is a great pleasure to write a Preface for this important, well-written, timely and authoritative book *Empowering Behavior Change in Patients: Practical Strategies for the Healthcare Professional*.

Behavior change provides the core and foundation of lifestyle medicine and, indeed, all of medicine. I recognized this fact as early as the first edition of my multi-authored *Lifestyle Medicine* textbook, which introduced this field in the academic literature in 1999.[1] Indeed, I have included substantial sections on behavioral medicine in all four editions of this *Lifestyle Medicine* textbook which has now grown to a massive tome with over 325 contributors. Behavioral medicine has comprised an important section in all four editions of this textbook.[2–4]

It is in this context that I came to know Drs. Beth Frates and Mark Faries. Dr. Frates has edited the superb behavioral medicine sections of the third and fourth editions of my *Lifestyle Medicine* textbook. Dr. Faries has contributed important chapters in each of these editions. These two healthcare professionals are acknowledged experts in both behavioral change and lifestyle medicine. You could not find better guides to lead you on your journey to understand the importance of behavioral change in lifestyle medicine and, indeed, in all of modern healthcare.

Drs. Frates and Faries have assembled an all-star cast of contributors, a veritable "who's who" of experts in virtually all aspects of behavioral medicine. These experts have, in turn, delivered an evidence-based and motivational compendium of virtually all aspects of behavioral change and seamlessly linked this evidence to the rapidly growing field of lifestyle medicine. The book is a *tour de force*!

This book contains important chapters in such diverse areas as coaching, stages of change, confidence building, motivational interviewing, health determination theory, the power of autonomy, and many other topics central to behavioral modification and essential to helping human beings make positive changes in their lives.

Empowering Behavior Change in Patients: Practical Strategies for the Healthcare Professional is the latest volume in the series of single topic *Lifestyle Medicine Series* textbooks where I have had the honor to serve as series editor. It joins previously published volumes in obesity prevention, cardiovascular medicine, women's health, nursing, diabetes, mental health, metabolic syndrome prevention, and many others. Additional volumes are intended in the next 2 years in family practice, psychiatry and health equity, geriatrics, and medical education. All of these books in the *Lifestyle*

Medicine Series are united by the central concept of how these diverse fields interact with lifestyle medicine.

In all of these books, I have challenged the editors to select the most capable and recognized experts in each field to deliver content which is evidence-based, practical and motivational. Drs. Frates and Faries and colleagues have delivered on this mandate with aplomb!

While there are diverse chapters in this book, the theme that unifies them is that in order to deliver impactful, behavioral change physicians and other healthcare workers must shed the mantle of "expert advice givers" and share that authority and perspective with their patients (referred to in this book as "clients") through the "coach" model After all, these "clients" are the true experts in their lives.

This is not to deny the hard-earned expertise that each of us has achieved through many years of rigorous training and/or practice in our chosen professions either as physicians or other healthcare workers. The mandate espoused in this book involves adopting a change in perspective to literally and figuratively reach out across the table to promote a passionate, genuine, and authentic dialogue with mutual respect and trust with our patients. This fundamental shift in attitude shows that we understand that true change will only come if the individual we are counseling embraces lifestyle changes in terms that are meaningful to the unique reality and challenges of each of their lives.

This shift in perspective will often require courage and commitment on the part of physicians and other healthcare workers. It requires adopting an openness and receptivity to dialogue. This will require us to shed many of the trappings of medical expertise we have worked so hard to master and adopt a fundamentally new, but still evidence-based, approach to helping our patients achieve their goals. We must overcome some of the perspectives that our careers have taught us. After all, as the legendary psychologist Dr. Abraham Maslow famously declared: "If all you have is a hammer, everything looks like a nail."[5]

The profound truth of Dr. Maslow's statement came home to me early in my career as a cardiologist. I had trained at some of the top medical institutions in America and was just launching my career. I had worked hard to master the difficult discipline of cardiology and truly saw myself as a "hammer" determined to impart this hard-earned expertise to my patients who, in essence, I was, unfortunately, in retrospect, treating as "nails." After all, I thought I could tell them all the important things I knew about the treatment of cardiovascular disease and anticipate that they would follow my advice.

Sometimes it worked, but in one particular case it did not, and I learned a profound lesson from it which I have attempted to embody throughout my subsequent career. In this particular patient encounter in cardiovascular clinic, I went through my litany of standard questions for an individual with stable angina to determine if he was experiencing additional symptoms that would require an adjustment in his medicines. When I finally turned away from him to write some new prescriptions, he suddenly blurted out with tears in his eyes "Doc, my wife has left me." I was ashamed that in my rapid-fire questions, I had missed the real reason for his appointment. It was an early example of using an "expert" mindset as opposed to more open "coaching" mindset. Since then, I have strived to do better. Although I am not perfect in this area, I think it has helped me a great deal to become a compassionate physician.

While every chapter in this book is filled with multiple aspects of state-of-the-art evidence, they also contain abundant practical strategies and motivational examples. Most importantly, these chapter authors infuse their discussions with not only expert knowledge but also profound compassion and humanity.

The thread that winds through virtually every chapter in this book is the difference between an "expert approach" and a "coaching approach." The expert approach, which is so prevalent in medical training, is based on offering factual advice with the expectation that the client will deferentially incorporate this expertise and automatically make recommended changes. This has led us to a situation where over 50% of medicines that we prescribe are not taken either accurately or *at all* by our patients. In contrast, the "coaching" approach offers a shared dialogue space where the physician meets the client where they are currently at and mutually examines ways to make meaningful changes.

Dr. Frates has previously developed the mnemonic "COACH" to underscore the personal traits such an individual must possess to effectively meet this mandate: Curious, Open Minded, Appreciative, Compassionate and Honest.

Those of us who have been fortunate enough to participate in youth athletics or have children who have participated in sports know how powerful and inspiring a great coach can be. Unfortunately, in medicine, our training seems to have moved us away from this important coaching mindset and model. We have moved away from this mindset to our own detriment and importantly that of our patients. Numerous studies have shown that physicians who truly reach out and understand their patients with compassion are more likely to achieve goals such as compliance with advice and even the likelihood that individuals will take their medicines as prescribed.

Behavior change is essential for most patients to improve their lifestyle and health. Life is complex and challenging. Old habits are hard to break. New ones may be difficult or anxiety provoking to accomplish. When I speak to young healthcare professionals about such issues as counseling their clients in areas such as regular exercise, improved nutrition, and weight loss, I challenge them to think about areas in their own lives where they know something that they should be doing and yet have found it hard to actually achieve. I often give an example from my own life, which is dental flossing. I have had excellent dental care since childhood, but for many years I found it hard to add flossing to my regular tooth brushing technique, despite knowing that I should. Finally, a new dentist managed to convince me, while she was cleaning my teeth, that teeth should last a lifetime and that my gums would stop bleeding if I added this simple procedure to the rest of the comprehensive routine I had been using for many years. Her framing of this practice to act in my own self-interest, as I was already doing in many other aspects of my life, finally got through to me. When I walked out of the office, I was able to embrace this simple procedure, much to the pleasure of my dentist and the improvement of my dental health! Without any formal training in behavioral medicine, my dentist displayed the fundamental principles outlined in many chapters of this book. She tapped into my "intrinsic motivation," helped me "overcome several obstacles" and "focused on my strengths."

One aspect of this important book that particularly struck me is the repeated mention that healthcare workers who adopt these behavioral changes for the benefit of their patients will also benefit themselves. This mindset gets us back to the reason we entered medicine in the first place...to truly make the lives of our patients healthier. It is also a powerful way to improve our own health and lower the risk of such important problems as physician burnout by deriving the satisfaction of helping our patients in these important, humane ways.

There is an additional reason why clinicians should consider adopting a "coach" strategy rather than an "expert" strategy. We are in a position to enormously influence the behavior of the students, residents and fellows who we train. Unfortunately, most medical education is geared to disparage people in training and make them feel less worthwhile than they did when they entered the profession. That is an enormous problem and carries implications for how they, in turn, will treat physicians in training under their supervision when they ultimately leave their own training. We need to be careful since we are trained as "hammers" not to see our students as "nails!" Most individuals who enter medical school have been at the top of their class in college and are accustomed to receiving kudos for their intelligence and drive. There is no reason to take this from them. It is destructive and often may lead to discouragement, self-doubt, and ultimately, burnout.

I want to close this Preface with an example from my own life which I believe underscores the power of the behavior change/coaching model which permeates this book.

Many years ago, between my third and fourth years in medical school, a series of circumstances arose in my life which fundamentally challenged my commitment to become a doctor. Many aspects of the training, at that point, had left me discouraged and doubtful about my initial commitment. Seeking some advice, I went to a senior physician who had been my mentor during two rotations in the coronary care unit. I told him that I was going to quit medical school because it clearly wasn't the right fit for me. He calmly and immediately closed the papers that he was working on and stood up and said: "You need to have somebody go out and get drunk with you." Now I am not suggesting that people go and get drunk during the course of the day, but this gesture from a senior physician, who I respected as a mentor, clearly underscored to me that my life and future meant more to him than any plans he had previously scheduled for that afternoon.

When we got to the bar and had each ordered a beer, my mentor let me start the conversation. He refrained from trying to convince me to stay in medical school and offered no judgment about my decision to quit. Instead, he listened carefully and occasionally offered his own viewpoints on issues at Harvard Medical School which made him uncomfortable and frustrated. His gesture of care and compassion made a profound difference in my life and essentially saved my medical career.

What this senior physician did came naturally for him. He exhibited great caring, allowed me to exhibit "personal autonomy" and helped me conclude with my own "self-determination." These are all principles that came naturally to him, but are outlined in considerable detail with enormous research backing in chapters in this book.

As physicians let's not forget that we are also mentors not only to our patients, but to individuals under our supervision who are in training. In fact, my first Chief of

Medicine when I started my academic career told me that every successful clinician needed to start with a good mentor and then carried the obligation to "pay it forward" by becoming a good mentor him or herself.

This is, in essence, the message reiterated over, and over again in chapters throughout this wonderful book. We all went into medicine to help change the lives of people that we care for and derive satisfaction from doing this. That is what this book is about…truly reaching out to patients and helping them make important changes in their lives. Nothing could be more timely or important.

I recognize that we all face challenges in multiple areas such as limited time to see patients, the burden of medical records, etc., but we need to find a way to blend those realities with the important mandate of helping people improve their lives. This is the essence of both behavior change and lifestyle medicine.

I hope every physician and other healthcare workers will read this book and benefit from the important lessons contained in it. Behavior change is what we should all be about and here is a beautiful map to guide us on this important journey!

James M. Rippe, MD
Founder and Director, Rippe Lifestyle Institute
Professor of Medicine, UMass Chan Medical School

REFERENCES

1. Rippe JM: *Lifestyle Medicine*, London: Blackwell Science, Inc., 1999.
2. Rippe JM: *Lifestyle Medicine* (2nd ed), Boca Raton: CRC Press, 2013.
3. Rippe JM. *Lifestyle Medicine* (3rd edition). Boca Raton: CRC Press, 2019.
4. Rippe JM. *Lifestyle Medicine* (4th edition). Boca Raton: CRC Press, 2023.
5. Maslow, AH. *Toward a Psychology of Being*. Princeton, NJ: Van Nostrand, 1962.

Editors

Beth Frates, MD, FACLM, DipABLM, is a trained physiatrist and a health and wellness coach. Dr. Frates has devoted the majority of her career to lifestyle medicine and health and wellness coaching. Teaching is a passion for her, and she has received multiple teaching accolades over the years from Harvard Medical School, where she is an assistant clinical professor, and also from Harvard Extension School, where she has taught Introduction to Lifestyle Medicine for a decade. Dr. Frates is a Fellow of the American College of Lifestyle Medicine and a Diplomate of the American Board of Lifestyle Medicine. In September 2020, Dr. Frates was voted president of the American College of Lifestyle Medicine, and she serves as president from November 2022 to November 2024.

Dr. Frates coauthored *The Lifestyle Medicine Handbook: An Introduction to the Power of Healthy Habits* with colleagues Dr. Jon Bonnet, Dr. Rich Joseph, and Dr. Jim Peterson. In addition, she co-authored *The Teen Lifestyle Medicine Handbook* and the *PAVING the Path to Wellness Workbook: A Guide to Thriving with a Healthy Body, Peaceful Mind, and Joyful Heart.*

In Dr. Rippe's *Manual of Lifestyle Medicine* textbooks, 3rd and 4th Editions, Dr. Frates served as editor for the Behavior Medicine section and Addictions section. She is passionate about lifestyle medicine and coaching people to adopt healthy habits.

Mark D. Faries, PhD, is an Associate Professor in Behavioral Medicine, with focus on *why* and *how* people initiate and maintain healthy behaviors, including theoretical, religious, and self-regulatory aspects of healthy lifestyles for chronic disease prevention. He has served on the Board of Directors for the American College of Lifestyle Medicine.

Contributors

Fraser Birrell
British Society of Lifestyle Medicine
Haddington, United Kingdom
Northumbria University
London, United Kingdom
Southern Cross University
Lismore, NSW, Australia
Northumbria Healthcare NHS
    Foundation Trust
Newcastle upon Tyne, United Kingdom
MRC-Versus Arthritis Centre
    for Integrated Research into
    Musculoskeletal Ageing (CIMA)
Newcastle University
Newcastle upon Tyne, United Kingdom

Sofia Chandler
Point Loma Nazarene University
San Diego, California

Monique Class
Yale School of Nursing
Orange, Connecticut

Amy Comander
Mass General Cancer Center
Harvard Medical School
Boston, Massachusetts

Marie Dacey
Massachusetts School of Pharmacy and
    Health Sciences
Boston, Massachusetts

Mark D. Faries
Texas A&M AgriLife Extension
Texas A&M School of Medicine
College Station, Texas

Peter Fifield
Wentworth-Douglass Hospital
Dover, New Hampshire

Beth Frates
Department of Physical Medicine and
    Rehabilitation
Spaulding Rehabilitation Hospital
Harvard Medical School
Department of Surgery
Massachusetts General Hospital
Boston, Massachusetts

Rachel Frye
Point Loma Nazarene University
San Diego, California

Erik Gnagy
University of Texas at Austin
Austin, Texas

Lyra Heller
Functional Medicine Coaching
    Academy
Chicago, Illinois

Marcus W. Kilpatrick
University of South Florida
Tampa, Florida

Hannah Lee
Massachusetts General Hospital
Boston, Massachusetts

Michael R. Mantell

Jessica A. Matthews
Point Loma Nazarene University
San Diego, California

Simon Matthews
Avondale University
Cooranbong, NSW, Australia

Tracie McCargo
Emory University School of Medicine
Atlanta, Georgia

Megan McClendon
Texas A&M AgriLife Extension
College Station, Texas

Katelyn Murphy
Texas A&M AgriLife Extension
College Station, Texas

James O. Prochaska
(August 6, 1942- July 9, 2023)
University of Rhode Island
Kingston, Rhode Island

Janice M. Prochaska
Consultant at ProChange Behavior
   Solutions

Sandra Scheinbaum
Functional Medicine Coaching
   Academy
Chicago, Illinois

Miquela G. Smith
Texas A&M AgriLife Extension
Lubbock, College Station, Texas

Joji Suzuki
Division of Addiction Psychiatry
Brigham and Women's Hospital
Boston, Massachusetts

An Introduction to the Book

*Beth Frates, MD, FACLM, DipABLM
and Mark D. Faries, PhD*

1. PURPOSE

Healthcare professionals face the tremendous challenge of helping their patients, clients, and/or students initiate and adopt a healthy lifestyle, perhaps through lifestyle prescriptions, coaching, counseling, or other patient–clinician relationships. Whether it is adopting healthy eating patterns, quitting smoking, or even flossing teeth before bed, behaviors can be challenging to change. Many people working toward behavior change have been struggling with seemingly insurmountable lifestyle patterns such as smoking, excessive alcohol intake, sleep deprivation, fast food consumption, eating sweets and processed foods, sitting most of the day and not moving around much, falling into P.A.D.D. (physical activity deficit disorder), or feeling isolated from friends or family. These lifestyle patterns lead to poor physical and mental health, highlighting the importance of a proper lifestyle prescription.

A common approach is to teach what to do, supported by guidelines and recommendations. This approach depends on our understanding that behavior begins with self-monitoring – becoming aware of the benefits of healthy living. Knowing the guidelines for a healthy lifestyle helps to set the stage for behavior change, and reflecting on how current habits and lifestyle practices compare to the guidelines can be motivating. However, knowing what to do, including an understanding of what is healthy for the body, is one step and only a part of the process of change.

A whole person approach to change involves much more than gathering facts. The response to one's comparison to guidelines or recommendations is complex. Some people learn new information and are motivated to change, but others are not. They may even be paralyzed by the facts. Change is hard, and counseling on lifestyle change can be a frustrating experience for healthcare professionals who truly want to help others succeed.

Why are some people more successful than others?

What can the clinician do to help others adopt a healthy lifestyle?

Likely, at least to some degree, this has been your experience. You have questions about how to help others adopt and sustain new, healthful patterns of living. This book was written to help answer such questions. Perhaps, you have also recognized that the process requires more than information and a lifestyle prescription. This book can help here too, as it is aimed to encourage and guide you beyond the *what* of healthy lifestyle change, into the meaning and values that lie behind motivation to change (the *why*), and the thoughts and behaviors that must be successfully performed while navigating within a complex, dynamic milieu of challenges and opportunities in everyday life (the *how*). More specifically, this book serves your needs by providing essential theories, techniques, strategies, and tips to help people adopt and sustain healthy patterns and practices. It is structured to provide a research-based, yet practical reference tool for clinicians to be used in practice.

2. AUDIENCE

This book was written for all clinicians who work in various aspects of healthcare and/or wellness care to empower people to change, which can span numerous titles and applications. So, if you are a physician, nurse, nursing aide, nurse practitioner, physician assistant, therapist, lifestyle medicine specialist, health coach, social worker, physical therapist, occupational therapist, speech therapist, dietician, nutrition specialist, recreational therapist, vocational therapist, sleep specialist, addiction specialist, mental health provider, fitness professional, behavior change expert, dentist, dental hygienist, music therapist, art therapist, or anyone else who is working to help patients regain their health, this book is for you.

This book is also useful for those in education. We hope that students, trainees, fellows, and residents will benefit from its structure and ease of use – being less like a traditional academic textbook and more like a manual or guide to better equip evidence-based healthcare professionals with behavior change strategies. Yet, there is enough depth to the content, its resources, and practical applications that educators in medical or other health professional schools who want to teach the future leaders in healthcare the basics of behavior change will also find this book helpful. The content is approachable to professors in undergraduate and graduate programs, medical schools, healthcare professional schools as well as teachers in high school and middle school, who could all benefit from the principles in this book. Course outlines can be formed around the content, and when this book is paired with lectures, case studies, and/or clinical practice, it can empower translation to real-world application, bringing the content to life and having a more direct impact on the individuals who seek our help in behavior change. Even caregivers, parents, and grandparents will be able to apply these theories and strategies in their own lives with their loved ones, thereby empowering change.

For ease, different terms are often used interchangeably throughout the book. The terms *provider, practitioner, clinician, healthcare professional* and *physician* may be used to label the person who is empowering the change. It would be difficult to consistently alternate between specific titles, such as physician, health coach, nurse, dietitian, therapist, professor, personal trainer, and parent throughout the book – although the concepts can apply to all of these. Also, the person who is working on changing is referred to in different ways. Individuals are often referred to as *clients* by health coaches, *patients* by clinicians, *students* by teachers, and so on. Given that the main target audience is healthcare professionals with people under their care, the language will reflect *patient* and *client* in most cases. Of course, we recognize that healthcare professionals are also patients and clients themselves.

3. APPROACH

Each chapter's topic and its expert authors were chosen to highlight theories and strategies that should be in any clinician's behavior change toolbox – a starter kit. We wanted to maintain a strong, research-based foundation, simplify the content to support knowledge and understanding, and structure for easier application in practice. We envision the clinician being able to pull the book from the shelf and flip to a specific chapter as a resource to directly help a specific patient issue in practice.

This was a difficult task, since behavior change is for people of all ages and stages of life. Many are steeped in unhealthy habits and have their own specific struggles and concerns that challenge general lifestyle recommendations. Yet, our authors recognize such complexities. They are experts not just in knowledge, but also in experience. They not only have passion, but also compassion. They understand that learning about the person who is struggling with unhealthy behaviors is a crucial first step toward empowering change. The more you know about the person, the easier it is to help them, because each individual is an expert in their own life – with insider knowledge of his or her own needs, values, desires, and fears. Each person has the capacity to recognize what has worked in the past, what has failed, what obstacles are in the way, and the possible solutions they have at their disposal.

This book was written by thought leaders in this field from around the world, including the United States, England, and Australia. The authors have years, often decades, of experience in teaching, research, and clinical practice. Each author is passionate and dedicated to sharing their knowledge, expertise, and insight, as evidenced by the countless hours each spent planning, preparing, writing, editing, and finally producing this book for you, the reader. We hope that you can feel their energy, excitement, and passion throughout the pages.

4. CONTENTS

To ease such challenges, this book approaches behavior change as a journey, rather than a destination. There are guideposts, but there is no real finish line. Humans are a "work in progress," and working on well-being and making changes to enhance life satisfaction is something people can do on a continual basis. Sometimes intensive lifestyle changes are required for people to manage and even in some cases reverse disease. There is a dose response to lifestyle medicine and lifestyle change. Some people respond to low intensity intervention such as reading a book or watching a movie with high intensity change. Others require high intensity interventions like inpatient stays at lifestyle medicine programs in order to make high intensity change. This book can be helpful in these two scenarios and everything in between. Behavior change toward healthy living can be enjoyable and does not need to be perceived as drudgery, overwhelming, or zapping autonomy and belief in oneself. The same can be said for clinicians who also face their own challenges, barriers, lack of confidence, and concerns in providing lifestyle recommendations. So, this book aims to help make the behavior journey easier and more enjoyable for everyone – clinician and patient/client alike.

Thus, consider the content of this book to be a road map. Each chapter shares insight into different, yet interconnected research-based theories, concepts, and strategies behind behavior change. The general outline for each chapter guides the reader through the following sections:

1. Brief Introduction
2. Evidence Summary
3. Practical Applications
4. Case Studies
5. Measurement Strategies
6. Key Takeaways and Resources

Real-life examples were encouraged. Tables and figures are used strategically to help ease understanding and application, while also encouraging quick access for reference when needed in practice. When possible, assessment tools are identified to help clinicians obtain a baseline level for the patients as well as allowing for monitoring progress. There is an emphasis on practical strategies and tips to help empower patients to change. The chapters do not need to be read in succession, one after the other. For example, if you are interested in *Motivational Interviewing*, jump to that chapter, first. If you are interested in the *Transtheoretical Model of Change*, you can start there. If you are currently working with a patient or client who is struggling with *building confidence*, *overcoming barriers*, or to *maintain motivation*, then thumb to the chapter that specifically covers those topics.

Yet, for maximum benefit, we suggest that you read all the chapters. You will notice that the authors often cite other chapters within the book, re-emphasizing that many of these theories and strategies do not exist in isolation, but rather overlap, encourage, and support each other. If each chapter is a new tool in your behavior change toolbox, in practice, each patient or client will benefit most from multiple tools and strategies that are individualized for each situation. The challenge for the clinician is to learn which tools to use and then to increase the effectiveness of chosen strategies through practice. In Table 1, you can see the list of chapters, key concepts, and probing questions to consider as you read the chapter.

TABLE 1

List of Chapters, Key Concepts, and Probing Questions to Consider during Reading

Chapter Title	Key Concepts	Guiding Questions
1. Introduction to the Book	The book is for anyone who wants to empower people to change	What can be learned?
2. Introduction to Behavior Change	Behavior change theories, coaching and key research	What are commonalities in these theories? What are existing theories?
3. Stages of Change	Identify stages	What indicators are there to help know which stage someone is in for change?
4. Motivational Interviewing	Evoke change talk	What questions will help evoke change talk? Why is change talk important?
5. The Power of Autonomy	Everyone wants choice	What techniques help to give people autonomy?
6. Appreciative Inquiry	Find the positive core	How does one identify what is working well? How can one build on what is working well?
7. Goal Setting & Planning	Goals put action into the process of change	What is a SMART goal? How does one set goals?
8. Maintaining Motivation	Motivators may change, staying the course takes effort	What can people do to maintain motivation?
9. Overcoming Obstacles	Obstacles are opportunities	How does one co-create solutions? How can people problem solve together?
10. Using Strengths	Everyone has strengths, not everyone uses them	How can someone bring out the strengths of the other? How can strengths help?
11. Accountabiliy	A sense of ownership and responsibility are key for sustainable change	Who is accountable for progress?
12. Five-Step Cycle of Collaboration	There are 5 steps from research and theory that help practitioners empower people to change	What is the importance of empathy, motivation, confidence, SMART goals, and accountability?
13. Group Healthcare Interventions in Lifestyle Medicine	People long to belong	How can one harness the power of a group to help people on their journey of change?
14. Lifestyle Medicine Practice	Describe the Six Pillars of Lifestyle Medicine. Identify the Guidelines Examine Trends	What are the six pillars? How are lifestyles impacting health?
15. Summary	There are evidence-based approaches to empower people	What did the reader learn? What will the reader do differently now?

5. BEFORE YOU BEGIN

Before you begin on this journey of behavior change with us, consider what you already know. Using Table 2:

1. List behavior change theories you know.
2. Identify behavior change strategies that work for you and those that do not.
3. List questions you currently have about behavior change.

You will complete this same exercise at the end of the book. Enjoy your learning journey!

TABLE 2
Knowledge Guide before Beginning the Book

Before you begin on this journey of behavior change with us, consider what you already know. List theories you are familiar with. Identify behavior change strategies you know work for you and those that do not. Then, list questions you currently have about behavior change here.

Behavior Change Theories I know now:

Behavior Change Strategies I know that work:

Behavior Change Strategies I know that do not work:

Questions that I have about Behavior Change:

You will be asked to complete this same exercise at the end of the book.

---

1 Introduction to Behavior Change

Beth Frates, MD and Tracie McCargo, PhD

1.1 INTRODUCTION

Empowering people to change is an essential element of practicing lifestyle medicine, whether in the clinic one-on-one with patients or in group consultations, either in person or virtually. Lifestyle medicine is a burgeoning new field of medicine that uses six pillars, including physical activity, a whole food plant predominant eating patterns, restorative sleep, stress resiliency techniques, positive social connections, and moderation or elimination of risky substances, to help patients prevent, treat, and in some cases even reverse conditions considered chronic diseases, such as heart disease, diabetes, obesity, metabolic syndrome, hypertension, and high cholesterol, to name a few. With these lifestyle-related conditions on the rise, there is an increasing need for counseling on behavior change that empowers people to adopt and sustain change. How healthcare professionals talk about change influences how people receive the information and whether or not they absorb it, digest it, and ultimately use it.

"No man walks in the same river twice," Heraclitus once said. This quote points out the fact that change is a part of life. We grow from child to adult. A river moves water and silt minute by minute. Our epithelial cells change daily.[1] Nothing remains the same. We are aging day by day. Some changes are out of our control, and others are in our control. What's out of our control? The COVID pandemic, hurricanes, waves, global wars, rain, other cars on the highway, jealousy of others, and other people's behaviors, for example. What is in our control? Our actions, our words, the speed of the car we are driving, our use of an umbrella, and our response to the behavior of other people are all examples of things in our control. One of the first things to identify is what is in our control and what is not. With behavior change, we focus on the things in our control.

1.2 CHANGE IS CONSTANT

What is behavior change? The American Psychological Association defines behavior change as

1. a systematic approach to changing behavior through the use of operant conditioning.
2. any alteration or adjustment of behavior that affects a patient's functioning, brought about by psychotherapeutic or other interventions occurring spontaneously.[2]

DOI: 10.1201/9781003161226-1

In lifestyle medicine, the focus is on addressing lifestyle behaviors, patterns, and practices. Lifestyle behaviors include physical activity, nutrition, sleep, stress management, social support, and the use of risky substances. Even the way we list these pillars and describe them can make a world of difference. For example, we can talk about joyous movement, delicious and nutritious foods, restorative sleep, positive social connections, and avoiding risky substances. Research indicates that chronic conditions are partly caused by these behaviors. Genetics plays a role in some diseases such as cancer, heart disease, stroke, obesity, and dementia. Even in the case of genetic susceptibility to a certain condition, lifestyle behaviors can often work to combat the development and progression of the disease. This phrase or one similar to it has been said by many people: "Genetics load the gun, and lifestyle behaviors pull the trigger." Lifestyle is that powerful. In some cases, lifestyle changes can prevent, treat, and even reverse some chronic conditions, including diabetes type 2, high blood pressure, and obesity.[3,4] For this reason, behavior change is a critical component of lifestyle medicine. The American College of Lifestyle Medicine (ACLM) revised its definition of lifestyle medicine in the spring of 2022 to read

> Lifestyle medicine is a medical specialty that uses therapeutic lifestyle interventions as a primary modality to treat chronic conditions including, but not limited to, cardiovascular diseases, type 2 diabetes, and obesity. Lifestyle medicine certified clinicians are trained to apply evidence-based, whole-person, prescriptive lifestyle change to treat and, when used intensively, often reverse such conditions. Applying the six pillars of lifestyle medicine—a whole-food, plant-predominant eating pattern, physical activity, restorative sleep, stress management, avoidance of risky substances and positive social connections—also provides effective prevention for these conditions.[5]

1.2.1 WHAT IS THE AMERICAN COLLEGE OF LIFESTYLE MEDICINE?

According to their website (https://lifestylemedicine.org),

> **ACLM** is the medical professional society for physicians and other professionals dedicated to clinical and worksite practice of lifestyle medicine as the foundation of a transformed and sustainable health care system.

Lifestyle Medicine research, education, and practice are all rapidly growing. As of 2023, the ACLM had over 11,000 members. To be certified in lifestyle medicine, physicians and other healthcare professionals need to demonstrate proficiency in exercise prescription, nutrition, sleep, social connection, stress management, and avoidance of risky substance use. In addition, they need to know about behavior change. Questions on the board exam are on behavior change theories and counseling strategies. That's because knowledge is powerful, but it's not powerful enough to instill lasting behavior change. Clinicians need to know the facts and figures, the data and the results of research studies, and they need to master the skills of empowering people to change behaviors. The American Board of Lifestyle Medicine (ABLM) is responsible for providing and grading the exam as well as giving certification certificates for MDs and DOs (https://ablm.org). The ACLM certifies other healthcare professionals after they pass the ABLM exam.

It is not just healthcare professionals who are interested in behavior change. Behavior change is often on the minds of people when they are patients, parents, clinicians, teachers, pet owners, people who have loved ones who smoke, drink in excess, or have substance use disorder, managers in companies, and partners in a relationship. In other words, this topic of behavior change is applicable to everyone.

In this book, all aspects of behavior change will be covered in detail, including the transtheoretical model of change, motivational interviewing, group consultations, self-efficacy, behavior-intention gap, and health coaching. In the first chapter, there is a basic summary of behavior change, important behavior change theories, health coaching information, and research on the topic of health coaching.

To be proficient in behavior change, people spend years reading research, performing experiments, and writing papers before earning their PhDs in behavior change. There are Master's degrees in psychology that focus on behavior change. Health and wellness coaches are educated on and become proficient in behavior change during their training and certification. Medical schools include lectures and workshops on motivational interviewing in the preclinical and clinical years. Nurses have behavior change as part of their education as well. Parents often work to better understand behavior change and take courses to help their children behave in a respectful, honest, and compassionate manner. Many people can benefit from learning more about behavior change.

Behavior change is a hot topic for researchers. In one research study exploring behavior change theories, it was determined that these theories focus on five main areas: (1) motives, (2) self-regulation, (3) resources, (4) habits, and (5) environmental and social influences.[6] In another study, 82 different theories of behavior change were identified. Most were described over two decades ago, and some as early as 1941 with Miller's Social Learning Theory, 1947 with Sutherland's Differential Association Theory, 1956 with Skinner's Operant Conditioning Theory, 1968 with Locke's Goal Setting Theory, 1977 with Bandura's Social Cognitive Theory, 1977 with Bandura's Self-Efficacy Theory, 1983 with Prochaska's Transtheoretical Model of Change, 1985 with Ajzen's Theory of Planned Behavior/Reasoned Action, 2000 with Deci's Self-Determination Theory, and 2006 with Panter-Brick's Social Ecological Model of Behavior Change.[7] Interestingly, many of these theories still guide behavior counseling efforts to this day. A 2021 review of behavior change techniques used to help oral health professionals with tobacco cessation counseling with their patients identified effective strategies including goal setting, providing written materials, using readiness to quit and ability assessment, tobacco-use assessment, providing self-efficacy boosts, listing reasons for quitting, action planning, and environment restructuring.[8]

Examining all the available research and utilizing the experience of the authors of chapters in this book on empowering people to change, there are 13 keys to behavior change that will be explored in detail in the following chapter. They are listed in Table 1.1.

TABLE 1.1

The 13 Keys to Behavior Change

The patient's agenda is the guide

Work with the patient's stage of change

Build self-efficacy and confidence

Tap into the patient's motivation

Honor the patient's autonomy

Appreciate the positive and what is working well

Co-create goals with the patient

Maintain motivation

Overcome obstacles

Identify and use the patient's strengths

Set accountability

Enjoy the process and five-step cycle of collaboration for behavior change

Use group interventions and social support to power behavior change

1.3 REVIEW OF MAJOR THEORIES

The Transtheoretical Model of Change created by Dr. James Prochaska and colleagues is outlined in detail in Chapter 2. It is an important theory to understand and be comfortable using. This is one important way that healthcare professionals can tailor their counseling and coaching to the individual patient who is sitting in front of them physically or by Zoom, Teams, or another virtual platform. In some cases of counseling, the patient might be on a treadmill side by side with the clinician. Or perhaps, the counseling will take place one-on-one outside during a quiet, private nature walk. There are times when counseling will take place in a group setting, and the individual's stage of change might be different than that of other members of the group. In this group setting, it is important to tailor conversations to the person who is receiving the one-on-one attention at that time. Group discussions can include strategies at multiple stages of change. This is covered in Chapter 13. As a reminder, there are five stages: pre-contemplation, contemplation, preparation, action, and maintenance. Table 1.2 might be beneficial to refer to during a clinic visit with a patient or during group visits. It reviews the five stages of change and provides a summary of feelings patients commonly report in those specific stages.

1.3.1 SOCIAL COGNITIVE THEORY

What we witness impacts our thoughts, feelings, and development. Dr. Albert Bandura's social cognitive theory examines how social influences impact personality development and also a person's behavior.[9,10]

The three areas of focus in social cognitive theory are as follows:

1. a person's cognition
2. their external environment
3. a person's behavior

TABLE 1.2
The Five Stages of Change and Patient's Feelings

	Pre-contemplation	Contemplation	Preparation	Action	Maintenance
Patient's feelings	Confusing	Considering	Getting ready	In motion	Steady
Patients' expressions	I won't I can't No way. Leave me alone	I may It's a good idea	I'm ready I need a plan	I'm doing it	I've been doing it, and I will keep doing it
Clinician's feelings	Frustrated	Hopeful	Excited	Satisfied	Inspired
Practitioner's expressions and questions	I hear you You are not ready I am here for you when you are ready Would you be interested in reading articles or watching videos on the topic of exercise and heart disease? Would you be interested in hearing about a patient who was just like you and made some major changes that improved her well-being?	I hear some ambivalence What are the pros and cons of change for you? How important is this for you right now? How would your life be different if you did start this new healthy habit?	What needs to be in place for you to get started? What are some of the barriers in your way?	Congratulations on your progress How do you feel? What seems different to you? What benefits are you noticing? What are your plans to continue?	Congratulations on your continued progress and commitment to this healthy habit! What are you doing that keeps you going? What's your motivation for maintaining this habit? What are your plans for the next month or two? How can I help you to keep going?

A person's social experience throughout life shapes much of who they are. What other people do and say around a person helps the individual to learn and grow without going through those experiences themselves. If an individual watches a sibling, cousin, or friend get in trouble for stealing or cheating, they may store that in their mind and use it when a situation like that manifests in their own lives. With group interventions, patients in the group listen to each other's strategies, successes, and failures, and they all learn together.

1.3.2 SELF-EFFICACY

People are more apt to change when they believe they can be successful. Self-efficacy is an individual's belief that they can be successful at a particular task. Confidence is an overarching feeling of empowerment and strength, whereas self-efficacy is specific to a task. Someone can be a confident person but not have self-efficacy in their ability to ballroom dance or fix a broken pipe. In behavior change to manage chronic conditions, an individual may be confident at work but not have self-efficacy about being able to exercise regularly or follow a healthy eating pattern.

Self-efficacy is essential to Bandura's social cognitive theory.[9] One can develop self-efficacy through four main sources: He first described self-efficacy in the 1970s.[10]

1. Mastery experiences – having opportunities to try new things, practice, and master them.
2. Vicarious experiences – interactions with others and watching others' success.
3. Social persuasion – listening to the stories and suggestions of others.
4. Emotional states – experiencing anxiety and depression impacts one's ability to feel that they are capable of performing a certain task and being successful.

Self-efficacy is important for behavior change because it leads to successful goal setting and attainment. People who have high levels of self-efficacy make progress in their healthy habit goals.

In Chapter 2, Drs. James and Janice Prochaska describe how dramatic relief can help someone in pre-contemplation. Listening to someone else's story, either another participant in a group setting, hearing about a patient who had a similar problem and overcame obstacles, or watching a powerful movie about someone else's change process all allow for these vicarious experiences, social persuasion, and emotional states. Chapter 7 on goal setting helps to highlight how mastery experiences are essential for sustained change.

During the consultation for behavior change, the clinician asks many open-ended questions to learn more about the patient. Motivational interviewing is covered in detail in Chapter 4. These open-ended questions are a critical part of motivational interviewing as they invite the patient to reflect and to dive into the recesses of their brains to think about circumstances, experiences, and thoughts with a fresh perspective. In fact, examining their own self-perceptions is an integral part of the process. Evaluating the patient's social connections and social interactions will help them to understand how people and past activities or events work to shape who they are today. How patients talk about their past to the clinicians and to themselves also shapes their reality. Self-talk is powerful. It can serve to build people up or tear them down. Someone's self-talk is a reflection of their own beliefs about themselves and their self-efficacy. Self-talk can lead to insecurity or build confidence. Confidence is built by previous successes and honoring the strengths and hard work it took to reach those successes. It is also created by rising from a fall and realizing that one mishap is not going to lead to perpetual failure. Confidence brings energy and empowerment. Self-talk can bolster both confidence and self-efficacy. If a person is constantly telling themselves, "I can't do that. I won't do that. That's impossible for me," they are keeping themselves in the pre-contemplation stage of change. If they are saying, "I may. I might. I could possibly do it," they are in the contemplation stage. This self-talk is often expressed to others in conversations. Asking someone about how confident they are about reaching a specific goal helps gauge their self-efficacy for that action step.

1.3.3 SELF-DETERMINATION THEORY

Self-Determination Theory was first described by Deci and Ryan in 1985.[11] According to this theory, the three main components required for volitional, sustained motivation include autonomy, competence, and relatedness.[12] When these three essential factors are in place, there is improved performance, creativity, and productivity. When working to help people adopt and sustain healthy patterns of living, it is important to make sure they have autonomy. The power of autonomy is addressed in detail in Chapter 5. Giving people choices and letting them choose the best fit for them is an impactful way to get buy in and engagement. People want a sense of control, and they want a sense of competence. When people feel competent, they are motivated to try new tasks and make progress. This helps people get out of their comfort zone. Self-efficacy, which was described earlier as the belief that one can be successful at a task, is linked to the competency aspect of self-determination theory. These theories build on each other and often support one another. The last component of the Self-Determination Theory is relatedness. Maslow's Hierarchy of Needs emphasizes this same concept in the third level of his hierarchy of needs.[13] Maslow explains that first of all people need food and water. Next, they need shelter. What do they need after that? They need a sense of belonging. People need people. Individuals long to belong. Providing people with social connections that are positive and supportive helps with behavior change and motivation to stay on track.

1.3.4 SOCIAL ECOLOGICAL MODEL OF CHANGE

Initially, in the behavior change process, there is a focus on the individual. Their beliefs, habits, strengths, goals, dreams, visions, past successes, past failures, fears, desires, wants, needs, self-efficacy, insecurity, obstacles, motivators, and attitudes. If behavior change counselors or coaches only focused on the individual then their ability to help people adopt and sustain healthy habits would be limited. People exist in communities, not in vacuums. It is a rare individual who is not associated with, living with, working with, or connected to another human being in some way. Most people live in apartments, condominiums, or houses in neighborhoods or other communities. There are laws and policies for individual cities and countries that people need to follow. And, there are cultural norms that people adhere to or, in some cases, rebel against. In all cases, there is an outside environment that influences each individual, the options, their choices, and their experiences.

The closest to home is the kitchen. What's in the kitchen and who is shopping for food? This is a question that will impact a person's ability to follow a healthy eating pattern. Who's cooking the food? A great question to ask in an interview is "What's in your refrigerator right now?" and "What's in your kitchen cabinetry?" These questions help the clinician better understand the person's homelife and its influence. In addition, knowing who the person lives with and what their lifestyle patterns include tell the clinician what exposure the individual is getting day to day. In some cases, there is someone at home who is knowingly or unknowingly acting as a saboteur by buying and bringing into the kitchen cookies, cakes, or ice cream. Understanding the people and the food items in the home helps equip the patient with the tools they need to have difficult conversations and to make difficult choices. Marking foods with red, yellow, or green colors with a pen, tape, or sticky note can be a first step in better understanding the kitchen. Red would indicate: Danger. Yellow would indicate: Caution. And Green would indicate: Go for it.

Many people spend the majority of their days at work, at least from 8 am to 5 pm. However, since COVID this is also changing for many people. In some cases, for those who commute to work, they spend more time at work than at home during the weekdays. And, for some, work events and dinners after hours are part of the job. In these cases, exploring the work environment is key. Is there a refrigerator or microwave available? Taking dinner leftovers to work for lunch is a great idea and saves money as well. When people are able to batch cook on Sundays and freeze food, they can bring homemade healthy lunch options into work and microwave them, if one is available. In some workplaces, there are still candy jars on desks and work meetings involve pizza delivery and soda or juices. In addition to these nutrition issues, there are physical activity issues too. Checking in on the desk set up at work is important. Encouraging people to use stand-up workstations, treadmill workstations, and stationary bike workstations can help people to increase the amount of minutes of physical activity they accumulate. Using a physioball as a desk chair is another option which can engage a person's core as they work. There are also portable peddlers people can use at work under their desks. Setting timers every hour to take standing breaks or walking breaks will help to break up the sedentary behavior.

A person's culture impacts their daily life and decisions. When growing up with parents who practice specific eating patterns and prefer certain dishes, one may become accustomed to that way of eating, healthy or not. As a child, there is not much choice. When people grow up and live on their own, they often fall back to what they knew as children. In addition, we may still participate in meals together with family. Understanding how to make healthy food within a variety of cultures is key. A recent review article on healthy eating pointed out how the Mediterranean, Japanese, Okinawan, and Nordic styles of diets can all be healthy.[14] Understanding the components of a healthy diet is the place to start. In this review article, the authors noted the healthful similarities in these diets from different cultures including the use of herbs, spices, and other natural seasonings. Protein intake was moderate, primarily from plants, lean meats, and fish, rarely from red or processed meat and consuming processed foods, sugar, and alcohol was minimal or avoided. On the other hand, these healthful diets encouraged the intake of mono- and polyunsaturated fats, such as olive oil and nuts.[14] In some cultures, it is common to see people jogging on the sidewalks, in other cultures jogging is rare. It is important to understand a person's culture while working on behavior change. Along these same lines, it may not be safe to walk in some neighborhoods around the world. Walking is a good form of physical activity and being outside in nature is healthy as well. However, this recommendation may not be feasible for some.

A person's physical environment is essential to factor into behavior change counseling. For example, when talking about the obesity epidemic, we do not just speak about willpower and an individual's choices. We must address the food environment in which they live. Some people live in food deserts where it is nearly impossible to buy fresh produce or food swamps where there are fast food restaurants on every corner. The food industry has created food products that are multi-colored, dye-infested, chemically laden, sugar-loaded, fat heavy, and excessively salty. These hyperpalatable foods hit the dopamine system in the brain in such a way that the person who eats them longs for the same food and that same reward. Helping people understand the healthy choices is one part of the journey to nutritious eating, and then providing ample opportunities to obtain these healthy choices is another. Even food pantries are now stocking their shelves with whole-food, plant-predominant options, recognizing the importance of plants for optimal health.

Knowing a person's background and their current circumstances will allow a clinician to co-create a plan that works for that specific individual. Behavior change does not work if the clinician simply provides the guidelines for exercise, nutrition, sleep, social connections, stress reduction, and avoidance of risky substances without knowing the whole person, their home environment, work environment, neighborhood, culture, and societal values.

Figure 1.1 depicts the Social Ecological Model of Change in enclosed circles ("Societal," "Community," "Social," "Individual").

1.4 SOCIAL DETERMINANTS OF HEALTH-SDOH

There has been a shift of focus not just on the individual but on the environment and how multiple forces impact an individual's lifestyle patterns and practices. In a 2021 article, the authors recommend using terms such as "eating practices and patterns" rather than food choices and decisions to better capture the intricate interconnectedness of individuals' diets with their environment.[15] Food availability, local grocery store inventory, whether someone can have their own garden, food advertising, the marketing of hyperpalatable foods which are high in sugar, fat, and salt, the number of fast food chains in the vicinity of someone's home, a person's income, a person's understanding of the impact of food on their health, and whether or not the person has a primary care physician or access to a nutritionist or health coach can all impact their food intake, patterns, and practices. Factors such as race, ethnicity, and age can also influence the

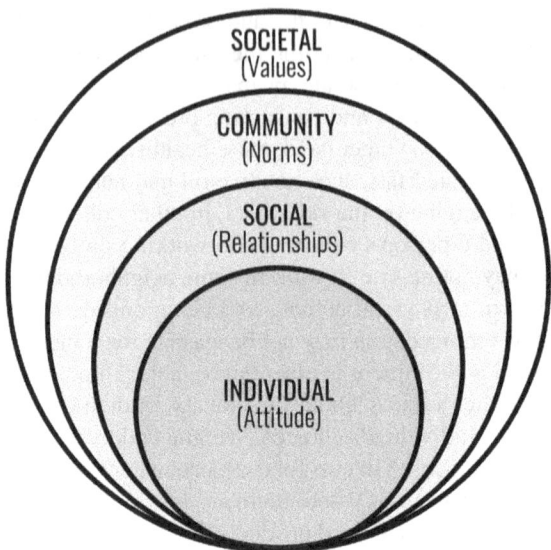

FIGURE 1.1 Social Ecological Model of Change in enclosed circles ("Societal," "Community," "Social," "Individual").

quality and variety of available food.[16] Those in underserved communities have less access to nutritious food and greater odds of experiencing food insecurity.[16] Behavior change is not just a matter of willpower. How is a person going to take a walk outside if there are gangs, drug deals, and shootings in their neighborhoods? They will need to find solutions for movement that work for them. A person's education level, economic status, family background, and neighborhood all influence a person's available options, decisions, and choices.[17] The social determinants of health are important to consider when counseling a patient about behavior change. They are depicted in Figure 1.2 and include economic stability, education access and quality, healthcare access and quality, neighborhood-built environment, and social and community context.

Figure 1.2 depicts the social determinants of health.[18] It is from Healthy People, United States Department of Health and Human Services.

Many of the studies in behavior change have a homogeneous subject pool. Including more minorities, people of color, immigrants, and individuals who are economically disadvantaged will be important for future investigations. The more information collected about current practices, patterns, and problems, the better equipped healthcare professionals will be to meet the needs of these populations. Encouraging people of color and minority populations to seek education and employment in the healthcare field will also help. It was noted that during the COVID-19 pandemic, some populations avoided hospitals because they felt a lack of trust, fear, and a disconnect with healthcare professionals.[19] This was experienced by people of color, minorities, immigrants, different genders, and people from economically challenged areas. Counseling on behavior change may open the door for individuals who are resistant or hesitant to seek medical attention and encourage them to take the step toward clinicians that they can relate to and may be able to trust more readily.[17]

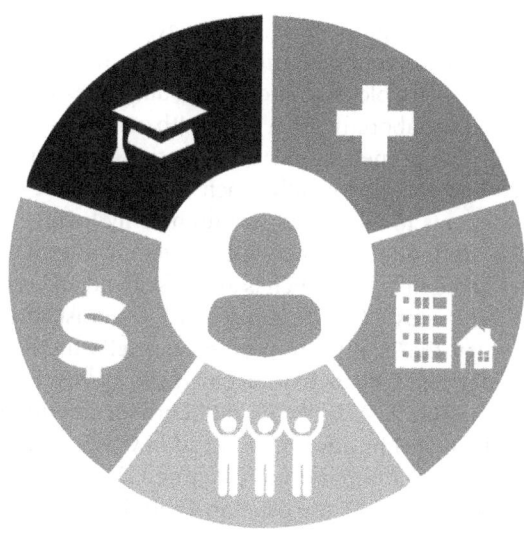

FIGURE 1.2 Social determinants of health (images of "graduation cap," "cross," "building," "people," "dollar sign," and "person") depicted inside of a circle. (Copy free image.)

1.5 WHAT IS HEALTH COACHING?

Health coaching is a profession that focuses on behavior change. There is a National Board of Health and Wellness Coaching,[20] which certifies individuals in health coaching after taking an exam, submitting a case study as well as a log of client interactions. The health coach training includes learning about behavior change theories and techniques as well as the research about coaching. Practicing coaching is key to becoming an effective coach. Many people are used to using the EXPERT Approach™ and telling people what to do. However, this tell-and-sell approach does not work for sustained behavior change. Every individual is different and requires a unique approach that suits their needs. Some people are concerned about their pre-diabetes. Others have BMIs in the obese range, carry extra adipose tissue in their abdomen, have a high waist circumference, and are worried about the plethora of conditions associated with obesity such as high blood pressure, heart disease, metabolic syndrome, sleep apnea, diabetes, and some cancers. And some people are struggling to quit smoking or drinking. Many struggle with similar unhealthy lifestyle patterns like eating fast food that is cheap and easy to acquire, skimping on sleep, drinking four to five glasses of wine, forgoing any exercise, and spending so much time working that social relationships are suffering. Though the unhealthy lifestyles may be similar, each individual will require a different approach. They may be in different stages of change for their behaviors. They may have tried several different strategies already. They may have a home environment that demands attention with a mother who has dementia or a child with Down's syndrome. No matter what the situation is or what the individual's personal struggles may be, a health coach can work with that person to adopt and sustain healthy habits by taking into account the person's personality, preferences, attitudes, education level, home environment, past successes and failures, their neighborhood, work environment, cultural influences, and more. A health coach helps co-create small goals that are compelling to the individual, doable, specific, measurable, action-oriented, and time-sensitive. It is through counseling, listening, and collaborating that the health coach can partner with clients to create powerful plans that propel people to take action and maintain it.

If you are a trained and certified health coach or a healthcare professional looking to help empower patients to adopt and sustain healthy habits, taking a COACH Approach will help. Dr. Beth Frates created this mnemonic almost a decade ago, and it continues to help people to this day, which is also discussed and used in Chapter 12.

Table 1.3 reviews the Frates COACH Approach™. Contrast this approach to the EXPERT Approach when the healthcare professional tells the patient what to do, how to do it, when to do it, and why to do it. In emergencies, this EXPERT Approach is essential for survival (Table 1.4). In the case of chronic conditions, this approach can build resistance, which will be covered in detail in Chapter 4.

Five specific domains of communication distinguish the COACH Approach™ from the Expert Approach™.[22] These are listed in Table 1.5.

TABLE 1.3
Frates COACH Approach™[21]

C-Curiosity

O-Openness

A-Appreciation

C-Compassion

H-Honesty

TABLE 1.4
EXPERT Mnemonic[21]

E = Examine the patient

X = X-ray and other imaging to efforts to diagnose the problem

P = Plan the resolution of the problem

E = Explain the problem, the solution, and the strategy

R = Repeat what you said multiple times

T = Tell the patient what to do. The "Tell-and-Sell" approach

TABLE 1.5
Frates' Five Specific Domains of Communication for Coaching

Sharing knowledge

Listening

Asking questions

Addressing problems

Taking responsibility

1.6   SHARING KNOWLEDGE

With the COACH Approach™, the coach works to share knowledge that is applicable to the patient, timely, resonates with the patient, matches the patient's stage of change, and answers a question the patient may have or provides honest feedback on the threat of the unhealthy behavior or the benefits of the healthy behavior. The key is that the patient is willing and able to listen to the information. One key question to ask after saying, "I have some information that could be really helpful to you." is "Would it be possible for me to share that with you now?" or "Would you be interested in this information?" By asking for permission from the patient, the clinician honors the patient's autonomy. This is a way of opening the mind and the ears of the patient. Patients are much more likely to pay attention when they are deciding to listen to the clinician. It is their decision. In an EXPERT™ approach, the clinician may launch into a lecture without checking in with the patient because the clinician has good intentions. The clinician wants the patient to know that their behavior is dangerous and that there are consequences to this type of unhealthy action, like smoking. The problem with sharing knowledge without checking in with the patient first is that the patient may not hear the clinician's words. The patient may be in precontemplation and decide to ignore the clinician. This is a waste of time for patients and clinicians alike. To use time wisely and effectively, considering how clinicians share knowledge is essential. Asking permission to share information sets the clinician up for success. The patient makes the choice to have the clinician share or not. If the patient says, "No. I don't want to hear about that. I already know all about it," that opens the door for the clinician to provide just-in-time information or information that is relevant and resonates with the patient. The clinician could ask, "What are you curious about with regard to your condition?" Then, the clinician will be meeting the patient where they are.

1.7   LISTENING

In the COACH Approach™, the clinician listens with their whole self and listens to the whole person in front of them. The clinician uses their eyes, ears, nose, and intuition to hear and understand where the patient is coming from. What can the nose do? Sometimes a clinician can smell alcohol, cannabis smoke, or cigarette smoke, which tells the clinician a great deal of information. The eyes look for body language, facial expressions, and eye movements to inform the clinician about the comfort level of the patient as well as the authenticity and vulnerability the patient is sharing. The ears hear more than the words. They hear tone of voice, velocity of speech, and volume changes. The intuition is where compassion comes in. When the clinician is fully mindful and in the present moment, they can often fully understand the patient in front of them and sense what they need. Listening is key to coaching. In the EXPERT Approach™, listening is also key, but the expert in the ER is often looking for red flags in a clinical history or on a physical exam like a murmur or wheezing in the lungs with the stethoscope. The listening aspect is important, but it is different. Most clinicians are not taught about the COACH Approach™ listening skills.

1.8   ASKING QUESTIONS

Asking questions is what a curious person does. Asking questions is how the expert using the EXPERT Approach™ in an acute care setting can solve the mystery of the symptoms plaguing a patient. There are a series of closed-ended questions like "Do you have a cough? Do you have blood in your stool? Do you have chest pain?" These questions help the expert to decipher the etiology of the signs and symptoms of disease the patient is displaying at that time. For the COACH Approach™, the questions need to be fueled by curiosity too. Curiosity is based on a desire to better understand the patient's motivators, obstacles, strengths, and strategies to succeed or MOSS™. Table 1.6 describes the Frates MOSS Mnemonic.

Asking open-ended questions is one of the staples of motivational interviewing. It is a powerful way to gain more knowledge and understanding of someone. It encourages the patient to speak, to talk about their situation, and to share their own expertise in their life and lifestyle. They know what they have tried before. They know what they want. They know what they are afraid of. They know what might work. They know the solutions and strategies that are available to them. Open-ended questions ensure that the patient does more talking than the clinician in the consultation. The behavior change counseling encounter is a chance for the patient to share their wisdom and experience, their desire and fear, and their strengths and possible strategies for success. "What makes you think about adopting this new healthy habit now? What do you see as the benefits? What scares you about making this change? What do you need to have in place to make this work for you?" All of these are examples of open-ended questions that can help propel a patient toward adopting and sustaining behavior change.

1.9   ADDRESSING PROBLEMS

In the EXPERT Approach™, the clinician is like Sherlock Holmes and finding the solution to the problem is the name of the game. The Expert is the one who asks the questions, directs the interview, and finds the solution to the patient's problem. In the acute care setting, this could be a matter of life or death. Time is of the essence, and the clinician knows this. Thus, finding the solution to the problem is the main goal of the clinician. With training in medicine, a physician feels that they have the answers or at least feels the responsibility to have the answers. After all, there was a lot of training, years of studying, and continued medical education to prepare the physician to have the answer to patient problems. In the COACH Approach™,

TABLE 1.6
Frates MOSS Mnemonic

M = Motivators

O = Obstacles

S = Strengths

S = Strategies

the coach works with the patient to find the solution to the problem when there is a chronic condition or behavior change that is contributing to the problem. The solution to the problem is not prescriptive in this case. It is usually multifaceted. With the COACH Approach™, the coach and client work synergistically to brainstorm solutions to problems. It is not that the coach has no solutions to offer. They may have effective and appropriate ideas. With a brainstorming session in which the patient and the coach come up with potential solutions, the patient can then have the autonomy to select the solution that is best for that patient. Problem solving is the job of the patient with the clinician there to help and to guide the conversation. Ultimately, the patient chooses what solution they will try and when they will try it.

1.10   TAKING RESPONSIBILITY

In the COACH Approach™, the patient is an active contributor in the process of change. The patient takes responsibility for their actions and for their change journey. By realizing it is the patient's choice to change or not and the patient's job to perform new behaviors, the patient becomes an active part of the transformation process. The patient can then feel a sense of pride when they feel better, when they improve their health, when they start to lose weight, when they start to feel less stress, when they quit smoking, or when they start sleeping more soundly. The patient knows that they had control, they took control, and their lives are improved because of it. In the EXPERT Approach™, the clinician has control of the medications, interventions, surgery and control over checking lab values as well as other biometrics like blood pressure and waist to hip circumference. The Expert takes full responsibility for the intervention and finding the solution to the problem. They feel it is their duty to heal and help the patient. Often in the ER or acute care setting, it is a surgery, intervention or medication that will save the patient's life. This happens with heart failure and the administration of IV diuretics, a hemorrhagic stroke and neurosurgery to remove the blood clot, or pneumonia and the selection of the correct antibiotic.

There is an entirely different process going on with chronic conditions and adopting new healthful behaviors. The Expert may know what behaviors the patient needs to adopt to enjoy improved health and well-being, but the coach is the one who can empower the patient to see the value of the change, find ways to make the change fit into their daily lives, and discover the motivation to take responsibility for this change to make it stick.

The most important part of behavior change counseling and the Frates COACH Approach™ is treating people with respect and honoring their beings including their desires, dreams, weaknesses, strengths, failures, and feelings at all times. Mishaps are opportunities to learn and grow, and people's past informs their futures. A coach or behavior change agent is there to help people learn and grow and make strides to their desired self. By embracing this Frates COACH Approach™ and this way of being with a focus on curiosity, non-judgmental behavior that is open-minded, appreciative, compassionate, and honest allows each individual patient to be fully seen and understood.

With diversity, equity, and inclusion work coming to be at the forefront, the COACH Approach is shining bright as a way to treat others right. Every person has the right to be heard, to be helped, and to heal. There are many recommendations for health coaches in order for them to enhance their equity skills. The Primal Health Coach website[23] clearly defines seven strategies as follows:

1. See each client as their own unique, exceptional being.
2. Co-discover each client's favorite ways to learn.
3. Meet your client with unconditional positive regard and believe in their unique ability to face challenges or try new behaviors.
4. Always meet the client where they are at, considering each client's ever changing readiness to change. (Discussed in Chapter 2.)
5. Demonstrate unfailing respect for each client's perceptions, past experiences, opinions, and emotions.
6. Practice autonomy-centered coaching.
7. Be culturally curious and responsive.

In terms of curiosity which has been emphasized with the Frates COACH Approach™ as it is the first C, curiosity is key. It is essential for health and wellness coaching and for health equity. Again referring to Primal Health Coach,[23] they recommend considering 10 specific areas with each person.

1. Race and ethnic identity
2. Location
3. Age
4. Gender identity
5. Sexual orientation
6. Socio-economic background
7. Cultural values
8. Religious/spiritual significance
9. Ability/accessibility
10. Neurodiversity (variety in brain/mood/social/learning behaviors and preferences)

1.11 LANDMARK STUDIES IN COACHING AND BEHAVIOR CHANGE

There is research that demonstrates that health and wellness coaching is a promising intervention for individuals looking to adopt and sustain healthy lifestyles. Some small randomized clinical trials demonstrate improvements in health outcomes with health coaching. Early studies about two decades ago showed positive effects in the areas of cardiovascular disease, diabetes, cancer pain, and asthma. Table 1.7 highlights some of the seminal studies that were randomized controlled trials (RCTs).

In 2003, Vale and colleagues studied 792 patients with cardiac disease to determine the impact of a coaching intervention Coaching on Achieving Cardiovascular

TABLE 1.7
Landmark Studies Chart

Study	Number of Participants	Primary Outcomes
Vale et al.[24]	Study on 792 patients with cardiac disease	Cholesterol lowered 21 vs. 7 mg/dL ($p < .0001$)
Whittemore et al.[25]	Study on 53 women with type 2 diabetes	Better diet self-management, less diabetes relates distress, higher satisfaction with care
Wolever et al.[26]	Study on 56 patients with type 2 diabetes	Significant reduction in Hemoglobin A1C among subjects with baseline ≥ 7
Fisher et al.[27]	Asthma outcomes in 191 children (parents and children coached)	Decreased re-hospitalization rates compared to controls 35.6% vs. 59.1% ($p < .01$)
Oliver et al.[28]	Study on 67 patients with cancer	Improved pain severity compared to controls ($p = .014$)

Health (COACH).[24] After five coaching sessions by telephone over a six-month period, subjects in the intervention group had a greater drop in cholesterol, lost more weight, reduced their fat intake, and were walking more compared to the patients in the control group.

In 2004, Whittemore and colleagues studied 53 women with type 2 diabetes.[25] They participated in six coaching sessions delivered by nurses. Results showed that those in the coaching group who were better able to manage their diets had less diabetes-related distress, had better exercise management, lowered their BMI, and were more satisfied with their medical care compared to the group in usual care.

In 2010, Wolever and colleagues studied the effects of coaching on 56 patients with type 2 diabetes who were randomly assigned to integrative care coaching for six months or usual care.[26] The coaching intervention included 14 sessions of telephonic coaching lasting 30 minutes. The subjects in the coaching group had lower Hemoglobin A1C when compared to those in the usual care group. In addition, those in the coaching group had less stress, better perceptions of their health, and better exercise adherence.

In 2009, Fisher and colleagues investigated children with asthma and their parents.[27] The subjects included 191 children and parents, and they were randomly assigned to the coaching group or usual care group. The coaching included telephone and in-person coaching to parents followed by bi-weekly calls for three months and monthly calls for two years. Children in the families who were coached had fewer hospitalizations (35.6%) than children whose families did not receive the coaching intervention (59.1%).

In 2001, Oliver and colleagues researched pain and coaching.[28] The study included 67 cancer patients with moderate pain. The subjects were randomly assigned to receive one 20-minute coaching session before seeing their oncologist or they were assigned to an education session which was usual care. The coach reviewed the World Health Organization pain control guidelines with the subject. They also discussed techniques to talk to and ask their oncologist questions about the treatment plan. Two weeks after the intervention in a follow-up phone interview, the subjects in the coach group reported significantly less pain than the usual care group.

1.12   REVIEW STUDIES IN COACHING AND BEHAVIOR CHANGE

Interest and research in coaching have grown significantly since the landmark studies were published in the early 2000s. Several reviews look at between 2 and 284 studies. They look at outcomes of patients with cardiovascular disease, chronic obstructive pulmonary disease, cancer, rehabilitation medicine, and those in retirement. The overall findings reveal that coaching is effective in these settings. There are gaps in the research including long-term effectiveness that need to be addressed in future studies. Table 1.8 highlights more recent studies in coaching.

TABLE 1.8
Review Studies Chart

Study	Number of Participants	Primary Outcomes
An and Song[29]	15 studies of adults with cardiovascular risk	Significant effect on physical activity, dietary behaviors, management of stress, health responsibility
Stara et al.[30]	Two studies with aging workers	Improved well-being based on physical criteria
Obro et al.[31]	Review of nine studies on chronic disease coaching	Patients prefer face-to-face coaching
Singh et al.[32]	12 studies on pharmacist coaching	Improved clinical and non-clinical outcomes
Long et al.[33]	Meta-analysis with 10 RCTs on COPD	Improved QOL and reduced COPD hospital admissions ($p = .0001$)
Dejonghe et al.[34]	14 studies in preventative and rehab settings	Improved outcomes in three studies in each group
Barakat et al.[35]	12 studies including 1,038 cancer survivors	Improved physical activity, mood, and QOL
Kivelä et al.[36]	13 studies on adults with chronic disease	Improved weight management, increased physical activity, improved health status (physical and mental)
Wolver et al.[37]	Review of 284 studies	Coaching operationalization of articles: Patient-centered 86%. Self-discovery/active learning 63%. Provides education and coaching 91%. Encourages accountability for behaviors 86%. Provides education and coaching 91%. Consistent ongoing relationship 78%

1.13   RECENT COACHING INTERVENTION STUDIES

In 2020, An and colleagues conducted a meta-analysis on the effects of health coaching on behavior in patients at risk for cardiovascular disease.[29] Fifteen randomized studies were included in the review. The review evaluated how coaching impacts patient responsibility, physical activity, dietary decisions, stress management, and smoking behaviors. Effect sizes of the coaching interventions were small but significant for four of the categories examined including physical activity, patient responsibility, stress management, and dietary decisions. Smoking behaviors did not reveal significance.

Stara and colleagues conducted a systematic review examining the use of digital health coaching for aging workers to help them adopt healthy behaviors and extend their time in the workforce.[30] The review consisted of examining only two studies that met the inclusion criteria out of 1931 identified. The digital health programs improved physical well-being in older workers, but social and psychological well-being was not discussed.

Obro and colleagues focused on the use of mobile health to help patients self-manage chronic diseases with health coaching. In this literature review, nine studies were included.[31] The authors found an important factor in developing self-management skills was patient engagement. According to the findings in this review, the patients preferred face-to-face coaching. Mobile health may be more efficient when it is used to assist the coach with telecommunication and to monitor disease.

Singh and colleagues examined the literature from 2000 to 2009 to identify studies investigating health coaching techniques utilized by pharmacists.[32] Twelve studies were included in this systematic review. The authors sought to determine whether face-to-face, telephone, or electronic communication was used to coach patients and assess coach training and health outcomes. Of the 12 studies selected, most used a combination of communication techniques, but four were just face-to-face and one was just by telephone. Review of the literature revealed that coaching by the pharmacist improved both clinical outcomes for subjects diagnosed with diabetes, hypertension, high cholesterol, and depression. There were improved non-clinical outcomes as well including medication adherence, attitude toward drug therapy, medical costs, and patient satisfaction toward the service.

Long and colleagues performed a meta-analysis on the use of health coaching to improve health-related quality of life (HRQoL) and reduce hospital admissions in patients with chronic obstructive pulmonary disease (COPD).[33] Ten RCTs that used motivational interviewing, goal setting, and health education on COPD were included in this review. Coaching was found to decrease hospital admissions related to COPD and to enhance the quality of life in this patient population.

Dejonghe and colleagues reviewed the long-term effects of health coaching on healthy individuals and patients with chronic disease in a systematic review.[34] Fourteen studies were included in the review: seven focused on prevention and seven focused on rehabilitation. The authors evaluated health coaching for prevention of disease and also for rehabilitation to assess how coaching influenced health outcomes. Three out of the seven studies in each group demonstrated a positive long-term effect of coaching on health outcomes at 24 weeks.

Barakat and colleagues performed a systematic review on the use of health coaching to build capacity to support cancer survivors.[35] Six randomized trials and six pre-post quasi-experimental studies were included, and with these studies, there were 1,038 cancer survivors in total. Research showed that coaching for patients with cancer increased quality of life, physical activity, social connections, and decreased pain and fatigue. Five out of the six studies included in the review revealed that coaching can improve mental health (depression/anxiety) outcomes. The authors identified future research topics as how coaching can improve self-efficacy and influence patient environments.

Kivelä and colleagues performed a systematic review investigating the impact of health coaching on patients suffering from chronic diseases.[36] Thirteen articles were included in the review out of the 1,696 articles published between 2009 and 2013. The authors reported that coaching improved the management of chronic disease by promoting positive psychological, behavioral, and physiological outcomes. Specifically, it was noted that coaching patients with chronic conditions helped to improve weight management, increase patient physical activity, and improve mental health conditions.

Wolever and colleagues performed a systematic review of 284 articles on health and wellness coaching available in 2014.[37] The goal of the review was to create a concrete definition of health coaching. The authors identified health coaching as a process performed by a health professional using behavior change theory and education in 91% of the studies. Coaching was considered a patient-centered process in 86% of the studies. And, in 71% of the studies coaching was offered to help patients set their own goals. Self-discovery was considered a component of coaching used to help the patient explore new ways of achieving their goals in 63% of papers. Seventy-eight percent of the research studies reviewed defined coaching as a reliable and consistent relationship between a patient and clinician.

1.13.1 RESEARCH ON EFFECTIVE BEHAVIOR CHANGE TECHNIQUES AND STRATEGIES ON SPECIFIC POPULATIONS

1.13.1.1 Retirement Age, Nutrition, and Physical Activity

According to a paper published by Lara and colleagues, clinicians can help aging adults adopt healthy eating habits and increase their physical activity by educating them on the benefits of these behavior changes.[38] These benefits may include disease prevention. Following an assessment of the patient's readiness to change, the clinician can help them identify goals and perceived barriers to success. This involves patient identification of what might stand in the way of adopting healthy habits and coaching them to explore ways to solve the problem. Using a patient-centric approach to brainstorming allows patients to decide how they may use social support to achieve their goals. This approach lets them plan solutions using friends, family, or social groups as support. This may entail changing social settings or selecting new group activities. The use of clinician follow-up prompts supports patient accountability and improves self-care. Providing feedback on performance helps to build and maintain a responsive clinician–patient relationship.

1.14   ADULT OBESITY

The literature on coaching for adult obesity discussed specific behaviors and strategies used to increase self-efficacy and physical activity. Coaching to increase the self-efficacy of the patient includes action planning of specific physical activity.[39] Remember, small successes build confidence for later success. This requires time management and self-monitoring of outcomes. The use of social support includes supervised and group activities or connecting with professional support such as a dietitian.

Coaching to increase healthy behavior prompts the patient to self-monitor. Clinicians teach patients to use prompts and cues. Coaching allows the patient to look at what they did right and replicate the behavior, or self-correct to ensure future success. Rewards that match the effort or progress are used to self-motivate.

Effective behavior change techniques to increase activity in obese adults address short- and long-term goals. Both short- and long-term behavior changes rely upon goal setting and self-monitoring of behavior. Long-term behavior change includes feedback on outcomes. In long term, clinicians may implement graded tasks with increasing levels of difficulty and add aides to the environment such as step counters or smartwatches.

Effective counseling strategies for behavior change in adults who are overweight change over time. Strategies that do not change include maintaining support for the patient's autonomy, a patient-centered approach, and the use of motivational interviewing.

1.14.1   BEHAVIOR AND WEIGHT CHANGE IN ADULTS

Several predictors of beneficial weight and behavior change were found in the literature.[40] Patients who were successful at increasing their physical activity were those with higher intrinsic motivation, self-efficacy, and self-regulation. Those who were better at weight control had positive body images and were more flexible with eating constraints.

1.14.2   CHILDHOOD OBESITY

Coaching to change physical activity and eating in children who have a BMI that puts them in the obesity category relies upon management and prevention interventions.[41] Management interventions are structured to provide information on the consequences of unhealthy behavior to the child and family. Families are prompted to restructure the environment to help the child adopt new behaviors. Prompting new behaviors is practiced with the family. Identification of family members as role models for healthy behavior creates an environment that supports the child's success. Family training on the management of emotional and stress eating becomes part of the coaching process as well as training on communication skills. Prevention intervention also includes prompting the family to generalize the behavior.

1.15 DIABETES AND BEHAVIOR CHANGE

A literature review on behavior change techniques for people with diabetes looked at 14 RCTs between 1975 and 2015.[42] This review found 4 out of 46 behavior change techniques to be effective: (1) instructions to carry out a behavior, (2) demonstration of the behavior, (3) behavior rehearsal, and (4) action planning. Strategies that worked for patients included: supervised physical activity, group exercise, and connecting with a physiologist and dietician. Studies that used increased frequency and intensity of physical activity had better patient outcomes.

1.16 SUMMARY

Behavior change is a science and an art. Many scientific journal articles have experimented with different methods to help people change their behavior, adopt healthy habits, and sustain them. Reviewing the science is essential. Many important psychological theories serve as the guiding principles for strategies and techniques used in behavior change counseling. These include but are not limited to Transtheoretical Model of Change, Social Cognitive Theory, Self-Determination Theory, and Social Ecological Model of Change. In addition to these theories, the social determinants of health are essential to take into consideration when counseling any individual on adopting and sustaining healthy habits.

One methodology of helping people change is to take the COACH approach™ which is different and in some ways opposite to the EXPERT approach™. The mnemonic COACH which highlights the use of curiosity, openness, appreciation, compassion, and honesty is the way of being when working with people and helping them adopt and sustain healthy behaviors. Anyone can use the COACH Approach™ and supplement their practice with this approach. There are certified health and wellness coaches who are trained to do this work for their profession. Working with health and wellness coaches and including them as members of a lifestyle medicine team or any healthcare team is a strategy that many clinicians are using. There are different behavior change experts, some with a PhD, some with Master's degrees. Some are psychologists, psychiatrists, and behavior health specialists. The key is that we include behavior change in our efforts to empower people to change.

Research supports the use of health and wellness coaching. More and more research is being performed in this area, and more is needed. Long-term studies with follow-up of 5–10 years or more, with thousands of patients enrolled in the interventions will help the field to better understand dosing of interventions, the most effective techniques and their mechanisms of action. Reporting on cases is helpful and useful, as clinicians can share best practices and strategies that work. Randomized clinical trials remain the gold standard.

Behavior change is a journey for patient and clinician. The exciting part is that no two journeys are the same.

1.17   TAKEAWAYS

1. Empowering patients to change involves behavior change theories, processes, and strategies that are evidence-based.
2. There are psychological theories that are foundational to behavior change.
3. The COACH Approach™ is a way of being that embodies and utilizes curiosity, openness, appreciation, compassion, and honesty.
4. The EXPERT Approach™ is a way of being that puts the responsibility of the outcome on the clinician. The clinician uses examining, x-raying, planning, explaining, repeating, and telling as a way to interact with the patient and solve the patient's problem.
5. Most healthcare clinicians were taught the EXPERT Approach™ in their healthcare professional schools and training.
6. To move from the EXPERT to the COACH Approach™ way of being the clinician needs to focus on five main areas: the way they share knowledge, listen, ask questions, address problems, and take responsibility.
7. Health and wellness coaching is a healthcare profession focused on behavior change.
8. There is research from randomized controlled studies that support the use of health and wellness coaching interventions with patients experiencing chronic conditions.
9. Asking questions is key to the behavior change process and empowering patients to change.
10. Identifying and addressing the patient's motivations, obstacles, strengths, and strategies (MOSS) is an important part of counseling/coaching patients for lasting behavior change.
11. This book will review in detail the 13 keys to behavior change.

REFERENCES

1. Duszyc K, Gomez GA, Schroder K, Sweet MJ, Yap AS. In life there is death: How epithelial tissue barriers are preserved despite the challenge of apoptosis. *Tissue Barriers*. 2017;5(4):e1345353. doi:10.1080/21688370.2017.1345353
2. Psychological Association. *APA Dictionary of Psychology*. 2022. https://dictionary.apa.org/behavior-change
3. Ozemek C, Tiwari S, Sabbahi A, Carbone S, Lavie CJ. Impact of therapeutic lifestyle changes in resistant hypertension. *Prog Cardiovasc Dis*. 2020;63(1):4–9. doi:10.1016/j.pcad.2019.11.012.
4. Almutairi N, Hosseinzadeh H, Gopaldasani V. The effectiveness of patient activation intervention on type 2 diabetes mellitus glycemic control and self-management behaviors: A systematic review of RCTs. *Prim Care Diabetes*. 2020;14(1):12–20. doi:10.1016/j.pcd.2019.08.009.
5. American College of Lifestyle Medicine. Spring. 2022. https://lifestylemedicine.org (accessed August 14, 2022). https://lifestylemedicine.org/overview/
6. Kwasnicka D, Dombrowski SU, White M, Sniehotta F. Theoretical explanations for maintenance of behaviour change: A systematic review of behaviour theories. *Health Psychol Rev*. 2016;10(3):277–296. doi:10.1080/17437199.2016.1151372.

7. Michie S. Theories of behaviour and behaviour change across the social and behavioural sciences: A scoping review. *Health Psychol Rev.* 2015; 9(3):323–344. doi:10.1080/17437199.2014.941722.

8. Moafa I, Hoving C, van den Borne B, Jafer M. Identifying behavior change techniques used in tobacco cessation interventions by oral health professionals and their relation to intervention effects—A review of the scientific literature. *Int J Environ Res Public Health.* 2021;18(14):7481. doi:10.3390/ijerph18147481.

9. Bandura A. *Social Foundations of Thought and Action: A Social Cognitive Theory.* Englewood Cliffs, NJ: Prentice-Hall. 1986.

10. Bandura A. *Self-Efficacy: The Exercise of Control.* W H Freeman/Times Books/Henry Holt & Co. 1997. New York, NY.

11. Deci EL, Ryan R. *Intrinsic Motivation and Self-Determination in Human Behavior.* New York: Plenum. 1985.

12. The Center for Self-Determination Theory (CSDT). https://selfdeterminationtheory.org. https://selfdeterminationtheory.org/theory/

13. Maslow AH. *Motivation and Personality.* 2nd ed. New York: Harper & Row. 1970.

14. Dominguez LJ, Veronese N, Baiamonte E, et al. Healthy aging and dietary patterns. *Nutrients.* 2022;14(4), 889. doi:10.3390/nu14040889.

15. Olstad DL, Kirkpatrick SI. Planting seeds of change: Reconceptualizing what people eat as eating practices and patterns. *Int J Behav Nutr Phys Act.* 2021; 18(1):32. doi:10.1186/s12966-021-01102-1.

16. Banks AR, Bell BA, Ngendahimana D, Embaye M, Freedman DA, Chisolm DJ. Identification of factors related to food insecurity and the implications for social determinants of health screenings. *BMC Public Health.* 2021;21(1):1410. doi:10.1186/s12889-021-11465-6.

17. Alcántara C, Diaz SV, Cosenzo LG, Loucks EB, Penedo FJ, Williams NJ. Social determinants as moderators of the effectiveness of health behavior change interventions: Scientific gaps and opportunities. *Health Psychol Rev.* 2020;14(1):132–144. doi:10.1080/17437199.2020.1718527.

18. U.S. Department of Health and Human Services, Office of Disease Prevention and Health Promotion. *Social Determinates of Health.* https://health.gov/healthypeople/priority-areas/social-determinants-health.

19. Kumar V, Encinosa W. Racial disparities in the perceived risk of COVID-19 and in getting needed medical care. *J Racial Ethn Health Disparities.* 2023 Feb;10(1):4–13. doi:10.1007/s40615-021-01191-5.

20. National Board for Health and Wellness Coaching. https://nbhwc.org.

21. Frates B, Bonnet J, Joseph R., Peterson J. *Lifestyle Medicine Handbook: An Introduction to the Power of Healthy Habits.* Healthy Learning. 2020. Monterey, CA.

22. Frates EP, Bonnet J. Collaboration and negotiation: The key to therapeutic lifestyle change. *Am J Lifestyle Med.* 2016;10(5):302–312.

23. Moon M. *7 Equity and Inclusion-Enhancing Skills for Health and Wellness Coaches.* Primal Health Coach Institute. https://www.primalhealthcoach.com/7-equity-and-inclusion-enhancing-skills-for-health-and-wellness-coaches/.

24. Vale MJ, Jelinek MV, Best JD, et al. Coaching patients on achieving cardiovascular health (COACH): A multicenter randomized trial in patients with coronary heart disease. *Arch Int Med.* 2003;163(22):2775–2783. doi:10.1001/archinte.163.22.2775.

25. Whittemore R, Melkus GD, Sullivan A, Grey MA. Nurse-coaching intervention for women with type 2 diabetes. *Diabetes Educ.* 2004; 30(5):795–804. doi:10.1177/014572170403000515.

26. Wolever RQ, Dreusicke M, Fikkan J, et al. Integrative health coaching for patients with type 2 diabetes: A randomized clinical trial. *Diabetes Educ*. 2010;36(4):629–639. doi:10.1177/0145721710371523.

27. Fisher EB, Strunk RC, Highstein GR, et al. A randomized controlled evaluation of the effect of community health workers on hospitalization for asthma: The asthma coach [published correction appears in *Arch Pediatr Adolesc Med*. 2009;163(5):493]. *Arch Pediatr Adolesc Med*. 2009;163(3):225–232. doi:10.1001/archpediatrics.2008.577.

28. Oliver JW, Kravitz RL, Kaplan SH, Meyers FJ. Individualized patient education and coaching to improve pain control among cancer outpatients. *J Clin Oncol*. 2001;19(8):2206–2212. doi:10.1200/JCO.2001.19.8.2206.

29. An S, Song R. Effects of health coaching on behavioral modification among adults with cardiovascular risk factors: Systematic review and meta-analysis. *Patient Educ Couns*. 2020;103(10):2029–2038. doi:10.1016/j.pec.2020.04.029.

30. Stara V, Santini S, Kropf J, D'Amen B. Digital health coaching programs among older employees in transition to retirement: Systematic literature review [published correction appears in *J Med Internet Res*. 2020 Dec 14;22(12):e25065]. *J Med Internet Res*. 2020;22(9):e17809. doi:10.2196/17809.

31. Obro LF, Heiselberg K, Krogh PG, et al. Combining mHealth and health-coaching for improving self-management in chronic care. A scoping review [published correction appears in *Patient Educ Couns*. 2021 Oct;104(10):2601]. *Patient Educ Couns*. 2021;104(4):680–688. doi:10.1016/j.pec.2020.10.026.

32. Singh H, Kennedy GA, Stupans I. Does the modality used in health coaching matter? A systematic review of health coaching outcomes. *Patient Prefer Adherence*. 2020;14:1477–1492. doi:10.2147/PPA.S265958.

33. Long H, Howells K, Peters S, Blakemore A. Does health coaching improve health-related quality of life and reduce hospital admissions in people with chronic obstructive pulmonary disease? A systematic review and meta-analysis. *Br J Health Psychol*. 2019;24(3):515–546. doi:10.1111/bjhp.12366.

34. Dejonghe LAL, Becker J, Froboese I, Schaller A. Long-term effectiveness of health coaching in rehabilitation and prevention: A systematic review. *Patient Educ Couns*. 2017;100(9):1643–1653. doi:10.1016/j.pec.2017.04.012.

35. Barakat S, Boehmer K, Abdelrahim M, et al. Does health coaching grow capacity in cancer survivors? A systematic review. *Popul Health Manag*. 2018;21(1):63–81. doi:10.1089/pop.2017.0040.

36. Kivelä K, Elo S, Kyngäs H, Kääriäinen M. The effects of health coaching on adult patients with chronic diseases: A systematic review. *Patient Educ Couns*. 2014;97(2):147–157. doi:10.1016/j.pec.2014.07.026.

37. Wolever RQ, Simmons LA, Sforzo GA, et al. A systematic review of the literature on health and wellness coaching: Defining a key behavioral intervention in healthcare. *Glob Adv Health Med*. 2013;2(4):38–57. doi:10.7453/gahmj.2013.042.

38. Lara J, Evans EH, O'Brien N, et al. Association of behaviour change techniques with effectiveness of dietary interventions among adults of retirement age: A systematic review and meta-analysis of randomised controlled trials. *BMC Med*. 2014;12:177. doi:10.1186/s12916-014-0177-3.

39. Samdal GB, Eide GE, Barth T, Williams G, Meland E. Effective behaviour change techniques for physical activity and healthy eating in overweight and obese adults; systematic review and meta-regression analyses. *Int J Behav Nutr Phys Act*. 2017;14(1):42. doi:10.1186/s12966-017-0494-y.

40. Teixeira PJ, Carraça EV, Marques MM, et al. Successful behavior change in obesity interventions in adults: A systematic review of self-regulation mediators. *BMC Med.* 2015;13:84. doi:10.1186/s12916-015-0323-6.
41. Martin J, Chater A, Lorencatto F. Effective behaviour change techniques in the prevention and management of childhood obesity. *Int J Obes (Lond).* 2013;37(10):1287–1294. doi:10.1038/ijo.2013.107.
42. Cradock KA, ÓLaighin G, Finucane FM, Gainforth HL, Quinlan LR, Ginis KA. Behaviour change techniques targeting both diet and physical activity in type 2 diabetes: A systematic review and meta-analysis. *Int J Behav Nutr Phys Act.* 2017;14(1):18. doi:10.1186/s12966-016-0436-0.

2 Stages of Change

James O. Prochaska, Ph.D. and
Janice M. Prochaska, Ph.D.

We are sad to report the untimely passing of Dr. James Prochaska. He was an important investigator in the area of behavioral medicine and mentored numerous psychologists and other healthcare workers in this area. We will miss him greatly.

2.1 INTRODUCTION

Health risk behaviors, such as smoking, unhealthy diets, inactivity, alcohol misuse, and ineffectively managed stress, significantly contribute to a population's morbidity, disability, mortality, reduced functioning and productivity, and escalating health care costs. In contrast, accumulating evidence suggests that a healthy lifestyle includes:

1. Abstinence from smoking;
2. Eating five servings of fruits and vegetables each day;
3. Adequate physical activity (e.g., moving 10,000 steps a day or doing 150 minutes of moderate exercise a week); and
4. Twenty minutes of daily stress management.

0–1-2–5–10–20–25

In addition, striving to maintain a body mass index (BMI) of less than 25 increases life expectancy by up to 14 years.[1–3] However, having a healthy lifestyle of 0 (smoking), 1 (drink per day for women, 2 for men under 65), 5 (fruits and vegetables), 10 (10,000 steps), 20 (at least 20 minutes of mindful breathing, meditation, or other methods for reducing distress), and 25 (<25 BMI) has been an elusive goal for 97% of the population.[4] The following formula can be a guide to a healthy lifestyle: 0, 1, 2, 5, 10, 20, and 25 for one's health.

Why are just five risk behaviors so critical for health? They represent the fundamental functions of life: breathing, drinking, eating, moving, and feeling. If we breathe toxins, we poison our bodies. If we drink alcohol to toxic levels, we do damage to both our minds and bodies. If we eat toxins like refined sugar, we seriously compromise our general well-being. If we don't move it, move it, move it enough, we don't push enough toxins out of our bodies. And, if we feel distressed, we are likely to

DOI: 10.1201/9781003161226-2

smoke more cigarettes, drink more alcohol, eat more unhealthy "comfort foods," and flop on the couch. Distress is also the number one reason why people relapse when they try to change unhealthy behaviors to healthy ones.

The fundamental functions of life are so important because they happen day, after day, after day for our whole lives. If the dysfunctional behaviors happen year after year, they build up the risk of producing diseases, disabilities, poor functioning, and premature death.

To have a significant and sustainable impact on attaining the healthy behaviors of 0, 1, 2, 5, 10, 20, and 25, a model of behavior change is needed to address the needs of entire populations, not just the minority who are motivated to take immediate action for better health. The Transtheoretical Model of Behavior Change (TTM) reframes change to equaling progress through a series of stages. The TTM is integrated around the stages of change which can identify segments of populations in different stages of change:

1. Precontemplation (not ready to take action)
2. Contemplation (getting ready)
3. Preparation (ready)
4. Action (meeting the healthy criteria behavior change)
5. Maintenance (keeping up the healthy criteria behavior change).[5,6]

Then, principles and processes are applied to facilitate engagement, reduce resistance, and prevent relapse through the stages of change.[5,6]

2.1.1 UNDERSTANDING THE STAGES OF CHANGE

Stage of change is the TTM's central organizing construct. Longitudinal studies of change have found that people move through a series of stages when modifying behavior on their own or with the help of formal interventions.[7,8] Understanding the stages of change allows one to appreciate change as a dynamic process and helps one to learn the variability in patients' responses to the uptake of health behavior interventions. The stage construct implies progress occurring over time. Traditionally, behavior change was often construed as an event, such as quitting smoking, drinking, or over-eating, but the TTM recognizes change as a process that unfolds over time and involves progress through a series of stages (see Figure 2.1).

2.1.1.1 Precontemplation (Not Ready)

Patients in the Precontemplation stage are not intending to take action in the foreseeable future, usually measured as the next 6 months. Being uninformed or underinformed about the consequences of one's behavior may cause a person to be in Precontemplation. Multiple, unsuccessful attempts at change can also lead to demoralization about one's ability to change. Both the uninformed and under-informed tend to avoid reading, talking, or thinking about their high-risk behaviors. They are often characterized in other theories as resistant, unmotivated, or not ready for interventions. The fact is that action-oriented programs are not ready for such individuals and are not developed to meet their needs. Messages like, "Wherever you are at, we

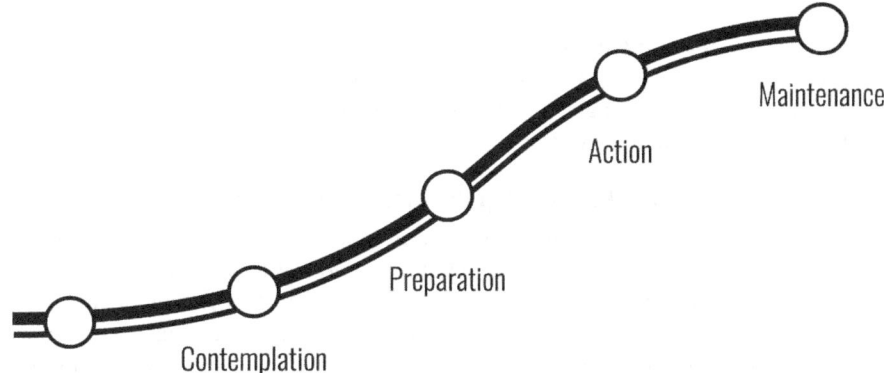

Maintenance

Action

Preparation

Contemplation

Precontemplation

FIGURE 2.1 The Transtheoretical Model (TTM) recognizes change as a process that unfolds over time and involves progress through a series of stages.

can work with that,"™ need to be delivered. Interventions need to be implemented that respect whichever stage individuals are in.

2.1.1.2 Contemplation (Getting Ready)

Contemplation is the stage in which patients intend to change in the next 6 months. They are more aware of the pros of changing but are also acutely aware of the cons. In a meta-analysis across 48 health risk behaviors, the pros and cons of changing were equal for people in Contemplation.[9] This weighting between the costs and benefits of changing can produce profound ambivalence that can cause people to remain in this stage for prolonged periods of time. This phenomenon is often characterized as chronic contemplation or behavioral procrastination. Individuals in Contemplation are also not ready for traditional action-oriented programs that expect participants to act immediately.

2.1.1.3 Preparation (Ready)

Preparation is the stage in which patients are intending to take action in the immediate future, usually measured as the next month. Typically, they have already taken some significant steps toward the healthier behavior in the past year. These individuals have a plan of action, such as joining an exercise class, consulting a nutritionist, talking to their physician, buying a self-help book, or relying on a self-change approach. These are the people who can be matched to action-oriented programs, such as nicotine replacement therapies or Weight Watchers.

2.1.1.4 Action (Doing the Healthy Behavior)

Action is the stage in which patients have made specific overt modifications in their lifestyles within the past 6 months. Since action is observable, the overall process of behavior change has often been equated with action. But in the TTM, Action is only one of the stages. Not all modifications of behavior count as action in this model. In most applications, people have to attain a criterion that scientists and professionals agree is sufficient to reduce the risk of disease. For example, reduction in the number of cigarettes or switching to low tar and nicotine cigarettes were formerly considered acceptable actions for smoking. Now the consensus is clear – only total abstinence counts, as those other changes do not necessarily lead to quitting and do not remove the risks associated with smoking.

2.1.1.5   Maintenance (Keeping Up the Healthy Behavior)

Maintenance is the stage in which people have made specific, overt modifications in their lifestyles for at least six months. They are working to prevent relapse but they do not apply change processes as frequently as do people in Action. They are less tempted to relapse, and grow increasingly more confident (have greater self-efficacy) that they can continue their changes. Based on self-efficacy and temptation data, researchers have estimated that Maintenance lasts from 6 months to about 5 years. Fitbit is a good example of a tool to help someone stay in Maintenance.

2.1.1.6   Termination

Termination is the stage in which people are not tempted; they have 100% self-efficacy. Whether depressed, anxious, bored, lonely, angry, or stressed, individuals in this stage are sure they will not return to unhealthy habits as a way of coping. It is as if the habit was never acquired in the first place or their new behavior has become an automatic healthy habit. Examples include people who have developed automatic seatbelt use or who automatically take their medications at the same time and place each day. In a study of former smokers and alcoholics, researchers found that less than 20% of each group had reached the criteria of zero temptation and total self-efficacy.[10] The criterion of 100% self-efficacy may be too strict or it may be that this stage is an ideal goal for population health efforts.

2.1.2   PRINCIPLES OF CHANGE

The principles of decisional balance and self-efficacy, alongside the Processes of Change, help patients move through the Stages of Change.

2.1.2.1   Decisional Balance

The weighing of the pros and cons of changing is decisional balance. Sound decision-making requires the consideration of the potential gains (pros) and losses (cons) associated with a behavior's consequences. For example, there are more than 65 scientifically established benefits of regular physical activity. A patient could be encouraged to make a list to see how many can be identified. They can then take a list of 65+ pros, from our book, *Changing to Thrive*, and see how many of the pros of changing are important to them. One can also list the cons. The more the list of pros outweighs the cons, the better prepared one will be to take effective action.

2.1.2.2   Self-Efficacy

Self-efficacy is the degree to which an individual believes they have the capacity to attain a desired goal (see Chapter 8).[11] With TTM-based interventions, self-efficacy is operationalized as confidence to make and sustain changes. Confidence is low in the Precontemplation stage and increases across the stages.[12] Given the importance of self-efficacy, it needs to be raised early by assisting patients in setting and achieving small goals that will build their confidence for taking on increasingly difficult challenges. If, for example, someone is not exercising at all but is intending to do so in the next 6 months, it would be helpful to have them set a reasonable and achievable goal to begin exercising slowly (e.g., 10 minutes, three times a week) and increase the frequency and intensity once that goal has been mastered.

2.1.2.3   Temptation

Temptation reflects the intensity of urges to engage in a specific unhealthy habit while in the midst of difficult situations. Typically, three factors reflect the most common types of tempting situations:

1. Emotional Distress
2. Positive Social Situations
3. Craving

People could ask themselves how they will cope with emotional distress (without relying on a cigarette or comfort foods) to help them cope more effectively, and thereby build their self-efficacy.

2.1.3   PROCESSES OF CHANGE

Figure 2.2 illustrates the Principles and Processes of Change by Stage. Processes of change are the experiential and behavioral activities that people use to progress through the stages. They provide important guides for intervention programs, serving

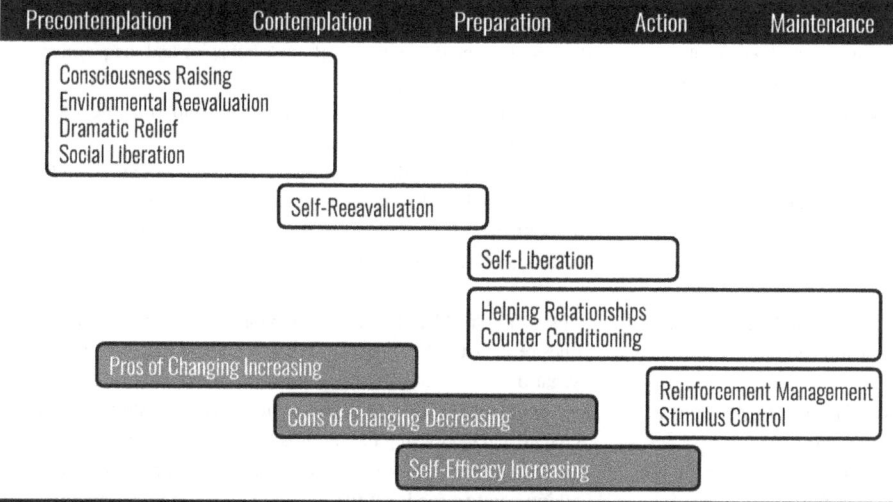

FIGURE 2.2   Integration of the stages (in black), principles (in gray), and processes of change (in white).

as activities that are applied to move from stage to stage. Ten processes have received the most scientific support to date. They are described in Table 2.1 and below.

2.1.3.1　Consciousness Raising (Get Informed)

Consciousness raising involves increased awareness about the causes, consequences, and cures for a particular problem behavior. Interventions that can increase awareness include feedback, interpretations, bibliotherapy (i.e., using self-help books or manuals), and media campaigns. Sedentary patients, for example, may not be aware that their inactivity can have the same risk as smoking a pack of cigarettes a day.

2.1.3.2　Dramatic Relief (Pay Attention to Feelings)

Dramatic relief initially produces increased emotional experiences followed by reduced affect or anticipated relief if appropriate action is taken. Personal testimonies, such as at Alcoholics Anonymous (AA), social networks, and sharing feelings with a friend or counselor are examples of techniques that can move people emotionally.

TABLE 2.1
Processes of Change

Consciousness raising (get informed)	Learning new facts, ideas, and tips that support the healthy behavior change
Dramatic relief (pay attention to feelings)	Experiencing negative emotions (fear, anxiety) that go along with old behaviors or the positive emotions (inspirations) that go along with healthy behavior change
Self-reevaluation (create a new self-image)	Looking back to how individuals think and feel about themselves and forward to how they will think and feel about themselves when free from their unhealthy habit
Environmental reevaluation (notice your effect on others)	Realizing the negative impact of one's behavior and the positive impact of change on others
Social liberation (notice social trends)	Realizing that social norms are changing to support the healthy behavior, e.g., not drinking to excess
Self-liberation (make a commitment)	Believing in one's ability to change and making a commitment to change based on that belief. Going public with one's commitment strengthens self-liberation
Helping relationships (get support)	Seeking and using social support to make and sustain changes
Counter Conditioning (use substitutes)	Substituting healthy alternative behaviors and thoughts for unhealthy ones (e.g., natural sugar in fruits and berries in place of processed sugar that is addictive)
Reinforcement management (use rewards)	Increasing the intrinsic and extrinsic rewards for healthy behavior change and decreasing the rewards for old behaviors
Stimulus control (manage your environment)	Removing reminders or cues to engage in the old behaviors (e.g., taking comfort foods off the shopping list), and using cues to engage in the new healthy behavior (adding fruits and berries to the list)

2.1.3.3 Self-Reevaluation (Create a New Self-Image)

Self-reevaluation combines both cognitive and affective assessments of one's self-image with and without a particular unhealthy habit, such as one's image as a couch potato versus an active person. Values clarification, identifying healthy role models, and imagery are techniques that can help patients apply self-reevaluation. One might ask, "Imagine if you were free from smoking – How would you feel about yourself?"

2.1.3.4 Environmental Reevaluation (Notice Your Effect on Others)

Environmental reevaluation combines both affective and cognitive assessments of how the presence or absence of a personal habit affects one's social environment, such as the effect of excessive drinking on others. It can also include the awareness that one can serve as a positive or negative role model for others. Empathy training and sharing memories can lead to such assessments.

2.1.3.5 Social Liberation (Notice Social Trends)

Social liberation involves realizing that social norms are changing to support the healthy behavior. Examples include recognizing how few places one can smoke, salad bars at restaurants, and walking paths.

2.1.3.6 Self-Liberation (Make a Commitment)

Self-liberation is both the belief that one can change and the commitment as well as re-commitment to act on that belief. New Year's resolutions, public testimonies, or a contract are ways of enhancing what the public calls willpower. The intervention could state, "Telling others about my commitment to take action can strengthen my willpower. Who am I going to tell?" Today with social networks, individuals can make commitments to many of their digital friends.

2.1.3.7 Counter Conditioning (Use Substitutes)

Counter conditioning requires learning healthy behaviors as substitutes for problem behaviors. Examples of counter-conditioning include mindful breathing as a healthy substitution for breathing smoke or walking as a healthier alternative than "comfort foods" as a way to cope with distress.

2.1.3.8 Stimulus Control (Manage Your Environment)

Stimulus control removes cues for unhealthy habits and adds prompts for healthier alternatives. Examples are removing all the alcohol from the house or removing high-fat foods from the shopping list.

2.1.3.9 Reinforcement Management (Use Rewards)

Reinforcement management provides positive consequences for taking steps in a positive direction. While contingency management can include the use of punishment, it was found that self-changers rely on reward much more than punishment. Reinforcements are emphasized since the philosophy of the stage model is to work in harmony with how people change naturally. People expect to be reinforced by others more frequently than is actually the case, so they should be encouraged to reinforce themselves through self-statements like "Nice going – you handled that temptation." They also can treat themselves at milestones as a reinforcement to increase the probability that healthy responses will be repeated.

2.1.3.10   Helping Relationships (Get Support)

Helping relationships combine caring, trust, openness, and acceptance, as well as support for healthy behavior change. Guiding people on how to get social support through support groups, social media, churches, and buddy systems can be sources of social support.

2.2   EVIDENCE SUMMARY

2.2.1   EVIDENCE-BASED STAGES OF CHANGE

TTM-based approaches result in increased participation and engagement because they appeal to the whole population rather than the minority ready to take action. TTM research across many behaviors and populations has demonstrated repeatedly that only a minority of any at-risk group are in Preparation (typically 20%) with 40% in Precontemplation and 40% Contemplation.[13,14] Yet, most behavior change messaging and treatments are action-oriented and assume readiness to participate in action-oriented programs. Such methods engage mostly the 20% or so of people who are ready to take action and misserve the majority of at-risk people who are not prepared to take action. TTM-based programs often achieve greater than 80% participation.[6,15] TTM approaches engage whole populations because they are perceived as more respectful, relevant, engaging, and appealing, thereby reducing resistance and reactance among early stage individuals.

2.2.2   RATES OF BEHAVIOR CHANGE

TTM-based approaches can dramatically increase rates of behavior change. While action-oriented programs may do well to help those ready to change, their impact is limited to the small percentage (20%) of people who are ready to take action. By using a stage approach, one not only increases participation, one also increases the likelihood that individuals will eventually take action. Research demonstrates that helping participants move forward at least one stage of change (such as moving from Precontemplation to Contemplation) can as much as double the likelihood that they will move to the Action stage in the next six months. Helping them to move two stages can triple their chances of taking action.[16]

2.2.3   STAGE-MATCHED INTERVENTIONS

TTM-based approaches have greater impacts. A large body of literature supports the increased impacts of stage-matched programs over action-oriented and one size fits all interventions (see Chart 1). Meta-analyses conclude that tailoring treatments on TTM constructs produces greater impacts than tailoring on most constructs of other behavior change theories.[17,18] TTM-based treatments have been found effective across dozens of behaviors and populations.[19-25] And have been found to surpass the average outcomes of other behavior change programs identified as benchmarks by a national task force.[26] Recent research demonstrates the additional impact TTM-based treatment can have on overall and specific domains of well-being, including happiness, joy, and thriving.[5,27]

2.2.4 MULTIPLE RISK IMPACTS

TTM-based approaches impact multiple risks. Several randomized clinical trials of TTM-based interventions have demonstrated the ability to impact multiple risks, even risks that were not specifically treated.[28,29] We call this transfer effect from a treatment to a non-treated behavior. This phenomenon reflects the synergy of TTM programs. This research includes areas such as adherence to anti-hypertension and lipid-lowering medication, weight management, obesity prevention, and prenatal care.[20–25,30,31] Through this research, the phenomena of coaction have been described as the increased probability that individuals who adopt one health behavior will adopt another health behavior. For example, in a randomized clinical trial of a TTM-tailored weight management intervention for overweight adults, the treatment group demonstrated a 2.5–5.2 increased likelihood of success on a second behavior. The control group demonstrated a 1.2–2.6 increase likelihood of success on a second behavior.[28] Given the vast differences in probability of additional behavior change between successful changers in the treatment group compared to control, it can be concluded that this is not a naturally occurring phenomenon. This is another example of synergy, where more changes are produced than are treated. Similar findings from other multiple behavior trials cumulate evidence that coaction occurs more in groups receiving TTM-tailored behavior change treatments. It can be hypothesized that by teaching individuals strategies that support the change process, they then apply those strategies successfully to other areas.

2.3 PRACTICAL APPLICATION

2.3.1 APPLICATION OF THE STAGES OF CHANGE FOR THE HEALTHCARE CLINICIAN

Within a practice setting, an important first step is to have the patient assessed for all relevant health behaviors via a Health Risk Assessment (HRA). This can be incorporated within electronic medical software or done in a patient interview with the healthcare professional.

In order to use the stage approach, it is necessary to identify which stage of readiness best classifies the patient for each relevant health risk behavior. A critical first component is clearly operationalizing the target behavior and action criteria. This can be thought of as what healthy behavior would one be doing if they were in Action. For example, the action criteria for smoking cessation is "no smoking."

In such areas as weight management, there may be multiple behaviors that are important to assess and treat – readiness to do healthy eating and regular exercise. In working with multiple risks, it's often beneficial to prioritize the at-risk behavior that the patient is most ready to change. If someone is in the Preparation stage, you can set goals and offer treatment options that will likely help them to fairly quickly reach

Action. Upon making that successful behavior change, they will have success under their belt and likely will have increased confidence and skills to make additional behavior changes.

2.3.2 Assessing the Stages of Change

There are several options by which stage of change can be assessed in clinical settings. For many health areas, reliable and valid assessment tools have been developed and can be found in published articles or online and are available in the public domain. Other times, measures can be licensed through the companies that developed them and then incorporated within your patient portal or electronic medical software. A list of companies with HRAs certified by the National Committee for Quality Assurance (NCQA) can be found at http://www.ncqa.org. Using certified assessment tools offers the most reliable and consistent way to monitor and report patient health behaviors and risks longitudinally. For those without the resources to implement standardized protocols, health care professionals can administer staging questions during their patient interview. In doing so, it is important to identify a specific and well-defined behavior and to ask their intention to do the behavior according to this sample:

Do you intend to {Insert Action criteria, e.g., start walking 10,000 steps a day}?

- **No.** I don't intend to do so in the next 6 months. (Precontemplation)
- **Yes.** I intend to do so in the next 6 months. (Contemplation)
- **Yes.** I intend to do so in the next 30 days. (Preparation)
- **Yes.** I have been doing so for less than 6 months. (Action)
- **Yes.** I have been doing so for more than 6 months. (Maintenance)

Once action criteria are identified and one understands the patient's intention to meet the action criteria, the next step is to use that knowledge to target the intervention strategy. Table 2.2 provides guidelines for considering the patient's stage and interventions by stage of change.

TABLE 2.2
Guidelines for Considering the Patient's Stage and Interventions by Stage of Change

Patient	Interventions
Precontemplation	
• Not ready to change/not intending to take action	• Engage them in a TTM change process, like the pros of changing
• May experience change as coerced	• Use motivational interviewing techniques (e.g., open-ended questions, reflection, evoking change talk, rolling with resistance)
• Might feel demoralized from multiple relapses	• Encourage thinking of relapse not as a failure, but as a learning experience. What mistakes did you make, what can you do differently next time

(Continued)

TABLE 2.2 (*Continued*)

Guidelines for Considering the Patient's Stage and Interventions by Stage of Change

Patient	Interventions
• May respond with denial, reactance, or resistance	• Ask them if they feel you are pressuring them to take action
• Under or unaware of the benefits of changing	• Facilitate movement to contemplation
• Identifies many cons to changing	• Suggest less intense treatment options
• Under-recognizes benefits of changing	• Discuss benefits of changing

Contemplation

• Aware that problem exists	• Increase the pros and decrease the cons to resolve ambivalence
• Expresses some interest in changing eventually	• Help problem solve around significant cons of changing perceived by patient
• Recognizes benefits of changing	• Increase benefits to changing (the longer the list the better)
• Marked by ambivalence	• Encourage reflection of how self-image would improve if behavior changed
• Lacks commitment to change	• Encourage progress rather than action
• Lacks confidence to change	• Encourage small steps
• Might feel stuck – not sure how to make progress	
• Acutely aware of the cons or barriers to changing	

Preparation

• Intending to make a change in the next month	• Goal is to encourage, excite, and empower patient
• Preparing to act	• Provide support
• Has taken some small steps	• Create an action plan that includes start date and steps to action
• Recognizes more benefits than cons to changing	• Ensure patient has necessary support systems
• Expresses commitment to change	• Encourage reflection on how self-image will change
• Has increased confidence in ability to change	• Problem solve barriers to change
• Developing a plan toward meeting action criteria	• Provide examples and inspiration of successful changers
	• Refer to more intense action-oriented treatment options

Action

• Recently made the behavior change	• Support action
• Still actively working (giving time and energy) to sustain the change	• Provide praise and recognition

(*Continued*)

TABLE 2.2 (*Continued*)
Guidelines for Considering the Patient's Stage and Interventions by Stage of Change

Patient	Interventions
• May experience strong urge to revert back to old behavior	• Encourage self-praise
• Identifying difficult times to stay adherent	• Communicate that sustaining action takes effort and commitment
• Slips and recycling to earlier stage common	• Encourage coping skills to handle urges to slip
	• Ensure their environment and routine support lasting action
	• Assist with strategies to prevent relapse
	• Intense treatment options still appropriate
	• Encourage coping skills to handle urges to slip
	• Think of relapse as slips rather than falls

Maintenance

• Maintaining the behavior change for at least 6 months	• Understand that change is dynamic and slips are the rule, not the exception
• High confidence	• Consult on ongoing challenge of ongoing doing the healthy behavior
• High commitment	• Focus on relapse prevention
• Slips still can happen but they don't have to be a fall	• Ensure good coping skills for times of distress and ongoing stress management
• Experience fewer temptations to slip back	• Assist with keeping confidence high
• Risk for relapse highest during times of distress	• Create plan for dealing with distress
	• Encourage patients to learn from slips and plan accordingly

2.3.3 INTERVENTIONS

The healthcare professional could also prescribe TTM computerized, tailored interventions online. With multiple behavior change, a combination of personal and online interventions could be beneficial. There is a comprehensive suite of programs available at Pro-Change Behavior Solutions, Inc. With online programs, patients are assessed on their pros and cons, confidence, and processes of change. They then receive feedback on strategies for increasing the pros, decreasing the cons, ideas for coping with temptations, what processes of change to use more, and strategies for taking small steps for progressing to the next stage. Patients are then able to assess a printed report as well as an online Personal Activity Center where they can find activities designed to reinforce their personal report.

Typically, 30 and 60 days after the first session, patients are prompted to return to complete a follow-up session. Here they are reassessed, given feedback on their progress, and receive an updated report. In addition, patients can receive tailored text messages every one to three days depending on their current stage of change. If a cluster of patients exist with a variety of risk behaviors, a group could be formed via video conference or in person and led by the healthcare professional to teach patients the stages of change and help patients support each other as they move through the stages. The primary care physician's role is to reinforce the use of online and group programs and to check on progress made through the stages of change.

2.4   CASE STUDY

Marilyn was asked to come into her primary care provider's office for an annual visit. She was offered a Health Risk Assessment (HRA) to take at home online which also staged her for any risks that were indicated. Before Marilyn arrived for her appointment, the health care professional on staff knew that Marilyn was in Precontemplation to stop smoking and Contemplation to do regular exercise (two risky health behaviors that can later contribute to chronic conditions). As part of Marilyn's office appointment, the health care professional met with her and gave Contemplation stage-matched messages for exercising regularly by encouraging her to recognize all of the pros of exercising and helping her to reduce the cons of changing (knowing where to safely walk, encouraging her to invite a walking partner). The healthcare worker also asked her to reflect on how her self-image would improve if she became a regular exerciser. She coached Marilyn to take small steps and to walk 10 minutes a day to start. With regards to smoking, the health care professional gave Marilyn an online link to a computerized, tailored, Transtheoretical Model of Change (TTM) smoking cessation program to take online.

One month later, the health care professional via Tele medicine checked in with Marilyn to track her progress with regular exercise and smoking cessation. She assessed what stage Marilyn was in for each and delivered stage-matched messaging for each. Marilyn moved to Preparation for exercise but was still in Precontemplation for smoking cessation. Marilyn was offered to attend a smoking cessation group for those in Precontemplation, recognizing that "wherever she was at, the leader would work with that."

One month later another contact was made. Progress was measured by treatment, stage, problem severity, and effort and was reported to the primary care provider. If Marilyn has progressed one stage, she has doubled her chances she will take action in the near future. If she has progressed two stages, she has tripled the chances she will take effective action. Such progress is very reinforcing for both the patient and the healthcare professional.

A helpful comparison of moving from traditional patient health to empowering patients is shown in Table 2.3.

TABLE 2.3

A Comparison of Moving from Traditional Patient Health to Empowering Patients

Traditional Patient Health	Empowering Patients
Passive, wait for patient to raise health risk	Proactive, assessing with an HRA
Acute Conditions	Prevention or better management of chronic conditions
Action-oriented	Stage-based
Clinic-based	Clinic or Home-based
Clinician-delivered	Clinician and technology delivered
Standardized	Tailored
Single target behavior	Multiple target behaviors
Fragmented	Integrated
Specificity (e.g., treat just one behavior)	Synergy (e.g., coaction)
Reducing Risks	Reducing risks and enhancing well-being

2.5   MEASUREMENT STRATEGIES

Using the HRA to measure progress over time generates reinforcing feedback for individuals and professionals (e.g., one stage progress doubles effective action and two stages triples it). One could also measure increases in the pros and decreases in the cons. Ultimately the measurement is whether there is an increase in the percentage of individuals who are reducing their health risk and enhancing well-being.

Blissmer et al. found that consistent treatment, stage, severity, and effort could measure long-term changes across risky behaviors of smoking, diet, and sun exposure.[32]

These four areas can be measured by:

- Whether or not individuals used the treatment-tailored interventions to help them change their behavior;
- Whether individuals express greater intentions to change and progress a stage;
- How wide is the discrepancy between an individual's current risk behavior and the criterion behavior; and
- How hard individuals are working at changing their behavior – how much are they using the processes of change which in turn influences their decisional balance (pros and cons) and confidence to perform the healthy behavior.

2.6   KEY TAKEAWAYS

These critical assumptions need to be taken into consideration when developing interventions for behavior change that can facilitate progress through the stages and enhance the health and well-being of individuals and populations.

1. Behavior change is a process that unfolds over time through a sequence of stages. Effective interventions need to match their help to patients' stage as they progress over time.

2. Stages can be both stable and subject to change, just as chronic, behavioral risk factors are both stable and subject to change. Health initiatives can motivate change by enhancing the understanding of the pros and diminishing the value of the cons.
3. The majority of an at-risk population is not prepared for action and will not be served by traditional action-oriented prevention programs. Helping individuals set realistic goals, like progressing to the next stage, will facilitate the change process.
4. Specific principles and processes of change need to be emphasized at specific stages for progress through the stages to occur.

Hopefully, you are progressing to incorporate a stage approach in your work with behavior change. Recognizing the unique needs of patients in different stages and seeing progress as movement to the next stage can assist in significantly increasing the impact of your interventions. They can also increase your confidence in assisting individuals at each stage of change.

Those who seek additional guidance can participate in an e-learning module titled "Become an Agent of Change; Applying the TTM of Behavior Change" (details at www.prochange.com\e-learning) or refer to the book *Changing to Thrive: Using the Stages of Change to Overcome the Top Threats to Your Health and Happiness* (2016).

There are many benefits to integrating a TTM stage approach including it:

• Prepares you to work with entire populations of patients wherever they are in the stages of change.
• Helps you reduce resistance among your patients.
• Allows you to see and appreciate how your patients are making progress in stages.
• Enables you to set stage-matched goals with patients.
• Gets you to offer and prescribe behavior change programs that are stage-appropriate.
• Teaches you the principles and processes of change that are applicable across all health behaviors.
• Shows you an approach that is successful at increasing engagement, increasing healthy behaviors, reducing multiple risks, enhancing multiple domains of well-being, and productivity.
• Helps you to change any of your health risk behaviors (e.g., to better manage stress).

A final question: How ready are *you* to integrate a stage approach in *your* work?

1. I don't intend to integrate a stage approach in my work in the next 6 months (Precontemplation).
2. I intend to integrate a stage approach in my work in the next 6 months (Contemplation).
3. I intend to integrate a stage approach in my work in the next month (Preparation).

4. I have been integrating a stage approach in my work for less than 6 months (Action).
5. I have been integrating a stage approach in my work for more than 6 months (Maintenance).

Some ideas to guide the next steps:

1. If you are in Precontemplation, look for more information (e.g., *Changing to Thrive*) in using a stage approach and consider how your work, your patient interactions, and your practice might benefit by adopting a stage approach.
2. If you are in Contemplation, make a list of the pros and cons of TTM and learn more about the pros of using a stage approach by talking with others who use it and seeking additional training in the approach at www.prochage.com/elearning. Identify what barriers might be in your way and consider ways to overcome them. Feel inspired by how the stage approach has helped so many others to more successfully engage patients. Recognize that there are evidence-based programs that are behavior medicines that parallel the biological medicines that individuals can apply at home.
3. If you are in Preparation, make a commitment to begin using a stage approach and share that commitment with others. Build your confidence by role-playing or practicing the approach with patients. Ask co-workers to support and assist your efforts, and notice the benefit.
4. If you are in Action *or* Maintenance, keep this chapter and other training materials visible to make it easy to use a stage approach. Appreciate the benefits TTM offers you and your patients. Boost your confidence by using the approach even with resistant patients. And, like your patients, you may have a slip but you don't have to fall all the way back to your old practice.

2.7 RESOURCES

- Prochaska, J. O., and Prochaska, J. M. 2016. *Changing to Thrive*. Center City, MN: Hazeldon Publishing.
- Prochaska, J. O., Norcross, J. C., and DiClemente, C. C. 1994. *Changing for Good*. New York: Morrow.
- www.prochange.com.
- www.jprochaska.com.

REFERENCES

1. Khaw, K. T., Wareham, N., Bingham, S., Welch, A., Luben, R., and Day, N. 2008. Combined impact of health behaviours and mortality in men and women: the EPIC-Norfolk prospective population study. *PLoS Medicine 5*: e12.
2. van den Brandt, P. A. 2011. The impact of a Mediterranean diet and healthy lifestyle on premature mortality in men and women. *The American Journal of Clinical Nutrition 94*: 913–920. https://doi.org/10.3945/ajcn.110.008250.

3. Pronk, N. P., Lowry, M., Kottke, T. E., Austin, E., Gallagher, J., and Katz, A. 2010. The association between optimal lifestyle adherence and short-term incidence of chronic conditions among employees. *Population Health Management 13*: 289–295. https://doi. org/10.1089/pop.2009.0075.
4. Reeves, M. J., and Rafferty, A. P. 2005. Healthy lifestyle characteristics among adults in the United States, 2000. *Archives of Internal Medicine 165*: 854–857. https://doi. org/10.1001/archinte.165.8.854.
5. Prochaska, J. O., and Prochaska, J. M. 2016. *Changing to Thrive*. Center City, MN: Hazeldon.
6. Prochaska, J. O., Norcross, J. C., and Saul, S. F. 2020. Generating psychotherapy break-throughs: transtheoretical strategies from population health psychology. *American Psychologist 75*: 996–1010.
7. DiClemente, C. C., and Prochaska, J. O. 1982. Self-change and therapy change of smoking behavior: a comparison of processes of change of cessation and maintenance. *Addictive Behaviors 7*: 133–142.
8. Prochaska, J. O., and DiClemente, C. C. 1983. Stages and processes of self-change of smoking: toward an integrative model of change. *Journal of Consulting and Clinical Psychology 51*: 390–395.
9. Hall, J. S., and Rossi, J. S. 2008. Meta-analytic examination of the strong and weak principles across 48 health behaviors. *Preventive Medicine 46*: 266–274.
10. Snow, M. G., Prochaska, J. O., and Rossi, J. S. 1992. Stages of change for smoking cessation among former problem drinkers: a cross-sectional analysis. *Journal of Substance Abuse 4*: 107–116. https://doi.org/10.1016/0899-3289(92)90011-l.
11. Bandura, A. 1982. Self-efficacy mechanism in human agency. *American Psychologist 37*: 122–147.
12. DiClemente, C. C., Prochaska, J. O., Fairhurst, S., Velicer, W. F., Velasquez, M., and Rossi, J. S. 1991. The process of smoking cessation: an analysis of precontemplation, contemplation and preparation stages of change. *Journal of Consulting and Clinical Psychology 59*: 259–304.
13. Velicer, W. F., Fava, J. L., Prochaska, J. O., Abrams, D. B., Emmons, K. M. and Pierce, J. P. 1995. Distribution of smokers by stage in three representative samples. *Preventive Medicine 24*: 401–411.
14. Wewers, M. E., Stillman, F. A., Hartman, A. M., and Shopland, D. R. 2003. Distribution of daily smokers by stage of change: current population survey results. *Preventive Medicine 36*: 710–720. https://doi.org/10.1016/s0091-7435(03)00044-6.
15. Prochaska, J. O., Velicer, W. F., Fava, J. L., Rossi, J. S., and Tsoh, J. Y. 2001. Evaluating a population-based recruitment approach and a stage-based expert system intervention for smoking cessation. *Addictive Behaviors 26*: 583–602.
16. Prochaska, J. O., Velicer, W. F., Fava, J. L., Rossi, J. S., and Tsoh, J. Y. 2001. Evaluating a population-based recruitment approach and a stage-based expert system intervention for smoking cessation. *Addictive Behaviors 26*: 583–602.
17. Krebs, P., Prochaska, J. O., and Rossi, J. S. 2010. A meta-analysis of computer-tailored interventions for health behavior change. *Preventive Medicine 51*: 214–221.
18. Noar, S., Benac, C., and Harris, M. 2007. Does tailoring matter? Meta-analytic review of tailored print health behavior change interventions. *Psychological Bulletin 133*: 673–693.
19. Evers, K. E., Prochaska, J. O., Johnson, J. L., Mauriello, L. M., Padula, J. A., and Prochaska, J. M. 2006. A randomized clinical trial of a population- and transtheoretical model-based stress-management intervention. *Health Psychology 25*: 521–529.
20. Johnson, S. S., Driskell, M. M., Johnson, J., Prochaska, J. M., Zwick, W., and Prochaska, J. O. 2006. Efficacy of a transtheoretical model-based expert system for antihypertensive adherence. *Disease Management 9*: 291–301.

21. Johnson, S., Driskel, N., Johnson, J., et al. 2006. Transtheoretical model intervention for adherence to lipid-lowering drugs. *Disease Management 9*: 102–114.

22. Johnson, S. S., Paiva, A. L., Cummins, C. O., et al. 2008. Transtheoretical model-based multiple behavior intervention for weight management: effectiveness on a population basis. *Preventive Medicine 46*: 238–246. https://doi.org/10.1016/j.ypmed.2007.09.010.

23. Levesque, D. A., Ciavatta, M. M., Castle, P. H., Prochaska, J. M., and Prochaska, J. O. 2012. Evaluation of a stage based computer tailored adjunct to usual care for domestic violence offenders. *Psycholoy of Violence 2*: 368–384. https://doi.org/10.1037/a0027501.

24. Mauriello, L. M., Ciavatta, M. M., Paiva, A. L., et al. 2010. Results of a multi-media multiple behavior obesity prevention program for adolescents. *Preventive Medicine 51*: 451–456. https://doi.org/10.1016/j.ypmed.2010.08.004.

25. Mauriello, L. M., Van Marter, D. F., Umanzor, C. D., Castle, P. H., and de Aguiar, E. L. 2016. Using mHealth to deliver behavior change interventions within prenatal care at community health centers. *American Journal of Health Promotion 30*: 554–562. https://doi.org/10.4278/ajhp.140530-QUAN-248.

26. Johnson, J. L., Prochaska, J. O., Paiva, A. L., Fernandez, A. C., DeWees, S. L., and Prochaska, J. M. 2013. Advancing bodies of evidence for population-based health promotion programs: randomized controlled trials and case studies. *Population Health Management 16*: 373–380. https://doi.org/10.1089/pop.2012.0094.

27. Prochaska, J. O., Evers, K. E., Castle, P. H., et al. 2012. Enhancing multiple domains of well-being by decreasing multiple health risk behaviors: a randomized clinical trial. *Population Health Management 15*: 1–11

28. Johnson, S. S., Paiva, A. L., Mauriello, L., Prochaska, J. O., Redding, C., and Velicer, W. F. 2014. Coaction in multiple behavior change interventions: consistency across multiple studies on weight management and obesity prevention. *Health Psychology 13*: 475–480.

29. Johnson, S., and Evers, K. 2015. Advances in multiple behavior change. *The Art of Health Promotion-American Journal of Health Promotion 29*: TAHP-6–TAHP-8.

30. Velicer, W. F., Redding, C. A., Paiva, A. L., et al. 2013. Multiple behavior interventions to prevent substance abuse and increase energy balance behaviors in middle school students. *Translational Behavioral Medicine: Practice, Policy and Research 3*: 82–93. https://doi.org/10.1007/S13142-013-0197-0.

31. Levesque, D. A., Johnson, J. L., and Prochaska, J. M. 2017. Teen choices, an online, stage-based program for healthy, nonviolent relationships: development and feasibility trial. *Journal of School Violence 16*: 376–385.

32. Blissmer, B., Prochaska, J. O., Velicer, W. F., Redding, C. A., Rossi, J. S., Greene, G. W., and Robbins, M. 2010 Common factors predicting long-term changes in multiple health behaviors. *Journal of Health Psychology 15*: 205–214.

3 Building Confidence

Mark D. Faries, PhD, Erik Gnagy, PhD,
Tracie McCargo, PhD, Megan McClendon, PhD,
and Katelyn Murphy, MPH

3.1 INTRODUCTION

If I believe I can, I might,
If I believe I can't, I probably won't.

This quote aptly describes the experience of many patients or clients who engage in a lifestyle prescription and who have low confidence in their abilities to change. In turn, the practitioner faces the challenge of building confidence in their patients – that behavior change is possible and it will produce expected outcomes (e.g., improved health or fitness, disease prevention).

Confidence, more formally recognized as *self-efficacy* (or *efficacy expectations*), "is the conviction that one can successfully execute the behavior required to produce the outcomes".[1] The principles outlined in this chapter provide a foundation of knowledge that the practitioner can leverage for modifying approaches to lifestyle prescriptions with a patient or client to help build confidence and subsequently increase the probability that the individual will be able to initiate and maintain the prescribed health behavior.

3.2 EVIDENCE SUMMARY

Summarizing the evidence for application of self-efficacy theory to practice is difficult. There is a tremendous breadth of research, innumerable ways in which it has been incorporated into behavior change theory, and large variability between research methodologies and interventions – with no best practice identified for lifestyle medicine prescriptions. Due to these complexities, we have taken a simple, theory-to-practice approach to the evidence summary, incorporating key examples of physical activity, healthy eating, medication adherence, and obesity prescriptions.

3.2.1 TYPES OF SELF-EFFICACY

Patients use perceptions of confidence in different ways and at different times when attempting to change or adopt a behavior. For example, a patient might need a level of confidence *before* starting a lifestyle prescription, *during* the lifestyle prescription dealing with barriers to keep behavior going, and *following* any setbacks, obstacles, or breaks from behavior (e.g., following a vacation or recovering from an injury or illness). While often mentioned as "types" of self-efficacy, they might be thought of as situational self-efficacy at different phases of the behavior change process.

DOI: 10.1201/9781003161226-3

Accordingly, the Health Action Process Approach (HAPA) provides a description of three separate, phase-specific constructs.[2–4]

1. Action self-efficacy
2. Maintenance self-efficacy
3. Recovery self-efficacy

3.2.1.1   Action Self-Efficacy

Action, pre-action, or *task self-efficacy* occurs *before* individuals act and helps individuals make judgments about their capacity to successfully perform the future behavior, such as being more physically active or eating more healthfully. Prior to behavior change, action self-efficacy supports the development of *intention* for health behavior change.

> *If high in action self-efficacy*: The patient and client are able to "imagine success, anticipate potential outcomes of diverse strategies, and are more likely to initiate a new behavior," (p. 92).[4]

Meta-analytic results revealed that action self-efficacy appears to have a larger effect on physical activity intention and behavior than dietary behavior, and it is important in helping support the building of confidence required *during* behavior changes (see next section).[5] Also, according to the HAPA, action self-efficacy is distinguished from, but works alongside, *outcome expectations* (or *expectancy*) – "a person's estimate that a given behavior will lead to certain outcomes," (p. 193).[1]

To build action self-efficacy, the practitioner aims to help the patient or client believe that he or she is capable of accomplishing the lifestyle prescription – which might require modifying the prescription to match one's beliefs and expectancies early in the change process (e.g., being physically active 2 days a week versus 5 days per week; see Section 3.3).

3.2.1.2   Maintenance Self-Efficacy

Maintenance or *coping self-efficacy* represents optimistic beliefs about one's capability to deal with barriers or obstacles that arise during the maintenance (or volitional) period of behavior, where the individual is in the process of enacting their intentions. A patient or client attempting a new lifestyle prescription, even if there is intention to change, might not have confidence in their abilities to overcome difficulties and challenges – many of which might be unknown due to inexperience with the prescribed behaviors. However, interventions that are designed to improve an individual's judgment of their capacity to perform a future behavior and then overcome potential barriers can have a pervasive effect on health behavior.[6]

> *If high in maintenance self-efficacy*: The patient and client are aware of and optimistic about coping with barriers, obstacles, and other challenges that might derail them from following a lifestyle prescription.

   Maintenance self-efficacy is generally considered the main type of confidence needed to follow a lifestyle prescription, and it might have a larger effect on dietary behavior than on physical activity intention and behavior.[6] Maintenance self-efficacy often predicts and supports the use of *coping planning* – imagining and making a plan for a scenario that might hinder them from performing an intended behavior (for more information, see Chapter 9).

   For examples in primary care, maintenance self-efficacy and coping planning education have been associated with improvements in:

- Diet and medication adherence in type 2 diabetes, 6-month post intervention[7]
- Physical activity in coronary or hypertensive patients, 12-month post intervention[8]
- Depression treatment adherence in subclinical depression, seven modules[9]
- Physical activity in inactive patients at risk of cardiovascular disease, 11 modules, web-based[10]
- Vaccination rates in patients with chronic obstructive pulmonary disease, four face-to-face meetings with an educational brochure[11]

3.2.1.3   Recovery Self-Efficacy

Recovery self-efficacy addresses the experience of failure, lapses, and setbacks. Like maintenance self-efficacy, recovery self-efficacy is theorized to have a direct effect on behavior and is related to action self-efficacy. When reviewed, recovery self-efficacy appears to have little to no effect on physical activity and dietary behavior,[6] but it has been found to provide some support for prediction of other health-related outcomes (e.g., body mass index[12]) or to mediate the effect of maintenance self-efficacy on health-related outcomes (e.g., breastfeeding[13]).

If high in recovery self-efficacy: The patient and client are confident in his or her abilities and capacity to overcome any setbacks or recover from any failed attempts to enact the lifestyle prescription, and they will try harder and persist longer.

3.2.2   Evidence for Patient Self-Efficacy

3.2.2.1   Physical Activity

Self-efficacy for physical activity generally describes the degree to which an individual believes he or she is capable of engaging in a *specific* physical activity behavior or situations, and it is theorized to be positively related to engaging in that behavior. Such confidence is based on the patient's current state, not their potential or future capability – so as to ensure distinction between self-efficacy and intention.[1,14,15]

   Relationships. In a systematic review done by Bauman and colleagues (2012), self-efficacy was a consistent positive correlate and determinant of physical activity in adults, adolescents, and children.[16] However, these positive relationships between self-efficacy and physical activity, although varying in effect, have been found across various chronic conditions. For example:

- Adult chronic disease patients, *self-efficacy in managing chronic disease*, $r=0.34$[17]
- Adults with chronic obstructive pulmonary disease (COPD), self-efficacy with various domains of physical activity, *weighted r=0.25*[18]
  - *Note*: This study further differentiates between domains of self-efficacy: *COPD symptom self-efficacy* (i.e., breathlessness), *exercise task self-efficacy* (i.e., confidence for performing physical movements, such as walking), *exercise barrier self-efficacy* (i.e., confidence for exercising under challenging situations), and *falls self-efficacy* (i.e., fear of falling during exercise activity).
- Adults with visual impairment, *self-efficacy for exercise* in moderate-to-vigorous physical activity, $\beta=0.26$[19]
- Adults with osteoarthritis, arthritis *self-efficacy scale*, whether exercised at home or supervised group[20]
- Further research is needed to examine the relationship between self-efficacy and physical activity for specific chronic diseases, such as diabetes mellitus, cancer, and chronic heart disease.

Interventions. Concerning physical activity interventions, a meta-analysis by Williams and French (2011) found that for healthy adults, there was a small but significant effect of various behavior change techniques (BCTs) on self-efficacy ($d=0.16$) and physical activity ($d=0.21$).[21] In adults with obesity, a review by Olander and colleagues (2013) also found a small effect on self-efficacy ($d=0.23$), but a moderate effect on physical activity behavior ($d=0.50$).[22] Similarly, Tang and colleagues (2019) found small intervention effects for post-intervention self-efficacy for physical activity ($d=0.26$).[23] However, the effect size of interventions on self-efficacy and physical activity appears to differ by the BCTs used within the intervention. The review by Tang and colleagues (2019) supported three BCTs for[23]:

Change in self-efficacy for physical activity:

- Demonstration of the behavior, positive effect ($d=0.47$)
- Behavioral practice/rehearsal, positive effect ($d=0.41$)
- Social support-practical (i.e., receiving advice or practical help from friends, family, and others), negative effect ($d=-0.40$)

Maintained changes in self-efficacy for physical activity, with interventions delivered:

- By health/fitness professional, positive effect ($d=0.67$)
- Within church/community settings, positive effect ($d=0.62$)
- In person, positive effect ($d=0.23$)
- In college/university/laboratory setting, negative effect ($d=-0.47$)

Also, the relationship of BCTs with building self-efficacy can also differ between populations, which should be considered when seeking to build individualized patient confidence in practice. For example:

Adults with obesity[22]

- Action planning – knowing what to do where and when
  - The patient creates a plan to partake in physical activity at a local park after they conclude their workday.
- Time management – control for potential obstacles
  - The patient includes action steps for unexpected changes in schedule.
- Self-monitoring of behavioral outcomes – keeping record of the specific outcome expected to be influenced by the behavior change
  - The patient self-monitors weight changes expected from physical activity.
- Plan for social support/social change
  - The patient gets involved with a support group focused on physical activity program adherence.
- In addition, two BCTs were associated with *decreased* self-efficacy.
  - Setting graded tasks – involves breaking behavior into smaller, manageable tasks
  - Prompting generalization of a target behavior – "encourages the individual to try the behavior in a different setting/situation after mastering it in one situation"

Nonclinical, community dwelling adults of 60 years or older[24]

- Setting graded tasks (in contrast to a *negative* relationship found in Olander et al.[22])
- Prompt self-monitoring of behavior
- Plan social support/social change
- Relapse prevention/coping planning (i.e., stimulus control techniques such as removing items associated with behavior that decreases self-efficacy, stress management, and meditation)

Patients with diabetes mellitus[25]

- Self-monitoring of exercise
- Exercise training (i.e., home-based resistance training, home-based walking, combination of resistance, and endurance training)

The evidence also suggests two final considerations:

1. The relationship between self-efficacy and physical activity behavior appears to be bidirectional – perceived confidence can impact intention and maintenance of physical activity, and in turn, direct personal experiences can influence one's belief in capability to complete the behavior.
2. The use of a combination of these strategies is likely to promote and sustain patient self-efficacy for physical activity, more so than using a single technique. As noted by Tang and colleagues (2019), "a significant positive relationship was found between number of BCTs and effect sizes for maintained

changes in self-efficacy for physical activity" (p. 812).[23] A comprehensive list of BCTs can be found in the delphi-type exercise done by Michie and colleagues (2013).[26]

3.2.2.2 Healthy Eating

Generally speaking, perceived self-efficacy is theorized to be positively related with healthy eating and dietary changes. However, there is a lack of systematic reviews to confirm the strength of this relationship, with variation in domain-specific measures of diet-related self-efficacy making such a review challenging (e.g., efficacy in eating particular foods, dietary behavior regulation, and self-regulatory effort to resist temptations[27]).

Relationships. Studies that are more easily applied to lifestyle practice show a *moderate* relationship of self-efficacy and dietary behavior. For example, in adult women within a weight-regulation program, self-efficacy for controlled eating was positively correlated with fruit and vegetables intake ($r=0.55$), while also mediating the effect of improved self-regulation (e.g., goal setting, identifying barriers, and reframing negative self-talk) on intake.[28]

Yet, mixed results are not uncommon. For example, in a study of young women, Simmonds and colleagues[29] found a statistically significant correlation between prudent eating (via food frequency questionnaire) and self-efficacy in healthy eating assessed with a novel 8-item scale (e.g., confidence to eat five portions of fruit and/or vegetables each day, to not eat or drink foods with added sugar, and to eat vegetable dishes or white meat instead of processed meat/red meat) with ($r=0.38, p<0.01$), but not when assessed using a global dietary self-efficacy measure ($r=0.25, p>0.05$).

Positive relationships between dietary self-efficacy and healthy eating have also been found across studies examining various, specific chronic conditions. For example:

- Type 2 diabetes and dietary self-efficacy[17,30]
- Adherence to gluten-free diet and celiac specific self-efficacy[31]
- Dietary adherence in patients receiving hemodialysis treatment and disease management self-efficacy, including dietary efficacy[32]

Interventions. Concerning dietary interventions, more research is needed. Overall effects from previous interventions, compared to control conditions, are small (Hedges' $g=0.24, p<0.001$).[33] Similarly, a systematic review found that automated digital health behavior change interventions had a small but positive effect on self-efficacy ($g=0.19$), and the effect did not differ as a function of the health behavior type – healthy eating ($k=4$), physical activity ($k=9$), and smoking ($k=4$).[34]

More moderate effects could be found in individual studies, such as Luszczynska and colleagues (2007) who implemented a self-efficacy intervention for fruit/vegetable consumption, consisting of three parts (p. 632).[35]

1. "Information on the importance of self-efficacy for goal pursuit and why it is necessary to enhance or maintain high self-efficacy."
2. "Feedback regarding a participant's results in a measure of self-efficacy."
3. "Information regarding ways to increase self-efficacy."

The researchers found that the intervention predicted changes in both self-efficacy to stick with or maintain a healthy diet ($\beta = 0.38$, $p < 0.001$, $R^2 = 0.14$) and fruit and vegetable intake ($\beta = 0.34$, $p < 0.001$, $R^2 = 0.12$). Prestwich and colleagues (2014) conducted perhaps the most complete meta-analysis of dietary interventions and highlighted the following BCTs positively associated with improved self-efficacy[33]:

- Incorporating self-monitoring (e.g., tracking one's own food-related behavior)
- Providing feedback on performance
- Prompting review of behavioral goals
- Providing contingent rewards (e.g., rewarding dietary successes)
- Planning for social support and social change

3.2.2.3   Medication Adherence

Patient self-efficacy for medication adherence appears to be less variable than that seen in physical activity and healthy eating behavior. A review by Náfrádi and colleagues (2017) found that high levels of various domains of self-efficacy were consistently associated with promotion of medication adherence, including[36]:

- Medication adherence self-efficacy (i.e., "a belief in the patient's capacity to follow the prescribed medical regimen in challenging situations")
- Disease management self-efficacy (i.e., a "patient's belief in their capacity to manage disease in general")
- General self-efficacy (i.e., "one's perceived competence across a wide array of life domains")
- Other domain-specific self-efficacy (e.g., coping self-efficacy)

More research is needed to distinguish which domains of patient self-efficacy might have the strongest relationship with medication adherence, as well as to distinguish these domains of self-efficacy from disease management confidence that commonly involves medicinal aids – such as in the management of chronic disease or sleep care.[37,38]

3.2.3   EVIDENCE FOR PRACTITIONER SELF-EFFICACY

Healthcare practitioners are a primary source of healthy lifestyle information due to their frequency of interaction with the public, and they are expected to have the skills and knowledge needed to approach discussions on lifestyle prescriptions. However, lack of confidence in providing lifestyle prescriptions can hinder the effectiveness of patient behavior change.

3.2.3.1   Barriers and Practitioner Self-Efficacy

Lack of confidence and knowledge are barriers to providing patients with physical activity and nutritional care,[39,40] and can result in the avoidance of these important lifestyle conversations. Concerning pediatric patients, practitioners who did *not* approach weight and lifestyle with patients[41]:

- Felt that it was not within their job description
- Did not know what words to use
- Did not have adequate training in communication strategies
- Had insufficient knowledge about the causes of obesity

These barriers express a lack of confidence in one's ability to provide lifestyle and weight discussions. As shown in Table 3.1, as the number of self-reported barriers increased, self-reported self-efficacy decreased. However, education to improve knowledge and skills in providing lifestyle prescriptions and barrier management can build practitioner confidence.

3.2.3.2 Building Practitioner Self-Efficacy

Nutrition Counseling. Sharour (2019) found that a prescription education program for nurses significantly improved self-confidence in providing nutrition care for oncology patients relative to those who did not attend the education program ($t = -10.25$, $p < 0.01$).[39] A similar result was found in faith community nurses' change in nutrition knowledge self-efficacy following a 3-hour educational intervention.[42] With the lack of counseling exposure during medical training,[43] enhancing continuing educational competencies in lifestyle medicine is theorized to increase self-efficacy in providing nutrition prescriptions.

Obesity Counseling. Similar suggestions can be made for obesity counseling. For example, over 500 U.S. non-physician health practitioners were asked, "How confident are you in your ability to help your obese patients or clients achieve a clinically significant weight loss (at least 5% of body weight)?"[44] The frequency (%) of those responding "pretty to very confident" varied by discipline (Table 3.2).

Interestingly, self-reported confidence did not appear to be related to prior success in helping patients achieve clinically significant weight loss. The authors hypothesize that the variation in confidence could be a result of the amount of training each

---

TABLE 3.1

Self-Rated Means (SD) for Self-Efficacy and Perceived Barriers to Lifestyle and Weight Discussions with Patients of Dutch Healthcare Professionals from Seven Disciplines

	Pediatricians	Dieticians	YHCPs	MHPs	YHCNs	Physio-therapists	GPs
Self-efficacy	8.1 (1.2)	7.5 (1.1)	7.4 (1.1)	7.2 (1.7)	7.1 (1.0)	6.9 (1.5)	6.8 (1.6)
No. of barriers	2.3 (2.0)	3.8 (2.1)	4.7 (2.7)	2.9 (2.0)	4.2 (2.1)	4.4 (2.7)	4.4. (2.5)

Source: Modified from van der Voorn et al.[41]

Self-efficacy (scale of 0–10); GPs, general practitioners; YHCPs, youth healthcare physicians; MHPs, mental health professionals; YHCNs, youth healthcare nurses; SD, standard deviation.

TABLE 3.2

Frequencies (%) of Health Practitioners Responding "Pretty to Very Confident" When Asked: How Confident Are You in Your Ability to Help Your Obese Patients or Clients Achieve a Clinically Significant Weight Loss (at least 5% of Body Weight)?

	Nursing (%)	Nutrition (%)	Behavioral/Mental Health (%)	Exercise (%)	Pharmacy (%)
Confident	61	88	51	52	60
Successful[a]	38	81	45	38	33

Source: Modified from Bleich et al.[44]

[a] Survey question: How successful are you at helping your obese patients or clients achieve a clinically significant weight loss (at least 5% of body weight)?

profession received on helping patients or clients achieve clinically significant weight loss, and they encouraged opportunities for continuing education.

To conclude, a large national study exploring self-efficacy in care for overweight and obese children found that "belief that pediatricians play an important role in addressing obesity was the strongest predictor of both assessment and counseling self-efficacy" (p. 1163).[45] Such findings instill confidence in healthcare practitioners (and students), demonstrating that they *do* have an important role in addressing obesity and other chronic conditions, and that they can pursue further education to build confidence in lifestyle prescriptions, improve practitioner–patient relations, and subsequently provide better support and care to patients.[46]

3.3   PRACTICAL APPLICATION

3.3.1   BUILDING PATIENT CONFIDENCE

Traditionally, there are four key principles or paths for building confidence: (1) mastery experience, (2) vicarious experience, (3) verbal persuasion, and (4) emotional arousal. The following is an expanded summary of Faries and Abreu.[47]

3.3.1.1   Mastery Experience

The first way to build confidence is through experiences of mastery, which arise from *effective* personal performance.[6] Simply doing or taking steps toward a behavior does not mean that an individual will gain mastery. Rather, the key is the patient's perception of *effective* personal performance (i.e., accomplishment). In other words, participating in a behavior in a way that helps the individual believe he or she is accomplishing and making progress is perhaps the most authentic proof of potential success, thus boosting self-confidence.

> **TIP:** Help patients choose behaviors that are perceived as challenging, *yet* attainable.

If the lifestyle prescription is perceived as too challenging or difficult, confidence can be diminished. At the same time, if the prescription is too easy, patients might not gain any confidence in their abilities. In addition, patient expectations of personal mastery can affect both their initiation and persistence with behavior, even in the face of challenges.[1]

Another key component of mastery experience is the *patient's perspective* (not the practitioner's) that the personal behavioral performance has been successful and is progressing. For example, a patient might say, "I *only* did 30 minutes of physical activity this week," not perceiving her effort to be successful – falling short of the prescribed 150 minutes per week. The practitioner could confirm this effort as unsuccessful since it did not meet the predetermined standard or "ideal" prescription, *or* the practitioner could help the patient see the 30 minutes as an accomplishment, especially in light of other challenges, and that progress is being made. The former approach would likely *undermine* an experience of mastery, while the latter approach would likely *enhance* an experience of mastery.

TIP: Help patients or clients see their behavior change, no matter how small, as a success, an accomplishment, and evidence that progress is being made.

Two additional factors that impact the patient's perception of success are: (1) perceived difficulty of the lifestyle prescription, and (2) whether or not they need any assistance. Patient confidence for a specific activity or behavior is modulated by their perception of how difficult it was to complete. Patients can misinterpret having to give their full effort as being incapable of or less skilled (i.e., physical debility). Likewise, if they felt that they needed too much help while completing the behavior, it is unlikely that their confidence will increase and can even decline.

If new to healthy lifestyle changes, patients might not understand the differences between normal levels of fatigue and pain that can arise during or after bouts of physical activity, or feelings of hunger with dietary changes. To help, the practitioner can explain that the common challenges they might experience or feel while performing the activity are normal, rather than a sign they are not performing the activity correctly or that they are simply not capable.

3.3.1.2 Vicarious Experience

Patients can perceive lifestyle prescriptions as intimidating or threatening, which can undermine their confidence. However, confidence can be built by seeing others perform the same behaviors and succeed through their own efforts, without the adverse consequences that they believe might occur.[6] Such vicarious experience can be found in modeling and testimonials.

Modeling: Other patients can serve as role models for successful behaviors, in turn building patients confidence that they can also be successful. In practice,

modeling commonly comes from interactions with patients who are similar to themselves, either individually, during educational session, or while participating in group
visits.

> **TIP:** Modeling can be strengthened when patients view models as credible,
> similar to themselves, valuing the same outcome, and someone they aspire to be.

There is also ample evidence to support that the health and behavior of the practitioner matter, affecting clinical attitudes and practices for lifestyle prescriptions.[48] In
turn, patients and clients can build confidence with practitioners who model ideal
behavior, "practicing what they preach."

> **TIP:** The practitioner does not have to be perfect with health behavior or free
> of barriers or struggles to maintain a healthy lifestyle – rather he or she should
> be simply open and humble about his or her own healthy lifestyle journey,
> strategies, and successes.

Testimonials: Testimonials of former patient's successes can also provide vicarious
experience. Group visits or training sessions can promote the sharing of personal
successes and strategies, and having a former patient come in to share his or her own
success story. However, it is important that the patient for whom you are prescribing
changes perceives those sharing their success stories to be similar to themselves. If
the patient does not perceive themselves to possess the same capabilities, they are
unlikely to believe that they too are capable of achieving the same results.

> **TIP:** Effective testimonials come from individuals who are similar to the
> patient in terms of ethnicity or gender, background or previous experience with
> healthy behaviors, and life demands (e.g., career, family dynamics).

3.3.1.3   Verbal Persuasion

With verbal persuasion, individuals can be prompted to believe that they are capable
of successfully handling, overcoming, and coping with challenges that occur while
changing a behavior that might have overwhelmed them in the past.[6]

> **TIP:** An encouraging word can go a long way.

The practitioner can help the patient locate and amplify the more positive, persuasive voice that says, "You can do it." The effectiveness of verbal persuasion will depend on whether or not the patient believes the person telling them that they can do it is credible. Thus, persuasions are more likely to increase the patient's confidence if they believe the person telling them is capable, truly knows what skills are required, and is competent at evaluating their capabilities. It is also important to teach patients to locate this inner voice when they need it, such as through *positive self-talk* and *positive reframing*. Imparting this skill has the added benefit of limiting the constant use of the practitioner, and it can be practiced for further mastery by the patient.

Lastly, verbal persuasion, alone, might not be enough to provide long-term benefits to self-efficacy.[49] The persuasiveness might come from constructive feedback on past performance rather than a simple reassurance.

> **TIP:** In-depth informative feedback can be used to clarify and provide rationale as to why some strategies to change and maintain behavior were successful while others were not.

3.3.1.4 Emotional Arousal

Emotions and feelings that come from stressful and taxing situations, such as lifestyle change, provide valuable information regarding one's sense of personal competency.[1] Emotions provide feedback and must be interpreted in a positive way to build confidence. A patient's current physiological and affective state can impair this judgment of competence. For example, patients experiencing negative feelings (e.g., stress, depression, fatigue) are more likely to underestimate their capabilities or overestimate the difficulty of the behavior.

> **TIP:** Help patients and clients see difficult situations in a more flexible, mindful, and nonjudgmental way. For example, fatigue and discomfort in exercise can be a sign that the patient is pushing themselves to improve their physical capabilities.

Also, high or aversive arousal can debilitate or undermine healthy behavioral efforts. For example, distress during and following bouts of physical activity, in the midst of dietary changes, or while monitoring one's body weight can affect confidence and resulting behavior.[50] The practitioner can be aware of how the patient is responding, help to discuss and positive reframe, and adjust prescriptions in order to maximize confidence and motivation.[2,51] Structuring lifestyle prescriptions in a way that maximizes both mastery experience and positive feedback, which will subsequently support self-efficacy.[52]

> **TIP:** Health behaviors can lead to negative feelings as well. See Chapter 10 to learn more on how responses to physical activity and healthy eating experience can shape behavior initiation and maintenance.

3.3.2 Building Practitioner Confidence

Practitioner self-efficacy can be built by translating theoretical knowledge and skills to the practitioner–patient interaction, patient barriers, and the modification of lifestyle prescriptions. Below are suggestions for building practitioner self-efficacy.[45]

3.3.2.1 Train in Motivational Interviewing

Using motivational interviewing to gather patient perspectives can build practitioner confidence in their lifestyle prescriptions. Consider adding an assessment questionnaire to your practice using motivational interviewing guidelines, and through practice, modify the questionnaire based on your level of comfort with discussion topics (covered in Chapter 4).

3.3.2.2 View Behavior Change as a Process

While confidence might be low in patients or clients when initiating a lifestyle prescription, self-efficacy can develop as they progress through the stages of change (see Chapter 2). Thus, approaching behavior change as a process can help practitioners build confidence that they are meeting the patients where they are, asking appropriate questions and providing appropriate information for each stage of change or phase of self-efficacy (see Section 2.1), and more actively working to move them to the next stage of readiness.

3.3.2.3 Self-Reflect and Explore

Building confidence to overcome barriers and motivate patient change starts with self-reflection and self-assessment. What is your readiness to learn new concepts and change your practice? The fact that you are reading this book indicates that you might be contemplating change already. Perhaps you are a planner. Mapping out a plan of attack can involve identifying several areas that you think might help your practice. If you enjoy research, you can build confidence by exploring existing research to find gaps or areas for future research. Building confidence simply requires getting involved and exposing yourself to the subject. You can ask your colleagues how they approach lifestyle prescriptions with their patients, or you can compare notes.

Also, research suggests that the practitioners' own health habits affect their counseling practices.[53] Doctors who exercised regularly counseled patients more often on physical activity[54] This suggests that, as a practitioner, your adoption of healthy habits improves your confidence in speaking with patients. Personal investigation of healthy lifestyle habits can improve your confidence and ability to help your patients explore solutions for themselves.

3.3.2.4   Seek Continuing Education

Research suggests that an acquired proficiency through educational interventions improves self-efficacy and builds confidence.[39,46] Gathering more information on the tools presented in this book will help build your confidence. Perhaps enrolling in continuing education courses in the areas that piqued your interest is the next step. Learning includes experimenting, so why not explore one concept from this book and approach a conversation with your patients next week? Practice will build confidence, and you will be able to add another concept of inquiry in a few weeks.

3.3.2.5   Refer to Community Partners

The practitioner does not have to feel that he or she must do everything, which can feel overwhelming and reduce confidence. Rather, it is important to consider community-based and public health programming that is designed to build confidence in patients and allows the community members to have a sense of ownership over the programs.[55] A review explained that referral to community-based partners gave patients more time and access to a health worker who was able to deliver health education, counseling, and social support.[56] Below are community-based partners who often provide free or low-cost behavior change programming:

- Cooperative Extension Service (state and county)
- Churches and Faith Communities
- County Coalitions
- Community Non-Profit Organizations
- State Health Departments
- County Health Departments
- Community Health Workers

Referral can also help relieve the burden of common barriers practitioners perceive in their patients or clients to completing a lifestyle prescription, and it can be a valuable supplement to the practitioner assisting the patient with barrier awareness and strategies (e.g., coping planning). However, such health education programs are not immune to the need for enhancing self-efficacy, as attendance can be impacted by a complex relationship with self-efficacy. For example, in uninsured patients participating in a health education program, self-efficacy increased perceived benefits and decreased perceived barriers to physical activity, while increasing perceived benefits and barriers for healthy food choice.[57]

TIP: Help patients find both awareness of and strategies for barriers. Start with, "What are some challenges you foresee with [lifestyle prescription]?" Follow with, "What do you think you can do in order to overcome these challenges?" Successful strategies can be used again to continue to build confidence.

3.4 CASE STUDIES

3.4.1 A CHALLENGE TO MASTERY

To achieve her physician's prescription for physical activity, Janet decided to join her local health club. Not knowing anything about exercise, she decided she would start by taking one of the free group exercise classes offered by the club. During the class, Janet struggled following along – so much so that the instructor, in an attempt to help, came over to correct her form. As a result, Janet's self-efficacy for physical activity plummeted. In this case:

- Identify new physical activity options that Janet feels confident she can perform.
- Reaffirm expectations and reassure Janet that it is normal to need assistance and not a sign that she is incapable.
- Encourage Janet to ask questions and to seek out help when needed.

3.4.2 A VICARIOUS MISS MATCH

Doug has been struggling to adhere to his lifestyle change prescription. Throughout his life, he has never really had an interest in physical activity. He never played sports and despised having to take gym class in high school. In an attempt to motivate and build his confidence, his physician shared with him how one of his other patients, who was a former All-American football player, had become sedentary, gained weight, and suffered from metabolic syndrome after his playing career ended – much like Doug. The physician shared how this patient, despite early reluctance to change, committed to start running three days per week, and after six months, no longer needed his hypertension or cholesterol medicine. Uninspired, Doug failed to gain confidence in his ability to accomplish the necessary changes he would need to make to obtain the same result. Doug thought that surely a former All-American athlete could do it, but he was no athlete, and there was no way he was that capable. In this case:

- Remember to share examples, models, and testimonies of success that possess similar characteristics and abilities to the patient.
- Converse with Doug to help identify another patient with more similarities and reassure him that he possesses the same abilities to succeed with the lifestyle prescription.

3.4.3 THE POWER TO PERSUADE

Mike refused to make changes to his lifestyle. Despite encouragement and assistance from his son, who held a PhD in the health field, he was adamant that medication was the *only* solution for his condition. After all, why would his physician put him on medication if that were not the best solution? He believed that if all it took was a little increase in physical activity and simple changes to his diet, surely his physician would have told him so. In this case:

- Remember that the practitioner is critical in being an active source for Mike's confidence in making lifestyle changes. You, more so than their family or friends, are a source that they will trust as credible.
- Do not hesitate in engaging in a conversation about Mike's level of confidence for accomplishing the prescribed changes.

    - Provide detailed, but concise and simple feedback as to why lifestyle changes, even if small, are effective in his disease prevention and management.
    - Encourage Mike's ability to succeed in implementing this critical lifestyle change.

3.4.4 MISINTERPRETING PHYSIOLOGY

Jackie was highly capable and fit. She had been participating in high-intensity interval training for several weeks, yet she was not feeling any more confident than when she first started. She felt that despite participating for weeks, her heart rate was always too high, and she was still feeling too much discomfort and fatigue. As a result, she was disappointed and felt like she was not getting any more "fit." Why was she not feeling more confident? In this case:

- Recognize that Jackie was not building confidence, because she was misinterpreting the physiological demands of the training as a sign of her incompetence.
- Explain to her that high-intensity training will always create the symptoms that she was experiencing (e.g., high heart rate, fatigue, and discomfort). Help her see that these feelings are not her failure to get better after weeks of training, but rather a normal physiological response to the demands of the training – a sign of accomplishment.
- Remember that it can be common for those new to physical activity to misinterpret minor discomfort or strain as signs of incompetence, undermining confidence and motivation to continue with the activity. As such, it will be helpful to prepare them by discussing these common experiences of physical activity.

3.4.5 FURTHER TIPS TO ENHANCE APPLICATION

To help build confidence through your patient or client interactions, consider the following questions from their perspective, and how you might respond.

- *Confidence:* Am I confident in my abilities to initiate and maintain this lifestyle prescription?

- *Outcome Expectancies*: Do I really believe doing this will lead to the outcome I want?
- *Valued Outcomes*: Do I really want or need to make this change?
- *Future Self*: Will my future self be thankful for making the sacrifice and commitment to these lifestyle changes? What are specific things my future self will be grateful for?
- *Planning*: Do I have a plan for overcoming my specific challenges, obstacles, and difficult situations that I will face in trying to make these lifestyle changes?

3.5 MEASUREMENT STRATEGIES

3.5.1 SELF-EFFICACY SCALES

3.5.1.1 General Self-Efficacy

The General Self-Efficacy Scale assesses optimistic self-beliefs used to cope with various demands in life (Table 3.3).[58]

TABLE 3.3
The General Self-Efficacy Scale[58]

	Not at all True	Barely True	Moderately True	Exactly True
1. I can always manage to solve difficult problems if I try hard enough	1	2	3	4
2. If someone opposes me, I can find means and ways to get what I want	1	2	3	4
3. It is easy for me to stick to my aims and accomplish goals	1	2	3	4
4. I am confident that I could deal efficiently with unexpected events	1	2	3	4
5. Thanks to my resourcefulness, I know how to handle unforeseen situations	1	2	3	4
6. I can solve most problems if I invest the necessary effort	1	2	3	4
7. I can remain calm when facing difficulties because I can rely on my coping abilities	1	2	3	4
8. When I am confronted with a problem, I can usually find several solutions	1	2	3	4
9. If I am in a bind, I can usually think of something to do	1	2	3	4
10. No matter what comes my way, I'm usually able to handle it	1	2	3	4

3.5.1.2   Exercise- and Diet-Specific Scales

Self-efficacy scales have been developed specific for exercise and diet, including confidence in regulating behaviors in the face of barriers. The key is finding a scale that works best for you and your practice. In addition to the exercise and diet self-efficacy scale examples in the appendix of Bandura,[14] we also recommend:

- The Self-Efficacy for Exercise Scale[59] or the Barriers to Self-Efficacy Scale (http://www.epl.illinois.edu/barse)[60] to assess confidence in exercising when faced with various barriers or challenges.
- The Scenario-Based Dieting Self-Efficacy Scale[61] to assess confidence in regulating scenarios of eating temptations, including those in response to high-caloric food, social and internal factors, and negative emotional events.

Other scales have also been developed for specific conditions and concerns, and they can be found in an online research search for "self-efficacy scales" or something similar. For example:

- Type 2 diabetes self-management[62]
- Osteoporosis[63]
- Arthritis[64]
- Cardiovascular management[65]
- Cardiac diet[66]
- Cholesterol-lowering diet[67]
- Mediterranean diet[68]
- Spinal Cord injury and exercise[69]

3.5.1.3   Specific Self-Efficacy

While previously validated scales are useful, they are not modifiable to help you meet specific patient needs and behaviors encountered in practice. Thankfully, Bandura (2006) provided instructions on building self-efficacy scales.[14] To highlight:

1. Content Validity
   a. The items you create must reflect the construct of self-efficacy or behaviour confidence – a judgment of perceived capability to execute or perform a behavior.
   b. Items should be phrased in terms of *can do*, rather than *will do*.
2. Content Connectivity
   a. The items you create should assess behaviors that your patients or clients can exercise some control and relate to a desired outcome.
   b. For example, assessing behaviors that relate to reduced cancer risk (desired outcome) – if *relaxation* does not affect cancer risk, then perceived confidence to relax will be unrelated to a reduction of cancer risk.

3. Content Specificity
   a. Discussion with patients or clients, and the items you create should be directed at specific performance components rather than general behavior.
   b. For example, instead of "How confident are you in your abilities to be physically active," use "How confident are you in your abilities to be physically active, *at a moderate intensity for 30 minutes on 5 of the next 7 days.*"
4. Instructions
   a. Efficacy beliefs are commonly assessed on a 100-point scale, with 10-unit intervals, from 0 (cannot do at all) to 50 (moderately can do) to 100 (highly certain can do).
   b. A 0–10 response format, with single unit intervals and the same descriptors, may also be used.
5. Examples
   Below are single-item examples for physical activity and dietary behaviors, but they can be modified to practitioner specificity and needs (Table 3.4).

3.6   SUMMARY

Self-efficacy, the confidence that one can achieve intended outcomes, is a key factor of behavior change to improve health or prevent disease. Patients' belief in their ability to change affects behavior and outcomes, and is therefore an area of practitioner focus. Self-efficacy changes based upon the patient's stage of change and

---

TABLE 3.4

Examples of Single-Item Scales for Physical Activity and Dietary Behaviors

Rate your degree of confidence in successfully performing the following behaviors by recording a number from 0 to 100 using the scale given below:

0	10	20	30	40	50	60	70	80	90	100
Cannot do at all					Moderately can do				Highly certain can do	

	Confidence (0–100)
Complete 150 minutes of moderate intensity physical activity this coming week	_____
Complete the prescribed resistance workout at the gym 2 days next week	_____
Eat five or more vegetables and fruits, each day, for the next 7 days	_____
Drink only three sodas over the next 7 days?	_____
Eat fast food only 2 days over the next week?	_____

Note: Modification can be made according to scale development instructions by Bandura (2006).[14]

---

the situation. Three types of self-efficacy (action, maintenance, recovery) provide information used by practitioners to help patients build confidence throughout the change process. This is helpful in identification of patients' intention to change and developing strategies to cope with barriers to change and setbacks.

Strategy development for healthy lifestyle behavior change is supported by research presented on the relationship between self-efficacy, chronic disease, and behavior change. Case studies and practical counseling tips are also provided throughout this chapter to build provider confidence in their ability to assist patients in adopting healthy behaviors to achieve positive lifestyle changes.

3.7   KEY TAKEAWAYS

- Confidence, or more formally *self-efficacy*, "is the conviction that one can successfully execute the behavior required to produce the outcomes" (p. 193).[1]
- Practitioners face a tremendous challenge, but they also play an important role in building confidence in their patients and clients – that behavior change is possible and will produce expected outcomes (e.g., improved health or fitness, disease prevention).
- Practitioners (and students) also face their own challenges in terms of confidence to successfully prescribe and monitor lifestyle prescriptions, which can be positively impacted by continuing education on how to conduct lifestyle prescriptions, self-efficacy, and behavior change techniques (BCTs).
- Patient self-efficacy is theorized to vary by situation, such as *before* initiating the lifestyle prescription to determine intention to change (i.e., action self-efficacy) and *during* the change process to overcome obstacles and challenges (i.e., maintenance self-efficacy).
- Traditionally, there are four key principles or paths for building confidence: (1) mastery experience, (2) vicarious experience, (3) verbal persuasion, and (4) emotional arousal.
- Detailed suggestions for patient and practitioner are provided in Section 3.3, supporting examples in Section 3.4, and measurement tips and examples in Section 3.5.

3.8   RESOURCES

- Guide for Constructing Self-Efficacy Scales[14]
- Healthy Eating and Exercise Lifestyle Program (HEELP) for promoting self-efficacy in patients[70]
- Recommendations for constructing messages to change self-efficacy[71]

REFERENCES

1. Bandura, Albert. "Self-efficacy: Toward a unifying theory of behavioral change." *Psychological Review* 84, no. 2 (1977): 191–215.

2. Faries, Mark D. "Why we don't "just do it" understanding the intention-behavior gap in lifestyle medicine." *American Journal of Lifestyle Medicine* 10, no. 5 (2016): 322–329.

3. Faries, Mark D., Wesley C. Kephart, and Devin Graham. "The intention–behavior gap." In *Lifestyle Medicine*, edited by James M. Rippe, 241–252. Boca Raton: CRC Press (in press; first print in 2019).

4. Schwarzer, Ralf. "Self-efficacy in the adoption and maintenance of health behaviors: Theoretical approaches and a new model." In *Self-Efficacy: Thought Control of Action*, edited by Ralf Schwarzer, 217–243. New York: Taylor and Francis, 1992.

5. Schwarzer, Ralf, and Kyra Hamilton. "Changing behavior using the health action process approach." In *The Handbook of Behavior Change*, edited by Martin L. Hagger, Linda D. Cameron, Kyra Hamilton, Nelli Hankonen, and Taru Lintunen, 89–103. Cambridge: Cambridge University Press, 2020.

6. Zhang, Chun-Qing, Ru Zhang, Ralf Schwarzer, and Martin S. Hagger. "A meta-analysis of the health action process approach." *Health Psychology* 38, no. 7 (2019): 623–637.

7. Ranjbaran, Soheila, Davoud Shojaeizadeh, Tahereh Dehdari, Mehdi Yaseri, and Elham Shakibazadeh. "The effectiveness of an intervention designed based on health action process approach on diet and medication adherence among patients with type 2 diabetes: A randomized controlled trial." *Diabetology & Metabolic Syndrome* 14, no. 1 (2022): 1–10.

8. Steca, P., L. Pancani, F. Cesana, F. Fattirolli, C. Giannattasio, Andrea Greco, M. D'Addario, D. Moonzani, E. R. Cappelletti, M. E. Magrin, M. Miglioretti, M. Sarini, M. Scrignaro, L. Vecchio, and C. Franzelli. "Changes in physical activity among coronary and hypertensive patients: A longitudinal study using the Health Action Process Approach." *Psychology & Health* 32, no. 3 (2017): 361–380.

9. Zarski, Anna-Carlotta, Matthias Berking, Dorota Reis, Dirk Lehr, Claudia Buntrock, Ralf Schwarzer, and David Daniel Ebert. "Turning good intentions into actions by using the health action process approach to predict adherence to internet-based depression prevention: Secondary analysis of a randomized controlled trial." *Journal of Medical Internet Research* 20, no. 1 (2018). https://doi.org/10.2196/jmir.8814.

10. Knittle, Keegan, Sarah J. Charman, Sophie O'Connell, Leah Avery, Michael Catt, Falko F. Sniehotta, and Michael I. Trenell. "Movement as medicine for cardiovascular disease prevention: Pilot feasibility study of a physical activity promotion intervention for at-risk patients in primary care." *JMIR Cardio* 6, no. 1 (2022): 1–20. https://doi.org/10.2196/29035.

11. Vayisoglu, Sumbule Koksoy, and Handan Zincir. "The health action process approach-based program's effects on influenza vaccination behavior." *The Journal for Nurse Practitioners* 15, no. 7 (2019): 517–524.

12. MacPhail, Mariana, Barbara Mullan, Louise Sharpe, Carolyn MacCann, and Jemma Todd. "Using the health action process approach to predict and improve health outcomes in individuals with type 2 diabetes mellitus." *Diabetes, Metabolic Syndrome and Obesity: Targets and Therapy* 7 (2014): 469–479.

13. Martinez-Brockman, Josefa L., Fatma M. Shebl, Nurit Harari, and Rafael Perez-Escamilla. "An assessment of the social cognitive predictors of exclusive breastfeeding behavior using the Health Action Process Approach." *Social Science & Medicine* 182 (2017): 106–116.

14. Bandura, Albert. "Guide for constructing self-efficacy scales." *Self-efficacy Beliefs of Adolescents* 5, no. 1 (2006): 307–337.

15. Bateman, Andre, Nicholas D. Myers, Sisi Chen, and Seungmin Lee. "Measurement of physical activity self-efficacy in physical activity-promoting interventions in adults: a systematic review." *Measurement in Physical Education and Exercise Science* 26, no. 2 (2021): 141–154. https://doi.org/10.1080/1091367X.2021.1962324.

16. Bauman, Adrian E., Rodrigo S. Reis, James F. Sallis, Jonathan C. Wells, Ruth J.F. Loos, and Brian W. Martin. "Correlates of physical activity: Why are some people physically active and others are not?" *The Lancet* 380, no. 9838 (2012): 258–271.

17. Daniali, Seyde Shahrbanoo, Firooze Mostafavi Darani, Ahmad Ali Eslami, and Mohammad Mazaheri. "Relationship between self-efficacy and physical activity, medication adherence in chronic disease patients." *Advanced Biomedical Research* 6, no. 63 (2017): 1–7. https://doi.org/10.4103/2277-9175.190997.

18. Selzler, Anne-Marie, Veronica Moore, Razanne Habash, Lauren Ellerton, Erica Lenton, Roger Goldstein, and Dina Brooks. "The relationship between self-efficacy, functional exercise capacity and physical activity in people with COPD: A systematic review and meta-analyses." *COPD: Journal of Chronic Obstructive Pulmonary Disease* 17, no. 4 (2020): 452–461. https://doi.org/10.1080/15412555.2020.1782866.

19. Haegele, Justin A., and Xihe Zhu. "Physical activity, self-efficacy and health-related quality of life among adults with visual impairments." *Disability and Rehabilitation* 43, no. 4 (2021): 530–536.

20. Olsson, Christina B., Jan Ekelund, Åsa Degerstedt, and Carina A. Thorstensson. "Change in self-efficacy after participation in a supported self-management program for osteoarthritis–An observational study of 11,906 patients." *Disability and Rehabilitation* 42, no. 15 (2020): 2133–2140.

21. Williams, Stephanie L. and David P. French. "What are the most effective intervention techniques for changing physical activity self-efficacy and physical activity behaviour—and are they the same?" *Health Education Research* 26, no. 2 (2011): 308–322. https://doi.org/10.1093/her/cyr005.

22. Olander, Ellinor K., Helen Fletcher, Stefanie Williams, Lou Atkinson, Andrew Turner, and David P. French. "What are the most effective techniques in changing obese individuals' physical activity self-efficacy and behaviour: A systematic review." *International Journal of Behavioral Nutrition and Physical Activity* 10, no. 29 (2013): 1–15. https://doi.org/10.1186/1479-5868-10-29.

23. Tang, Mei Yee, Debbie M. Smith, Jennifer McSharry, Mark Hann, and David P. French. "Behavior change techniques associated with changes in post intervention and maintained changes in self-efficacy for physical activity: A systematic review with meta-analysis." *Annals of Behavioral Medicine* 53, no. 9 (2019): 801–815. https://doi.org/10.1093/abm/kay090.

24. French, David P., Ellinor K. Olander, Anna Chisholm, and Jennifer McSharry. "Which behaviour change techniques are most effective at increasing older adults' self-efficacy and physical activity behaviour? A systematic review." *Annals of Behavioral Medicine* 48, no. 2 (2014): 225–234. https://doi.org/10.1007/s12160-014-9593-z.

25. Hamidi, Sajjad, Zahra Gholamnezhad, Narges Kasraie, and Amirhossein Sahebkar. "The effects of self-efficacy and physical activity improving methods on the quality of life in patients with diabetes: a systematic review." *Journal of Diabetes Research* 2022 (2022): 1–14. https://doi.org/10.1155/2022/2884933.

26. Michie, Susan, Michelle Richardson, Marie Johnston, Charles Abraham, Jill Francis, Wendy Hardeman, Martin P. Eccles, James Cane, and Caroline E. Wood. "The behavior change technique taxonomy (v1) of 93 hierarchically clustered techniques:

Building an international consensus for the reporting of behavior change interventions." *Annals of Behavioral Medicine* 46, no. 1 (2013): 81–95. https://doi.org/10.1007/s12160-013-9486-6.

27. Warner, Lisa Marie, and Ralf Schwarzer. "Self-efficacy and health." In *The Wiley Encyclopedia of Health Psychology*, edited by Kate Sweeny, Megan L. Robbins, Lee M. Cohen, 605–613, Hoboken: John Wiley & Sons, Ltd, 2020.

28. Annesi, James J. "Effects of self-regulatory skill usage on weight management behaviours: Mediating effects of induced self-efficacy changes in non-obese through morbidly obese women." *British Journal of Health Psychology* 23, no. 4 (2018): 1066–1083.

29. Simmonds, Gregory, Tannaze Tinati, Mary Barker, and Felicity L. Bishop. "Measuring young women's self-efficacy for healthy eating: Initial development and validation of a new questionnaire." *Journal of Health Psychology* 21, no. 11 (2016): 2503–2513.

30. Yang, Li, Kun Li, Yan Liang, Qiuli Zhao, Dan Cui, and Xuemei Zhu. "Mediating role diet self-efficacy plays in the relationship between social support and diet self-management for patients with type 2 diabetes." *Archives of Public Health* 79, no. 1 (2021): 1–8.

31. Fueyo-Díaz, Ricardo, Rosa Magallón-Botaya, Santiago Gascón-Santos, Ángela Asensio-Martínez, Guillermo Palacios-Navarro, and Juan J. Sebastián-Domingo. "The effect of self-efficacy expectations in the adherence to a gluten free diet in celiac disease." *Psychology & Health* 35, no. 6 (2020): 734–749.

32. Oquendo, Lissete González, José Miguel Morales Asencio, and Candela Bonill de Las Nieves. "Contributing factors for therapeutic diet adherence in patients receiving haemodialysis treatment: An integrative review." *Journal of Clinical Nursing* 26, no. 23–24 (2017): 3893–3905.

33. Prestwich, Andrew, Ian Kellar, Richard Parker, Siobhan MacRae, Matthew Learmonth, Bianca Sykes, Natalie Taylor, and Holly Castle. "How can self-efficacy be increased? Meta-analysis of dietary interventions." *Health Psychology Review* 8, no. 3 (2014): 270–285.

34. Newby, Katie, Grace Teah, Richard Cooke, Xinru Li, Katherine Brown, Bradley Salisbury-Finch, Kayleigh Kwah, Naomi Bartle, Kristina Curtis, Emmie Fulton, Joanne Parsons, Elsie Dusseldorp, and Stefanie L. Williams.. "Do automated digital health behaviour change interventions have a positive effect on self-efficacy? A systematic review and meta-analysis." *Health Psychology Review* 15, no. 1 (2021): 140–158.

35. Luszczynska, Aleksandra, Maciej Tryburcy, and Ralf Schwarzer. "Improving fruit and vegetable consumption: A self-efficacy intervention compared with a combined self-efficacy and planning intervention." *Health Education Research* 22, no. 5 (2007): 630–638.

36. Náfrádi, Lilla, Kent Nakamoto, and Peter J. Schulz. "Is patient empowerment the key to promote adherence? A systematic review of the relationship between self-efficacy, health locus of control and medication adherence." *PLoS One* 12, no. 10 (2017): e0186458.

37. Peters, Michele, Caroline M. Potter, Laura Kelly, and Ray Fitzpatrick. "Self-efficacy and health-related quality of life: A cross-sectional study of primary care patients with multi-morbidity." *Health and Quality of Life Outcomes* 17, no. 1 (2019): 1–11.

38. Rutledge, Carolyn M., Amanda C. La Guardia, and Daniel Bluestein. "Predictors of self-efficacy for sleep in primary care." *Journal of Clinical Nursing* 22, no. 9–10 (2013): 1254–1261.

39. Sharour, Loai Abu. "Improving oncology nurses' knowledge, self-confidence, and self-efficacy in nutritional assessment and counseling for patients with cancer: A quasi-experimental design." *Nutrition* 62 (2019): 131–134. https://doi.org/10.1016/j.nut.2018.12.004.

40. O'Brien, Sarah, Lucia Prihodova, Mairéad Heffron, and Peter Wright. "Physical activity counselling in Ireland: A survey of doctors' knowledge, attitudes and self-reported practice." *BMJ Open Sport & Exercise Medicine* 5, no. 1 (2019): e000572.

41. van der Voorn, B., R. Camfferman, J. C. Seidell, and J. Halberstadt. "Talking with pediatric patients with overweight or obesity and their parents: Self-rated self-efficacy and perceived barriers of Dutch healthcare professionals from seven disciplines." *BMC Health Services Research* 22, no. 1 (2022): 1236. https://doi.org/10.1186/s12913-022-08520-2.

42. Gotwals, Beth. "Self-efficacy and nutrition education: A study of the effect of an intervention with faith community nurses." *Journal of Religion and Health* 57, no. 1 (2018): 333–348.

43. Smith, Samantha, Eileen L. Seeholzer, Heidi Gullett, Brigid Jackson, Elizabeth Antognoli, Susan A. Krejci, and Susan A. Flocke. "Primary care residents' knowledge, attitudes, self-efficacy, and perceived professional norms regarding obesity, nutrition, and physical activity counseling." *Journal of Graduate Medical Education* 7, no. 3 (2015): 388–394.

44. Bleich, Sara N., Sachini Bandara, Wendy L. Bennett, Lisa A. Cooper, and Kimberly A. Gudzune. "US health professionals' views on obesity care, training, and self-efficacy." *American Journal of Preventive Medicine* 48, no. 4 (2015): 411–418.

45. Liebhart, Janice L., Alyson B. Goodman, Jeanne Lindros, Catherine Krafft, Stephen R. Cook, Alison Baker, and Sandra G. Hassink. "Key predictors of primary care providers' self-efficacy in caring for children with overweight or obesity." *Academic Pediatrics* 22, no. 7 (2022): 1158–1166. https://doi.org/10.1016/j.acap.2022.02.017.

46. Sturgiss, Elizabeth, Emily Haesler, Nicholas Elmitt, Chris van Weel, and Kirsty Douglas. "Increasing general practitioners' confidence and self-efficacy in managing obesity: A mixed methods study." *BMJ Open* 7, no. 1 (2017): e014314. https://doi.org/10.1136/bmjopen-2016-014314.

47. Faries, Mark D., and Alyssa Abreu. "Medication adherence, when lifestyle is the medicine." *American Journal of Lifestyle Medicine* 11, no. 5 (2017): 397–403.

48. Frank, Erica, Jason Breyan, and Lisa Elon. "Physician disclosure of healthy personal behaviors improves credibility and ability to motivate." *Archives of Family Medicine* 9, no. 3 (2000): 287–290.

49. Ashford, Stefanie, Jemma Edmunds, and David P. French. "What is the best way to change self-efficacy to promote lifestyle and recreational physical activity? A systematic review with meta-analysis." *British Journal of Health Psychology* 15, no. 2 (2010): 265–288.

50. Faries, Mark D., and John B. Bartholomew. "Coping with weight-related discrepancies: initial development of the WEIGHTCOPE." *Women's Health Issues* 25, no. 3 (2015): 267–275.

51. Mancuso, Serafino G. "Body image inflexibility mediates the relationship between body image evaluation and maladaptive body image coping strategies." *Body Image* 16 (2016): 28–31.

52. Jerome, Gerald J., David X. Marquez, Edward McAuley, Steriani Canaklisova, Erin Snook, and Melissa Vickers. "Self-efficacy effects on feeling states in women." *International Journal of Behavioral Medicine* 9, no. 2 (2002): 139–154.

53. Lobelo, Felipe, John Duperly, and Erica Frank. "Physical activity habits of doctors and medical students influence their counselling practices." *British Journal of Sports Medicine* 43, no. 2 (2009): 89–92.

54. Belfrage, Anna Sofia Viktoria, Kjersti Støen Grotmol, Reidar Tyssen, Torbjørn Moum, Arnstein Finset, Karin Isaksson Rø, and Lars Lien. "Factors influencing doctors' counselling on patients' lifestyle habits: a cohort study." *BJGP Open* 2, no. 3 (2018). https://doi.org/10.3399/bjgpopen18X101607

55. Scott, Kerry, S. Wilson Beckham, Margaret Gross, George Pariyo, Krishna D. Rao, Giorgio Cometto, and Henry B. Perry. "What do we know about community-based health worker programs? A systematic review of existing reviews on community health workers." *Human Resources for Health* 16, no. 1 (2018): 1–17.

56. Kim, Kyounghae, Janet S. Choi, Eunsuk Choi, Carrie L. Nieman, Jin Hui Joo, Frank R. Lin, Laura N. Gitlin, and Hae-Ra Han. "Effects of community-based health worker interventions to improve chronic disease management and care among vulnerable populations: A systematic review." *American Journal of Public Health* 106, no. 4 (2016): e3–e28.

57. Kamimura, Akiko, Maziar M. Nourian, Allison Jess, Alla Chernenko, Nushean Assasnik, and Jeanie Ashby. "Perceived benefits and barriers and self-efficacy affecting the attendance of health education programs among uninsured primary care patients." *Evaluation and Program Planning* 59 (2016): 55–61.

58. Schwarzer, Ralf, and Matthias Jerusalem. "Generalized self-efficacy scale." In *Measures in Health Psychology: A User's Portfolio. Causal and Control Beliefs*, edited by J. Weinman, S. Wright, & M. Johnston, 35–37. Windsor: NFER-Nelson, 1995.

59. Resnick, Barbara, and Louise S. Jenkins. "Testing the reliability and validity of the self-efficacy for exercise scale." *Nursing Research* 49, no. 3 (2000): 154–159.

60. McAuley, Edward. "The role of efficacy cognitions in the prediction of exercise behavior in middle-aged adults." *Journal of Behavioral Medicine* 15, no. 1 (1992): 65–88.

61. Stich, Christine, Bärbel Knäuper, and Ami Tint. "A scenario-based dieting self-efficacy scale: The DIET-SE." *Assessment* 16, no. 1 (2009): 16–30.

62. Strychar, Irene, Belinda Elisha, and Norbert Schmitz. "Type 2 diabetes self-management: Role of diet self-efficacy." *Canadian Journal of Diabetes* 36, no. 6 (2012): 337–344.

63. Horan, Mary L., Katherine K. Kim, Phyllis Gendler, Robin D. Froman, and Minu D. Patel. "Development and evaluation of the osteoporosis self-efficacy scale." *Research in Nursing & Health* 21, no. 5 (1998): 395–403.

64. Lorig, Kate, Robert L. Chastain, Elaine Ung, Stanford Shoor, and Halsted R. Holman. "Development and evaluation of a scale to measure perceived self-efficacy in people with arthritis." *Arthritis & Rheumatism: Official Journal of the American College of Rheumatology* 32, no. 1 (1989): 37–44.

65. Steca, Patrizia, Andrea Greco, Erika Cappelletti, Marco D'addario, Dario Monzani, Luca Pancani, Giovanni Ferrari, Alessandro Politi, Roberta Gestra, Gabriella Malfatto, and Gianfranco Parati. "Cardiovascular management self-efficacy: Psychometric properties of a new scale and its usefulness in a rehabilitation context." *Annals of Behavioral Medicine* 49, no. 5 (2015): 660–674.

66. Hickey, Mairead L., Steven V. Owen, and Robin D. Froman. "Instrument development: cardiac diet and exercise self-efficacy." *Nursing Research* 41, no. 6 (1992): 347–351.

67. Burke, Lora E., Jacqueline Dunbar-Jacob, Susan Sereika, and Craig K. Ewart. "Development and testing of the cholesterol-lowering diet self-efficacy scale." *European Journal of Cardiovascular Nursing* 2, no. 4 (2003): 265–273.

68. Cuadrado, Esther, Tamara Gutiérrez-Domingo, Rosario Castillo-Mayen, Bárbara Luque, Alicia Arenas, and Carmen Taberneroa. "The self-efficacy scale for adherence to the Mediterranean diet (SESAMeD): A scale construction and validation." *Appetite* 120 (2018): 6–15.
69. Kroll, Thilo, Matthew Kehn, Pei-Shu Ho, and Suzanne Groah. "The SCI exercise self-efficacy scale (ESES): Development and psychometric properties." *International Journal of Behavioral Nutrition and Physical Activity* 4, no. 1 (2007): 1–6.
70. Alharbi, Muaddi, Robyn Gallagher, Ann Kirkness, David Sibbritt, and Geoffrey Tofler. "Long-term outcomes from healthy eating and exercise lifestyle program for over-weight people with heart disease and diabetes." *European Journal of Cardiovascular Nursing* 15, no. 1 (2016): 91–99.
71. Latimer, Amy E., Lawrence R. Brawley, and Rebecca L. Bassett. "A systematic review of three approaches for constructing physical activity messages: What messages work and what improvements are needed?" *International Journal of Behavioral Nutrition and Physical Activity* 7, no. 1 (2010): 1–17.

4 Motivational Interviewing

Peter Fifield, Ed.D LCMHC, MLADC
and Joji Suzuki, MD

Daring as it is to investigate the unknown, even more so, it is to question the known.

Kaspar

4.1 INTRODUCTION

Most of us can claim we are experts in something. If you are reading this book, you may even claim to be an expert in some specific health-related field. Up front, we would like to acknowledge your years of hard work and effort put into this expertise. You have most likely invested endless hours studying, practicing, and honing your skills – testing and validating your knowledge. This has been no easy feat. With all honesty and sincerity, we acknowledge and thank you for your hard work and expertise in your field and/or specialty. Now that we have recognized this fact, we want to ask you to leave that person – that expert – behind. The person we would like to invite to read this chapter is the layperson, the raw human – not the expert – but the beginner. You will struggle with this request and not all will succeed; however, for the intent of this lesson, the closer you get to leaving the expert behind, the closer you become to understanding the reason for this request.

We forget that we quite often ask our clients to change – take this medication, lose that weight, do this exercise, go to this referral – we are constantly requesting a "next step" or change behavior from our clients. For some, change is easy; however, for others, making changes requires a level of vulnerability, humility, and acceptance that we are entering the unknown but are willing to go there anyway. We clinicians may not remember what it feels like to be vulnerable – to commit to something when we don't *know* the outcome or to act when we don't really *want to*. The act of being vulnerable allows us to balance the interaction with our clients – knowing we are the expert in a certain field and they are the expert in themselves. The key to Motivational Interviewing (MI) is to combine these two entities – you are bringing your expertise in *health* and the client bringing their expertise in *self*.

In general, managing complex chronic medical concerns could be called "wicked problems";[1] problems that are so complex that they have no straightforward solution, only better or worse strategies. There is no one-size-fits-all approach. For years, we relied on the directive approach where the clinicians would tell clients what to do and the motivated client would follow those instructions. The clinician would play the expert role and the client would play the novice, the empty vessel, awaiting the

DOI: 10.1201/9781003161226-4

clinician to impart upon them their infinite wisdom. Often, these seemingly straight-forward plans were not successful, and subsequently, the client was seen as non-compliant or unmotivated. Providing different solutions to the same problem is a version of first-order change. This approach is very linear and incremental; if you do "A," then "B" will happen. Management of behavioral changes however is too complex to generally be approached in such a linear fashion. Another option is to use a non-linear approach and attempt what some System Theorists would call second-order change;[2] abandoning a transactional or incremental approach and taking on a radical, transformational approach instead.

MI can facilitate second-order change for it allows us to see a change through a transformational lens as a non-linear process. We know that we can expect with some regularity that a standard prescription for one client will not work for the other. We also know that clients approach behavioral change with different levels of readiness. MI (Miller and Rollnick, 2013)[3] is a clinical tool that offers a shift in focus; a view into the client's world that we had not seen before. It offers an approach that is evidence-based, client-centered, and proven to be effective in getting clients closer to and planning for change.[4] We can use MI as a more effective strategy to address these *complex problems* in hopes to increase the odds of successfully assisting the client in the process of change.

This process involves working with the client to investigate options for increasing intrinsic motivation. It also includes facing the challenge of sitting in the discomfort of not being the expert in what may work best for the client – fighting the reflex to fix the problem. A common pearl of wisdom in the MI world is to "be responsible for the interaction and not the outcome." If we do our best at committing to the interaction of change, it allows us to then resign to the fact that the outcome is the client's responsibility. This acceptance is rooted in the fundamental truism that clinicians can do very little to **make** their clients implement sustained behavior change unless they want to do so. Clinicians can, however, assist them in increasing and strengthening their internal motivation and preparedness for change. As Miller and Rollnick (2013)[3] put it, MI "involves a collaborative partnership with clients, a respectful evoking of their own motivation and wisdom and a radical acceptance recognizing that ultimately whether change happens is each person's own choice, an autonomy that cannot be taken away no matter how much one might wish to at times."

4.2 EVIDENCE BASE IN SUPPORT OF MOTIVATIONAL INTERVIEWING

Since the time that MI was adopted in clinical settings as a tool to help patients change behavior, the rigor in which this intervention was both implemented and evaluated stand out among many of the psychotherapeutic approaches currently in use in health care settings. There have been hundreds of controlled and uncontrolled trials of MI for a wide range of target behaviors, such as unhealthy substance use, exercise, diabetes management, weight-related outcomes, physical activity, diet, medication adherence, and self-care. Of note, both genders among adult and adolescent populations are well represented in these trials, as well as diverse racial and ethnic patient populations. Given the enormous volume of research that has been published over the decades, a review of all the evidence base is beyond the scope of this chapter.

Nevertheless, we can summarize the available evidence by reviewing systematic reviews and meta-analyses that have been published. In 2018, the most comprehensive systematic review of reviews was published which included 104 systematic reviews and 38 meta-analyses of MI.[5] The overall quality of the evidence was rated as low, but the authors concluded that MI appears to be most effective in stopping or preventing unhealthy behaviors such as unhealthy alcohol use, smoking, and other substance use. The results also indicated that evidence to support MI in helping to reduce weight among obese and overweight adults is generally lacking, although the evidence does point to MI helping to increase physical activity.

Since then, additional reviews for a variety of target behaviors have been published to further clarify the role of MI in helping patients improve health-related behaviors and outcomes. These studies now confirm that MI has robust empirical support in improving medication adherence,[6] weight-related outcomes in adolescents,[7] diabetes management,[8] physical activity,[9] and self-care among individuals with heart failure.[10] Similar to the conclusion of the 2018 systematic review of reviews, the most recent systematic review of MI for adult obesity failed to show a statistically significant benefit on weight-related outcomes such as weight or BMI among adults.[11] Taken together, the most up-to-date evidence base continues to support the effectiveness of MI in a wide range of target behaviors with a particular impact on reducing and preventing unhealthy behaviors, but MI may be more challenging when improving weight-related outcomes for adults who are obese or overweight. Therefore, clinicians need to recognize that MI alone will not be the most effective strategy in impacting weight-related outcomes in overweight adults.

4.3   KEY POINTS

- MI is a strengths-based approach that focuses on evoking the client's inherent strengths and capabilities to successfully navigate lifestyle changes.
- MI recognizes and accepts the fact that every client enters the process of lifestyle changes at different levels of readiness and willingness to change their behavior.
- Ambivalence is normal behavior that should be expected when anyone considers making a change in their lives. The client can see both the reasons for and against change.
- Before discussing the next steps or "plans," clinicians should first focus their attention on creating therapeutic rapport with the client then increasing change talk and decreasing sustain talk.

4.4 WHAT IS MOTIVATIONAL INTERVIEWING

Working Definition: "Motivational interviewing is a collaborative goal-oriented style of communication with particular attention to the language of change. It is designed to strengthen personal motivation for and commitment to a specific goal by eliciting and exploring the person's own reasons for change within an atmosphere of acceptance and compassion".[3]

MI was first perceived during a clinical trial comparing treatment approaches for individuals who reported problem drinking. Originally, the researchers noted that empathic statements made by the clinicians had a stronger effect on reducing problem drinking behaviors than other interventions such as directive comments. Although this was only the beginning, this led to Miller creating the structural framework that would later become MI. The first edition of MI was published in 1999. Now in its 3rd edition, this communication model continues to focus on the intentional application of specific techniques, designed to increase change talk and decrease sustain talk.

MI is very useful in navigating ambivalence – a phase in which a person may feel two ways about something – I could change or I could not change and stay the same – both could be equally acceptable. Most likely, MI would not be used when a person is in the action phase because excessive processing, talking, and contemplation may just reverse their current level of motivation and action. However, MI is most effective in negotiating this ambivalence within the individual and is often present in the pre-contemplative or contemplative phase of change. See Chapter 2 on the Stages of Change for more detail on this topic.

The Four Processes: MI has four processes; all of which are fluid and intertwined. The four processes are engaging, focusing, evoking, and planning. Although we do not always complete all the stages, we will always approach them in sequential order. First, we engage with the individual, then we focus on a change behavior, and finally, we evoke the change talk that will bring us to creating a plan. In practice, behavior change often requires that these processes be repeated over weeks, months, or even years.

4.4.1 ENGAGING

Client engagement is fundamental to the change process. MI seeks to create an appropriate interpersonal environment that sets the stage for the possibility of change to occur by intentionally working to create a strong and collaborative relationship between the client and the clinician. In psychotherapy, one meta-analysis showed a moderate and reliable relationship between a good therapeutic alliance and positive therapeutic outcomes;[12] said otherwise, there is the progress made simply by creating a solid relationship between therapist and client. The goal of engagement is to establish an effective relationship with the client that allows for agreement on treatment goals and collaboration regarding reaching them. As noted earlier, this is in contrast to some approaches where the clinician plays the role of the authoritative educator or expert.

Individuals that enter the health-related fields are often "help" oriented. We want to help reduce pain and suffering, and ultimately, we want people to heal and get better. Without the right tools, however, we can often get distracted from helping by getting stuck in the process of fixing the problem instead. MI recognizes this act as the Righting Reflex – a concept we will talk more about later. The popular psychologist and social icon Brown[13] posits that "Rarely can a response make something better. What makes something better is connection." The understanding is that if the individual knows they can share with you, that is, on its own, a start to resolving the problem. This illustrates the fundamental concept of engagement which is to establish a safe zone for clients to share their vulnerability – a place where true transparency may occur. Without this safe zone, all we typically get is a perception of communication with the truths and facts safely hidden away and protected elsewhere. The Spirit of MI is a core component of the engagement process.

Metaphorically speaking, MI Spirit is the music that accompanies the words in a song. The artistic environment accompanies the technical framework of the interaction. MI Spirit or the Key Principles are what differentiates MI from a simple trick or a ruse, and without it, interactions between clinicians and clients can regress to "another version of the righting reflex".[3] Before we continue, it may help to understand that the Spirit of MI can be used anytime, anyplace, and anywhere and can be simply seen as a way to humanely interact with another person. To familiarize you with the importance of MI Spirit, we must first understand the four disparate components that, together, create the Gestalt of MI Spirit.

Partnership is the notion and understanding that MI is done *with* the client not *to* the client. It is the collaborative process that occurs between a clinician and client that maintains the central concept that there are two experts in the room: the clinician and the client. The clinician is the expert in the content area (e.g., weight management, treating depression, and substance use recovery coaching), while the client is the expert on themselves. The client may know the most effective ways to integrate the clinical interventions into their own lives. Therefore, the clinician must work alongside the client to best help them. A frequently used metaphor for MI is an opportunity to dance with a client, not wrestle. The clinician should guide the session in a goal-oriented fashion; however, they should not attempt to convince or force the client to make any choices. Another distinction of this collaborative partnership is that, because clients have their strengths and motivations, clinicians must understand that they are not solely responsible for having all of the answers and solving all of the problems. Because we are often indoctrinated to think we, as professionals, should know the right answer, to right a wrong or to fix a problem, it is sometimes hard for clinicians to internalize that they may be more responsible for the intervention than the outcome. This perspective change alone could have a profound impact on reducing burnout[14] and compassion fatigue – knowing when and where to focus the most concerted efforts.

Acceptance is made up of four key components and is rooted in Rogerian concepts. First and foremost, Acceptance has nothing to do with the clinician's approval or disapproval of the client's behaviors, situation, or intentions. We do not have to approve of a person using intravenous heroin or endorse the poor eating habits of a person living with diabetes to work with them toward a recovery plan. There are four components of Acceptance:

- *Absolute Worth*, as identified by Carl Rogers, is the Unconditional Positive Regard for an individual. Absolute worth allows the clinician the ability to create a place of trust, a zone of safety in which the client is willing to step into that is free of judgment, contempt, and instruction.
- *Affirmation* is the clinician's ability to appreciate the efforts made by the client thus far. Many times, clinical professions focus on the deficiency or absence of a skill set – a disease state, a fracture, or tumor – something that is broken or un-whole. The focus is on what is wrong and needs to be righted. The use of Affirmations in MI is intended to be the exact opposite. They intend to identify and reflect the client's existing resilience, strength, and accomplishments with hopes to build confidence within the client.
- *Autonomy* – As noted in Chapter 5, there is power in Autonomy. In MI, the clinician fully accepts and appreciates the individual's perspectives and decisions. As Victor Frankl once said, "Everything can be taken from a man but one thing: the last of the human freedoms – to choose one's attitude in any given set of circumstances, to choose one's own way".[15] Honoring personal autonomy and their internal locus of control, as well as showing respect for their ability to self-direct, is in contrast to a directive approach in which the clinician plays the expert. Ultimately, regardless of the clinical approach, the client chooses their own path and will decide what changes to implement, and if they are maneuvered toward a direction they do not agree with, they will advocate for the opposite behavior as a way of demonstrating their free will. Respecting autonomy from the beginning can shorten the time it takes to select the most effective route.
- *Accurate Empathy* is another "critical condition" for change according to Rogers. In art appreciation, empathy was the viewer's ability to project themselves into the piece of artwork. In MI, the clinician can project themselves into the life of the client. Accurate empathy is seeing that your client is stuck in a deep, dark, and frightening hole and appreciating the severity of their situation without actually being in the hole with them. The clinician's job is to reside at the top of the hole, looking down, and helping from up above. Although MI does not officially differentiate, there are two types of empathy worth mentioning here: cognitive and affective empathy.[16] Simply put, it is the difference between understanding what a situation must be like (cognitive empathy) versus what it must feel like (affective empathy) in any given situation.

Compassion: Compassion goes beyond having positive regard for another – in a way that it has an action element to it – to include purposely prioritizing what is in the best interest of the client. The other three aspects of MI's spirit (Partnership, Evocation, and Acceptance) can be employed to serve the interests of the clinician, but with compassion, the emphasis is always placed on doing what is best for the client. Compassion is being aware of the clients suffering and putting their interests as the number one priority in a situation. If done successfully, compassion allows us to focus solely on what is best for the client, underscoring the idea of selflessness and creating a communication structure intent on satisfying the client's personal goals rather than our own.

Evocation: A basic tenet of MI is that the client intrinsically possesses almost all of what it will take to actualize the desired change goal. Our job as MI professionals is to strategically evoke that latent expertise and illuminate a plan for moving forward. If we successfully navigate this process, eliciting more and expounding on the client change talk, ambivalence can often be resolved. Working through the ambivalence moves us closer to the preparation and planning phase – getting us one step closer to sustained change.

Motivational Interviewing Skills: MI clinicianclinicians use several tools or skills to assist with the change process. As noted by Gordon,[17] there are many potential places of miscommunication; what the person says, what the listener hears, what the listener thinks the speaker means, and what the speaker actually means. Specific MI skills can play a role in clarifying this miscommunication.

Open-Ended Questions (OEQ): Closed-ended questions have a finite and limited potential for response. Examples of closed-ended questions are: "Do you smoke?," "Have you ever quit smoking?," or "Have you ever tried Nicotine Replacement Therapy to quit smoking?" All three of these questions ask for a very specific, finite amount of information. Closed-ended questions are very clinician-centric and are used to get specific bits of information. However, OEQs tend to feel more personal and patient-centric. OEQs are used to inquire in a much broader way; they ask the client to provide a narrative – a deeper, more personal response. They add fluidity to the conversation by avoiding a "check-list" questioning type approach and, if used strategically, can answer multiple closed-ended questions at once. For example, if the clinician asked, "so I understand you have smoked in the past, tell me about how you were successful trying to quit." With this one inquiry, the clinician could potentially get all three of the aforementioned closed-ended questions answered all at once. Additionally, open-ended questions ask for feedback that is pertinent, relevant, and important to the client, something many closed-ended questions do not address. Some examples of each closed-ended and open-ended questions are given in Table 4.1.

TABLE 4.1
Open-Ended vs. Closed Ended Question Examples

Open-Ended Questions	Closed Ended Questions
What are some reasons you would want to quit smoking?	Is it correct that you would like to quit smoking?
What is important to you about changing your diet?	How many times have you tried to go on a diet?
Tell me a little bit about your health habits	Do you mind if I ask you a few questions about your health habits?
If you had to quit smoking, how would you do it?	Do you want to try the nicotine patch?

Affirmations: Affirmations are statements or reflections of an individual's strengths or efforts and they can be simple ("You did it") or complex ("You are a resourceful person for dealing with this stress for so long"). By making affirmative statements to the client, the clinician is playing the cheerleader role, attempting to increase the client's self-esteem and self-efficacy. Increasing an individual's confidence and control has shown to be a key predictor of positive health outcomes.[18] It is important that affirmations, as with any emphatic statement, are expressed genuinely. Also, it is best to avoid making statements focused on your approval or praise of a client's behavior, which is considered compliments rather than affirmations. In the end, this puts undue pressure on the client to perform for the clinician in the future. Additionally, with approval or compliments, there also exists the opposite: disapproval. If we demonstrate approval, then the individual may stop being authentic due to fear of receiving disapproval one day. Take for example a client who has unmanaged diabetes with a high A1C, is overweight, eats poorly, does not exercise, and, albeit is late every visit, yet continues to show up. An affirmation for this individual could be, "You were determined to make it here today." Sometimes, we as clinicians must dig deep and look very hard to identify a positive trait for our most difficult clients. A fun way to imagine this however is to put on *glasses* that only show you their strengths. It may take a while however with some practice, affirmations, even for our most difficult clients, will become easier and easier to conjure (Table 4.2).

Reflections – Reflections are the number one *go-to tool* for the MI clinician. They technically should be used more often than any of the other skills. Generally, we start a conversation and fill in the gaps by asking OEQs. Affirmations are used to keep the momentum and the tempo of the conversation up. Reflections, however, are used to maximize efficiency in clarifying information that has been gathered as well as offer a certain hypothesis regarding the assumed situation so far. One goal for using reflections is to convey empathy and compassion to the client. A second and perhaps more unique goal is to use reflections to intentionally guide the discussion toward change talk – to enhance motivation for change.

There are several types of reflections, but they are broken down into three main groups: simple, complex, and reflections of emotion. Those who are just beginning to practice MI may choose to focus on simple reflections until they become more proficient. To best illustrate different types of reflections, let us first look at a case example.

TABLE 4.2
Affirmation Examples

"You are very good at caring for others"

"You enjoy adventure and having fun"

"It is hard to get you down for long"

"You are resilient"

"You were determined to get here"

"You don't see the value in this plan"

Clinician: *"Thank you for coming in today Mr. Smith. Your care clinician shared with me that you might be interested in using weight loss to help control your diabetes, but why don't you tell me in your own words what brings you in today."*

Client: *"Well, I'd like to lose weight and I've been thinking about it for a while, but I'm not sure I can. My doctor has mentioned several times that this would be a good idea but between work and raising my children, I'm unsure if I can find the time or the energy."*

Simple: Considering the case above, a simple reflection would be to repeat back either exactly or close to what the client just stated,

Rephrase 1:

Client: *"Well, I'd like to lose weight and I've been thinking about it for a while, but I'm not sure I can."*

Clinician: "You'd like to lose weight and you've been thinking about it for a while."

Although this can be useful, simple reflections are best used in moderation for it may become tiresome for both clinician and client to hear the same message repeated multiple times. Simple reflections might also involve the clinician reflecting a statement very close to what the client said but substituting synonyms or slightly rephrasing what the client offered. For example:

Rephrase 2:

Client: *"Well, I'd like to lose weight and I've been thinking about it for a while, but I'm not sure I can."*

Clinician: "Your doctor wants you to lose weight, and as you said, you don't have a lot of time or energy at the end of the day."

Clinicians might also utilize paraphrasing, which is when the clinician is listening for ways to infer the underlying meaning of what the client is saying and to reflect that meaning back to the client. When this is done well, it helps the client to continue their own thought process rather than starting a new one. Paraphrasing in this example might look like this.

Paraphrase:

Client: *"Well, I'd like to lose weight and I've been thinking about it for a while, but I'm not sure I can."*

Clinician: "Tackling something like losing weight seems difficult as a single parent, and part of you recognizes that this is an important part of your health."

Complex: In complex reflections, clinicians are reflecting on the feeling that highlights the emotional underpinnings of the discussion. These are often more complex versions of paraphrases. As clinicians become more skilled at this type of reflection, they use both feeling statements ("you are worried") and metaphors ("you feel like you are constantly pushing uphill"). In this example, the clinician might reflect (Table 4.3),

Client: "Well, I'd like to lose weight and I've been thinking about it for a while, but I'm not sure I can."

Clinician: "You are really stressed and worried about not being able to actually be successful at this."

Amplified reflections tend to exaggerate a situation, whereas double-sided reflections enhance both sides of the argument. When using double-sided reflections, note the use of "and" and not "but" in these examples. This is done intentionally because oftentimes, everything that comes before the "but" is canceled out by what comes after. For example, "you did great on the work but there is still room for improvement." We also have reflections that rely on metaphor to prove the point, as well as ones that reflect an emotion or affect. Reflections of emotion are often very powerful, so do not be surprised if the individual emotes after deploying such a technique. Other options are continuing the sentence, which is used when the client makes a significant pause – here, the clinician simply finishes what the client was ponderous to say. In some difficult situations, when progress seems to have stalled, the clinician can strategically utilize the emphasis on personal choice as well as siding with the negative. These may backfire, so be careful, however if used skillfully, they can provide a safe space for the reticent individual to expand the conversation into.

Roadblocks for engaging. Despite our best efforts and intentions, there are often barriers to engaging with clients that are important to be aware of. In addition to the righting reflex described earlier in this *chapter*, the 12 common roadblocks listed

---

TABLE 4.3
Reflection Examples

Amplified: Here, the clinician intensifies the aspect of the situation	"You are really unsure what to do"
Double-Sided: Both sides are compared side by side with the use of "and". Notice you always end the comparison with the positive	"Stopping all of this will be hard **and** you realize how it will improve your health"
Affective: Reflecting more on the emotion present	"It is upsetting to even think about this"
Metaphor: Skillful use of metaphors can be very powerful	"It feels like you are treading water"
Continuing the sentence: Used when the person may fade off and not complete a sentence. The clinician provides a hypothesis on the continuation	"and you have wanted to say that out loud for a long time now"
Emphasizing personal choice: Often used when there seems to be a stagnation in the movement forward	"and you know you are the only one who can take control of this"
Siding with the negative: An approach that can be useful although there is potential for backfire here. Use this carefully	"and then there is always the choice to do nothing about it right now"

in Table 4.4 may hinder effective communication. The list below is adapted from Thomas Gordon's 12 Roadblocks.[17] MI is an approach that may help navigate these roadblocks. The communication styles outlined here rely on being directive, educative, or judgmental rather than collaborative and supportive of autonomy, which are approaches fundamental to MI.

Summaries – Like reflections, summaries are used to provide clarification regarding information that has been gained thus far, but they are not used as frequently as reflections. Also, like reflections, the clinician must resist giving advice or trying to solve the problem. Consider using summaries at the end of different sections or periods in the conversation, summing up one major concept before moving on to the next. Summaries can use collateral information from outside sources such as information gathered from the chart review, external evaluations, or input from family or loved ones in your summaries. Some examples of summaries are given in Table 4.5.

Putting it all Together: Beginner MI clinicianclinicians may get overwhelmed and often have questions regarding the general structure of an MI-based conversation. What do I say? How do I begin the conversation? When do I use reflections vs. open-ended questions? Etc.? A helpful guiding structure for beginner clinicianclinicians is the Elicit-Provide with Permission-Elicit model (see Table 4.6). In this model, the

TABLE 4.4
The 12 Roadblocks

1. Ordering, directing, or commanding
2. Warning, cautioning, or threatening
3. Giving advice, making suggestions, or providing solutions
4. Persuading with logic, argument, or lecturing
5. Telling people what they should do; moralizing
6. Disagreeing, judging, criticizing, or blaming
7. Agreeing, approving or praising
8. Shaming, ridiculing, or labeling
9. Interpreting or analyzing
10. Reassuring, sympathizing, or consoling
11. Questioning or probing
12. Withdrawing, distracting, humoring, or changing the subject

TABLE 4.5
Summary Examples

Summary Starters

"Let me understand if I have everything correct so far"
"So far, what I'm hearing is"

Summary Clarifiers

"From what I have shared back with you, is there anything else you would like to add"
"Have I missed anything so far"

TABLE 4.6
Elicit, Provide with Permission, Elicit Model

Elicit	Listen/Reflect	Provide	Listen/Reflect	Elicit

clinician would first *elicit* what the client already knows about condition X. While the client is sharing, the clinician is actively listening and providing affirmations and reflections to guide the conversation. When the client is done with sharing, the clinician then asks the client if they are interested in learning more about condition X and if the clinician could share more information. This approach respects client autonomy by asking permission and assessing interest. If permission is given, the next step would be to provide affirmations, feedback, advice, or one or two pieces of relevant information to the client. There is no implicit permission to provide education just because the client is present in the exam room. Although it may sound strange, if permission is not granted, do not continue with educating. Continuing to educate without permission can potentially damage the relationship you have created to this point. If this occurs, simply state "if you change your mind, I have plenty of information on topic X that I would be happy to share."

For the last step, the clinician would again *elicit* reactions and questions, and possibly plan for the next steps. Depending on how many cycles are completed, summaries can be used intermittently to assure that a basic understanding of the information shared is accurate. This model transitions easily into the plan-making phase that could sound something like this: "thank you for sharing your thoughts with me today. I feel that we have a clear direction to follow, and I heard two options we could choose from. Tell me which one you feel the most confident with and a first step you would like to take towards this goal."

4.4.2 Focusing

Focusing on an identified problem is essential to the MI process because it narrows the scope of the conversation. Remember that MI is not an unintentional conversation about change but more of a communication approach designed for personal motivation and commitment to a specific goal. Focusing on a specific target can be facilitated by the clinician and can assist in quickly getting on track with the client to allow for more time to engage in the MI process. An importance ruler is a tool used within the MI setting that helps elicit the next steps in the progression of identifying and moving toward a changed behavior. First, you ask if the change is important to the person (scale of 1–10, 10 being the highest). If the score is below 7, spend clinical time working on investigating the importance. This could be done by asking the client "so tell me a little bit more about why you would want to make this change." By asking this question, the clinician is most likely to elicit more change talk related to building importance. If the score is 7 or above, we know that the topic is relatively important so we can next ask the confidence question. Using the same scale (1–10, 10 being the highest), ask "how confident are you that you can complete this task?" If they are below 7, continue working on increasing confidence by asking "what would it take to increase your confidence just a little bit, say an increase of ½ or 1 point?" Responses from the client will vary, but they typically focus on small changes the client could make to increase their confidence in completing the change. If the score is 7 or above, continue with the conversation edging toward the next stage of planning. Although this is not strictly an MI initiative, the practice of using these questions holds to the spirit and provides a structure that can assist in guiding the progression through the four phases of MI (Tables 4.7 and 4.8).

4.4.3   EVOKING

Responding to Change Talk and Sustain Talk is elemental to the process of MI. Change talk builds on the client's confidence (see Chapter 3) and is simply the idea that the client is self-promoting reasons to make a change. Sustain talk is the opposite, where the client is providing arguments for the status quo. The bulk of the research that suggests that MI is an effective intervention is centered around the increase of change talk and how it relates to making a behavior change. As Moyer et al.[4] discovered, increased change talk leads to increased confidence. Lorig et al.[18] also showed that one of the key predictors of change is the confidence and control related to a behavior change rather than the change itself. Said differently, the number of collective steps made toward a specific goal is not as important as the confidence that the individual can control the progress toward the next step. Therefore, focusing on strategies to enhance change talk and facilitate an increased sense of confidence and control are essential objectives of the MI clinician.

Taking a closer look at change talk, we see that there are two types: Preparatory and mobilizing change talk. The chart below elucidates the differences through a few pointed examples. When the clinician hears one or more of the concepts mentioned below, it behooves the clinician to facilitate more of this change talk by either providing a reflection or asking an open-ended question. *Note the acronym of DARN CAT to help remember the different elements.

TABLE 4.7
Importance Ruler

0<-->10
Not important at all   extremely important

TABLE 4.8
Confidence Ruler

0<-->10
Not confident at all   extremely confident

Preparatory Change Talk:

Desires	Client:	"I really wish things were different."
	Clinician:	"You have thought about this change for a long time. How might things be better if you did complete this goal?"
	Client:	"I have made changes like this before...I know I can do it."
	Clinician:	"You have experience with this and because of that you feel a bit more
Ability		confident that you can do it again."
Reason	Client:	"If I could just lose a few pounds, I know my A1C would decrease, and I know how bad for me smoking is."
	Clinician:	"You know quite a bit about what changes might impact your health the most."
Need	Client:	"I must do this for me and my family. My wife said I need to quit."
	Clinician:	"You want to be around for them."

Mobilizing Change Talk:

Commitment	Client:	"I'm going to look into how to do this."
	Clinician:	"You really have put a lot of thought into this. I have some ideas if you would like to hear them."
	Client:	"I've been thinking about how to change all of this and I think I'm ready to start."
Activation	Clinician:	"You really are motivated. What do you think you will do first?"
Taking Steps:	Client:	"I called the gym and left a message about how to get a membership."
	Clinician:	"Wonderful job. What can I do to help move this forward?"

Discord is also a concept worth discussing. Historically, MI clinicians used the term "resistance" when describing a client who is struggling with change and it was thought that resistance was a conflict between changing and staying the same. In the 3rd edition, Miller and Rollnick (2013)[3] focused less on resistance and more on the concepts of change and sustain talk. Although discord is a phenomenon that impacts the movement toward change, it is not an internal conflict with self, but more often a conflict between the clinician and the client. Discord can present in many different ways including defensiveness, arguing, interrupting, and ignoring. If discord is present, time and attention must be directed back to the beginning, revisiting the concept of engagement. At this point, due to any given number of reasons, the relationship between the clinician and the client has been jeopardized, and time and attention must be paid to repairing it before you can move on.

As noted in Chapter 2, weighing the pros and cons of changing is one way to negotiate ambivalence. In the Focus phase, the clinician and the client could use the decisional balance to sift through some of the ambivalence and hopefully make their way toward a clearer target behavior. Noting that the pros of changing are not always equal to the cons of staying the same. After making this list, the clinician could do two things next. First, ask the client to "name this change," and second,

---

TABLE 4.9
Decision-Making Matrix

	Benefits/Pros	Costs/Cons
Making a change		
Not making a change		

---

to identify the next step in the process. If motivation continues to be transitory, this tool can also be used to enhance change talk by only focusing on the pros of changing and the pros of staying the same. This strength-based approach is one way to clarify the wants and needs of the client without being weighed down or distracted by obstacles (Table 4.9).

4.4.4 PLANNING

Exploring a change plan is integral to the process but not always achieved. Assuring that it is not done too soon, and only when change talk presents more continuously, it may be appropriate to investigate a plan. Creating a change plan is an ongoing and ever-changing process that requires the clinician to assess potential approaches to addressing the target behavior. First, the clinician offers the client a summary to assure that mutual agreement and understanding have been achieved. This can be followed by a simple question such as, "Where should we go from here?" This combination of a summary followed by an invitation can assist with the transition from processing to planning. Typically, this question results in one of the following: (1) a step forward with no clear path, (2) a multitude of options forward, or (3) a clear step forward.

First, there is a scenario where there is no clear plan at all. As with all three options, the clinician initially offers a summary and then attempts to clarify the plan. At this point, you want to work with the client's ideas from general to specific in a brainstorming session, collecting any plausible option. As the saying goes "throw it all against the wall and see what sticks." Because there is no clear way forward, motivation may wane, and the discussion may ebb and flow from any of the preceding phases, engaging, evoking, or focusing. Remember to use the CATS mnemonic under mobilizing change talk to guide you as you continue working toward commitment, action, and taking a few next steps.

Sometimes, the path forward has many branches; the motivation is present, but there are multiple options to choose from. Whether it is choosing between multiple good options or trying to choose the least "bad" option, this scenario may take some time. In these situations, after you have provided the summary and asked the "what next question," it becomes very important to clarify and confirm the specific goal. Some questions that help investigate client preferences are "If you could imagine being most successful in this task, which three options seem most likely to move you forward?" or simply, "Which one appeals to you most?" Then from here, continue evoking change talk and troubleshooting further tasks.

When there is a clear path to change, it is helpful to clarify the goal and then summarize your current understanding of the progress. From here, you begin troubleshooting hurdles and speed bumps impeding progress and narrowing down the details to attain more specific details regarding the plan. Notice that we defer focusing on the obstacles until we have established a solid understanding of the individual's readiness. Although not MI-specific, the acronym SMART is often helpful when creating goals. Chapter 7 of this book delves deeper into the SMART format; however, below you may find a basic outline useful.

Specific: Define the goal as much as possible including interrogatives such as what, where, and when will the goal/behavior occur.

Measurable: **Assure that the goal/behavior is trackable. For example, "I will drink 72 ounces of water every day."**

Attainable: Assure that the goal can be accomplished. Try to make the goal not too high or too low below their standard performance.

Relevant: **Is the goal in line with other goals you have as well as your overall priorities and values?**

Timely: Goals should have a start time and a time limit to accommodate for evaluation. For example, after a certain amount of time, such as one week, one month, or one year, the goal will be evaluated for success.

CASE STUDY

A 52-year-old African American male lives with his wife and is the father of three adult children. Mr. Smith works full-time in a security management role at a local hospital. He has a history of bilateral ankle fusions and mild to moderate reported right knee pain.

Clinician:	Good afternoon, thank you for coming in. We do have the results of your labs here, and I would like to discuss them with you. (Start of agenda setting) Would that be, OK? (Asking for permission)
Client:	Sure, that would be fine.
Clinician:	Your cholesterol levels are out of range – the HDLs are low and the LDLs are high. (Giving information)
Client:	Does that mean I have high cholesterol? (Asking you for information)
Clinician:	Yes it does. Your HDL is 27 mg/dL and your LDL is 121 mg/dL. Technically, we like the HDL to be above 40 mg/dL and the LDL to be less than 100 mg/dL. This condition is also called hyperlipidemia. (Giving information) What are your thoughts about this? (Asking open question)
Client:	I don't know, I don't feel that it could be high but then again, how would I know?
Clinician:	It's true, this condition often goes unnoticed by many people, because in the short term, there are very few symptoms. Most people report feeling just fine! (Basic reflection back, giving information, and validating the client's experience)

Client:	I actually do feel pretty healthy, so I'm surprised to hear that I'm not. I know I am a little overweight and I don't exercise much, but I don't smoke. I don't know what to make of this. (Ambivalence)
Clinician:	You know something about the risks of high cholesterol already! (Reflection reinforcing client's knowledge about risk behavior)
Client:	I guess I do but knowing and doing are two very different things. (Ambivalence and minor sustain talk)
Clinician:	Of the things you mentioned, your weight, perhaps your level of physical activity, I wonder if you could tell me which of these, if any, concerns you most? (Open question)
Client:	Interesting question and timely. My wife just asked me the other day if I wanted to go on walks with her in the morning. I told her may be because my feet and ankles have been hurting a lot lately. I used to love to walk, run, and hike, but my ankles have gotten so bad over the years I basically have just given up on it. (Ambivalence)
Clinician:	You loved being outdoors, walking, hiking, running, doing whatever? (Reflection of emotion) Tell me what about it you enjoyed (Asking open questions)
Client:	I just really liked being out of doors. Yah know, my wife and I met while hiking. Over the years, we have hiked quite a few mountains together her and I. I really do miss it. I'm not that young anymore though...I can't hike like I used to, and running is definitely out of the question. (Still, some sustain talk).
Clinician:	We know running is out of the question and maybe even some of the harder hikes, however, there seems to be a lot of passion for being active outdoors with your wife. That is something you enjoyed. (reflection).
Client:	Yes, I really do, and I'd love to do it again to be honest (change talk – Want/Desire)
Clinician:	Okay then, what are some options you could pursue that meet this criterion: activities done outside with your wife? (Open-ended question)
Client:	Well, I guess I could start with those walks she invited me on. I have said "no" all of these times, because well basically because I feel like I can't "do it like I used to." It does bother her though... me saying no when she asks me. I can tell she is disappointed.
Clinician:	She would approve of this and that makes you happy.
Client:	She really would love me to join her.
Clinician:	You sound excited about this. I wonder how confident you are regarding following through with this. On a scale from 0 to 10 – where 0 is not at all confident and 10 is completely confident – how confident are you? (Assessing readiness and motivation for change)
Client:	I think it will work out. I would say I'm about 6 or 7. Yah know, I'm sick and tired of the same old routine and I do miss spending time with my wife outside.

Clinician:	So a 6.5. That's great. Let's imagine she asks you tomorrow if you want to go for a walk with her. What would you need (equipment or plan) to feel comfortable saying "yes," maybe increasing your confidence level to a rounded 7? (building confidence)
Client:	I would need to find my old sneakers. I would probably have to get some new ones, but those old ones would do for now, I would just have to find them, I guess. I also would have to find a pair of jogging pants or just something comfortable to walk in. The weather has been great lately, so I don't think I'd need much.
Clinician:	Okay, So let me see if I understand so far, what has to be done next is for you to find some workout clothes and your sneakers... then wait for the ask? That sounds attainable. (Summary followed by reflecting on ability).
Client:	Actually, I think I'm going to see if I can find these things tonight after I leave here. Then maybe, just maybe, tomorrow morning, I'll ask her.

Measurement Strategies: Coding a MI session is one way to measure the validity or MI consistency of a conversation. Coding, as it is called, is completed by several different companies and organizations worldwide. One broadly used approach is the Motivational Interviewing Treatment Integrity (MITI) which was developed by Moyers, Manue, and Ernst (2015). Currently, MITI's most recent manual is version 4.2.1. The MITI focuses on assessing the clinician's MI skill in two domains. First, it provides you with a Global Rating Score ranging from 1 to 5, with five being the highest and one being the lowest, and second, it provides a Behavioral Count Score. Each Global Rating score will have four subscores. One score will be given for each of the following dimensions – Cultivating Change Talk, Softening Sustain Talk, Partnership, and Empathy. The Global Rating Score is designed to assess the total "Gestalt" (Moyers, Manue, and Ernst, 2015) of the conversation and to give a general feel of how well the session adhered to the Spirit of MI. One key element of the recording is an identified change goal. With an identified change goal, the MITI rater can focus on the direction of the change talk relative to a specific goal.

Another often used tool is the MISC (Motivational Interviewing Skills Code) which is currently in version 2.1. Like the MITI coding system, there are several domains, however the ratings with the MISC are done in "passes." Rated on a five-point Likert scale, these passes include Global Ratings, Parsing, and Behavior Coding. Pass one offers a Global Rating where the rater looks at the recording as a whole and provides a rating based primarily on the counselor's behavior during the observed session. Concepts that are evaluated are autonomy support, empathy, direction, collaboration, and evocation. The second part of this global rating is the client behavior score where the rater looks at the level of client self-exploration and sharing of personally relevant material. Pass two, Parsing, is used to identify different utterances within a sentence, whereas client change language should be parsed into separate utterances. Pass three is Behavior Coding. This pass has a significant level

TABLE 4.10

Coding Instruments

MISC	The Motivational Interviewing Skills Code (MISC) 2.1. This system is used to measure the quality of MI as well as the impact of training and assess overall client language
CACTI	CASSA Application for Coding Treatment Interactions (CACTI). This open-source application assesses digital recordings with downloadable software and a user manual. CACTI is used specifically for qualifying treatment interactions
CLEAR	The CLEAR is formally known as MISC 1.1 and is used specifically to identify client change talk or counter-change talk
MISO	The Motivational Interviewing with Significant Others is an instrument designed to assess the language of the client's significant other(s) who are also participating in the session
SCOPE	The Sequential Code for Observing Process Exchanges is used to assess the relationship between the behaviors of the interviewer and those of the client during the session
GROMIT	Global Rating of Motivational Interviewing Therapists is used to broadly measure therapist skill responsiveness and overall competence in MI

of sophistication associated with it and includes evaluation of constructs such as the use of facilitative language, advice-giving, use of affirmations, confrontation, use of various types of questions, emphasizing control and summaries.

What would the measurement tool be used for and when? The coding process can be deployed for both refining initial skills as well as ongoing maintenance. The first step is for the clinician to get permission from the client to record a short session (typically in the 20–30-minute range). After recording, the clinician would then send this recorded session to a selected coding company (see Table 4.10) which would code it for MI consistency and then send feedback back to the clinician. This is typically done several times in a row – to meet a certain level of proficiency in succession. After this initial proficiency is achieved, the MITI coding could be used periodically throughout their career to verify ongoing adherence to MI.

There are several coding options other than the MITI tool. Although not completely exhaustive, Table 4.10 provides a list of several more commonly used coding resources. Specific details regarding costs and deliverables are beyond the scope of this document. If you are interested in pursuing coding for MI fidelity, the University of Mexico's Center on Alcohol, Substance Use, and Addictions can be very helpful.

4.5 SUMMARY

MI is a client-centered, therapeutic approach designed to help clients with the process of change. Evoking change talk and reducing sustain talk is one of the main objectives of this approach. The Spirit of MI includes partnership, acceptance, compassion, and evocation. The Four Processes of MI include engaging, focusing, evoking, and planning. When a client is ambivalent about change, MI is one of the best approaches to take for counseling on behavior change. It takes knowledge, skill, and practice to perform MI. People who use MI in their practices are reviewing their interviews and constantly working to improve their adherence to the model. Scales such as the MITI and MISC are used to help clinicians gauge their fidelity to the MI process. Learning how to use MI is one of the best things one can do to help clients make progress during their change journeys. It also makes the counseling sessions more enjoyable and productive for all involved.

4.6 KEY TAKEAWAYS

4.6.1 WHAT DO YOU WANT THE READER TO REMEMBER FROM YOUR CHAPTER?

Although ultimately it comes from being compassionate – wanting to help the other – we must resist the righting reflex. If we don't, it typically leads to frustrating conversations and unproductive outcomes. If we don't internally embrace the fact that we are not able to directly change another, we will continue to be frustrated and have poor outcomes.

Taking responsibility for the intervention rather than the outcome allows us to be better at performing MI by being an active listener, exploring ambivalence, and enhancing change talk thus coming closer to truly understanding the client's motivations.

MI is often an auxiliary approach and can be combined with other clinical concepts such as Cognitive Behavioral Therapy and Acceptance Commitment Therapy.

The philosophical underpinnings of MI align well with current Patient-Centered Medical Home and Trauma Informed Care efforts.

4.6.2 HOW WILL THE READER CHANGE THEIR COUNSELING TECHNIQUES AFTER READING YOUR CHAPTER?

They may abandon the expert role, utilize listening over speaking, and focus on the moment they are with the client (investing in the interaction) and not so much on what happens (the outcome).

They will practice seeking strengths instead of deficiencies, and in doing so, they will see the opportunities more readily. Affirmations will come more easily. They will be able to balance seeing the problem and the solution.

4.6.3 WHAT'S YOUR MAIN POINT?

MI is an effective communication strategy for increasing change talk and subsequent positive behavior when executed correctly and discussing a specific behavioral change.

The Spirit of MI can be used in any situation with anyone at any time. It can be seen as just being a "good human."

The clinician must take a humble stance to understand the client which requires the clinician to drop the expert role and resist making assumptions about the potential outcome or the motivations of the client. They must be humble and journey together with the client side by side.

TABLE 4.11
Additional Resources

Title	Authors	Source	Year	Key Findings
Motivational Interviewing in Health Care	Rollnick, S., Miller, W.R., Butler, C.C.	Book	2022	Specific Health Care related examples, topics, and discussions
Motivational Interviewing for Leadership: MI Lead	Wilcox, J., Kersh, B.C., Jenkins, E.	Book	2017	Integrating MI concepts into organizational leadership
Building Motivational Interviewing Skills (2nd Ed.)	Rosengren, D.B.	Book	2017	Workbook to help develop skills in MI, either used alone or in group settings
Motivational Interviewing in Schools (2nd Ed.)	Herman, K.C., Reinke, W.M., Frey, A.J.	Book	2020	Utilizing MI to engage parents, teachers, and students
Casaa.unm.edu	University of New Mexico	Website	2022	UNM Center on alcohol, substance use, and addictions

4.7 RESOURCES

See Table 4.11.

REFERENCES

1. Rozario D. Burnout, resilience and moral injury: How the wicked problems of health care defy solutions, yet require innovative strategies in the modern era. *Canadian Journal of Surgery*. 2019;62(4):EE6`E8. doi:https://doi.org/10.1503/cjs.0028191.
2. Watzlawick P, Weakland JH, Fisch R. *Change: Principles of Problem Formation and Problem Resolution*. W.W. Norton & Co; 2011.
3. Miller WR, Rollnick S. *Motivational Interviewing: Helping People Change*. 3rd ed. The Guilford Press, Cop; 2013.
4. Moyers TB, Martin T, Christopher PJ, Houck JM, Tonigan JS, Amrhein PC. Client Language as a Mediator of Motivational Interviewing Efficacy: Where Is the Evidence? Alcoholism: *Clinical and Experimental Research*. 2007;31(s3):40s47s. doi:https://doi.org/10.1111/j.1530-0277.2007.00492.x
5. Frost H, Campbell P, Maxwell M, et al. Effectiveness of Motivational Interviewing on adult behaviour change in health and social care settings: A systematic review of reviews. Moitra E, ed. *PLOS ONE*. 2018;13(10):1–39. doi:https://doi.org/10.1371/journal.pone.0204890
6. Aubeeluck E, Al-Arkee S, Finlay K, Jalal Z. The impact of pharmacy care and motivational interviewing on improving medication adherence in patients with cardiovascular diseases: A systematic review of randomised controlled trials. *International Journal of Clinical Practice. Published online* July 2021. doi:https://doi.org/10.1111/ijcp.14457
7. Amiri P, Mansouri-Tehrani MM, Khalili-Chelik A, et al. Does Motivational Interviewing Improve the Weight Management Process in Adolescents? A Systematic Review and Meta-analysis. *International Journal of Behavioral Medicine. Published online* July 15, 2021. doi:https://doi.org/10.1007/s12529-021-09994-w

8. McDaniel CC, Kavookjian J, Whitley HP. Telehealth delivery of motivational interviewing for diabetes management: A systematic review of randomized controlled trials. *Patient Education and Counseling.* 2021;105(4). doi:https://doi.org/10.1016/j.pec.2021.07.036
9. Nuss K, Moore K, Nelson T, Li K. Effects of Motivational Interviewing and Wearable Fitness Trackers on Motivation and Physical Activity: A Systematic Review. *Am J Health Promot.* 2021;35(2):226–235. doi:10.1177/0890117120939030
10. Ghizzardi G, Arrigoni C, Dellafiore F, Vellone E, Caruso R. Efficacy of motivational interviewing on enhancing self-care behaviors among patients with chronic heart failure: a systematic review and meta-analysis of randomized controlled trials. *Heart Failure Reviews. Published online* April 17, 2021. doi:https://doi.org/10.1007/s10741-021-10110-z
11. Makin H, Chisholm A, Fallon V, Goodwin L. Use of motivational interviewing in behavioural interventions among adults with obesity: A systematic review and meta-analysis. *Clinical Obesity.* 2021;11(4). doi:https://doi.org/10.1111/cob.12457
12. Ardito RB, Rabellino D. Therapeutic Alliance and Outcome of Psychotherapy: Historical Excursus, Measurements, and Prospects for Research. *Frontiers in Psychology.* 2012;2(270). doi:https://doi.org/10.3389/fpsyg.2011.00270
13. RSA. Brené Brown on Empathy. YouTube. *Published online* December 10, 2013.https://www.youtube.com/watch?v=1Evwgu369Jw
14. Pollak KI, Nagy P, Bigger J, et al. Effect of teaching motivational interviewing via communication coaching on clinician and patient satisfaction in primary care and pediatric obesity-focused offices. *Patient Education and Counseling.* 2016;99(2):300–303. doi:https://doi.org/10.1016/j.pec.2015.08.013
15. Frankl VE. *Man's Search for Meaning.* Beacon Press; 2006.
16. Healey ML, Grossman M. Cognitive and Affective Perspective-Taking: Evidence for Shared and Dissociable Anatomical Substrates. *Frontiers in Neurology.* 2018;9. doi:https://doi.org/10.3389/fneur.2018.00491
17. Dr. *Thomas Gordon.* Parent Effectiveness Training. Harmony; 2008.
18. Lorig K. *Living a Healthy Life with Chronic Conditions: Self-Management of Heart Disease, Arthritis, Diabetes, Depression, Asthma, Bronchitis, Emphysema and Other Physical and Mental Health Conditions.* Bull Pub. Co; 2012.

5 The Power of Autonomy

Jessica A. Matthews, DBH, NBC-HWC, DipACLM, FACLM, Sofia Chandler, MS, NBC-HWC, Rachel Frye, MS, BSN, RN, and Michael R. Mantell, Ph.D

Everything can be taken from a man but one thing: the last of the human freedoms—to choose one's attitude in any given set of circumstance, to choose one's own way.

Viktor Frankl
Man's Search for Meaning (1962)

5.1 INTRODUCTION

As revealed in self-determination theory (SDT), a primary human psychological need, across cultures, is the need to feel autonomous and not controlled.[1] Yet with time constraints often placed on patient visits and the need to address multiple agenda items within a limited time frame, clinicians tend to rely on a more directive style of communication in which instructions, advice, and education are readily offered, often with minimal input from the patient. This "expert approach," while necessary at times, fails to foster a positive and productive patient-clinician partnership rooted in trust, empathy, and respect – key components of a successful therapeutic relationship. In addition, this approach falls short of satisfying the basic psychological needs of patients, as in order to enact meaningful and lasting lifestyle changes, patients must feel in control, confident, and connected. The EXPERT Approach was introduced in Chapter 1.

With the core components of autonomy, competence, and relatedness in mind, clinicians have the opportunity to adopt a more effective style of collaborative communication – known as a "coach approach" – to meet patient needs and support them in fostering more intrinsic and self-determined forms of motivation. This chapter aims to equip clinicians with an understanding of the theoretical underpinnings of SDT and the spirit and skills of a coach approach to foster autonomy-supporting care environments in which patients are empowered to enact and sustain health-promoting behaviors. The COACH Approach was discussed in Chapter 1.

5.2 SELF-DETERMINATION THEORY

SDT was first theorized by Deci and Ryan.[2] This theory puts forward the idea that there are two main types of motivation that powerfully shape how we act – intrinsic motivation and extrinsic motivation. Intrinsic motivation originates from within the patient, where the behavior is pursued with genuine interest, enjoyment, and inherent satisfaction. This type of motivation requires little to no self-regulation, and the behavior itself is often in concert with the patient's personal values. Extrinsic

DOI: 10.1201/9781003161226-5

motivation, on the other hand, is anchored in external sources such as rewards, goals, or extrinsic outcomes that govern the behavior. SDT highlights how the type of motivation a patient has could reveal more about future actions toward health behavior change as opposed to overall motivation.[2] As such, this theory further delineates more refined subtypes of extrinsic motivation to self-regulate behavior, ranging from other-determined (controlled) motivation to more self-determined (autonomous) motivation. This continuum will be further discussed in the next section.

At the core of SDT lies the understanding that in order for high-quality intrinsic motivation to occur, three basic psychological needs must be met – autonomy, competence, and relatedness.[2,3] These psychological needs, when satisfied, help facilitate lasting lifestyle change and improved health and well-being.

5.2.1 AUTONOMY

Autonomy is the need to feel one has personal choice and control over their behaviors. This innate need to feel in the "driver's seat" of one's own life is paramount to achieving long-lasting behavior change.[4] Clinicians can provide autonomy support by cultivating care environments that acknowledge patient feelings, nurture patient values and interests, as well as enhance patient choice through the use of collaborative conversation skills. Autonomy support has been implicated as key in several lifestyles and clinically relevant behaviors, such as medication adherence and fruit and vegetable consumption in patients with diabetes.[5,6]

5.2.2 COMPETENCE

Competence is the need to feel effective or capable in one's experiences.[7] The more competent one feels in terms of having the knowledge, skills, and abilities needed to succeed, the more self-determined motivation can flourish. Competence is enhanced through optimal challenges and detailed, positive feedback and undermined by excessive challenge, and nonexistent, underdeveloped, or negative feedback.[8] Tailoring the task level appropriate to the individual patient and working with them to identify barriers to changing their behavior are helpful strategies to increase competence.[9,10]

5.2.3 RELATEDNESS

Relatedness is one's feeling of connectedness with others and the world around them.[7] Social connection is a foundational pillar of lifestyle medicine, and the clinician and patient relationship plays a key role in initiating sustained behavior change. When clinicians take time to connect with patients and learn more about them on a personal level, patients are more likely to rate their medical care as excellent.[11] In addition, fostering a patient-clinician relationship rooted in trust, empathy, and respect – key components of a successful therapeutic relationship – has been shown to have a small yet statistically significant effect on healthcare outcomes.[12]

5.2.4 ENJOYMENT

In addition to these three psychological needs, clinicians should also consider enjoyment as another important fact, as patients can experience difficulty in overcoming certain biases and predetermined attitudes about healthy lifestyles. Although enjoyment is not a specific construct of SDT, the upward spiral theory of lifestyle change suggests that when patients experience positive affect when engaging in positive health behaviors it can fuel intrinsic motivation by cultivating nonconscious and increasing motives for these behaviors which, in turn, are more likely to become sustained lifestyle practices.[13]

With the acronym CARE in mind – competence, autonomy, relatedness, and enjoyment – clinicians can help patients foster more autonomous motivation, as behavior change anchored in meeting these important needs is more likely to be better internalized and retained.

5.3 MOTIVATION TYPE

While motivation is often viewed broadly as a singular construct, SDT posits a continuum ranging from amotivation to intrinsic motivation, with a multitude of refined subtypes of extrinsic motivation in between.

5.3.1 AMOTIVATION

Amotivation contradicts intrinsic motivation and often leaves an individual feeling out of control. Amotivating events are marked by a lack of perceived competence and are experienced as the inability to master a given task or activity.[14] Individuals experiencing amotivation lack any intention to act or change their behavior.[4]

5.3.2 EXTRINSIC MOTIVATION

Extrinsic motivation occurs as a result of external influences. This type of motivation is unlikely to lead to long-term behavior change[9]; however, it can play an important role in the initial adoption of an activity.[3] Introjected regulation and external regulation are both considered forms of controlled motivation where external rewards or punishments are the primary stimuli for behavior change.[14–16] The transformation that occurs from controlled forms of motivation to more autonomous forms of regulation is called "internalization".[4]

5.3.3 INTROJECTED REGULATION

Introjected regulation is a form of motivation that occurs intrinsically; however, an individual takes action because of feelings of guilt, shame, or worry should they not engage in a given behavior. This is inherently different from purely intrinsic motivation where an individual engages in a behavior with genuine interest and enjoyment.[9] Utilizing rewards and punishments may yield short-term results but again, is unlikely to contribute to long-lasting behavior change.[3,9] Ultimately these forms of motivation are driven by a sense of responsibility or tied to a motive (i.e., "I have to go on a run to lose weight") rather than enjoyment (i.e., "I want to go on a run because it's fun").[3]

5.3.4 IDENTIFIED AND INTEGRATED REGULATIONS

Next, identified and integrated regulations demonstrate autonomy to an extent; however, behaviors that are driven by these forms of regulation are not typically perceived as enjoyable to the individual.[9] Instead, identified regulation is marked by an individual consciously identifying with an activity and experiencing a willingness to act because of the personal endorsement tied to a behavior.[15,17] Research suggests that identified regulation predicts short-term adoption of exercise more so than intrinsic motivation; however, long-term exercise adherence is more closely associated with intrinsic motivation.[3] Lastly, along the continuum of autonomy, integrated regulation is the most autonomous form of extrinsic motivation where an individual identifies with a behavior and recognizes that it aligns with one's core values or beliefs.[15,17]

5.3.5 INTRINSIC MOTIVATION

At the far end of the continuum, intrinsic motivation is defined as the most autonomous form of motivation,[9] and for this reason, it is understood as the most powerful and reliable form of motivation when undertaking behavior change. Behaviors that are driven by intrinsic motivation are done for the pure enjoyment, exploration, or curiosity of a given activity. In addition, intrinsic motivation is free of external pressures influencing behavior.[17]

5.4 EVIDENCE REVIEW

The powerful role of autonomy in behavior change is well documented. For example, Teixeira et al.[3] identified that individuals with higher autonomous motivation consistently exercised for more minutes each week compared to those with lower autonomous motivation. Ryan and Deci[17] found that more autonomous forms of motivation led to increased engagement and learning among students. Yet, the type of motivation and level of motivation can vary from person to person as well as fluctuate and evolve within the same individual. For example, studies show that autonomous motivation increases as a person progresses through the stages of change,[3] a topic further discussed in Chapter 2. Other factors that influence the type and level of motivation a patient may experience include exposure to external pressures, enjoyment of an activity (or lack thereof), identifying with a given behavior, perceived barriers, and health limitations.[15]

Research suggests that SDT-based interventions, to a certain extent, can positively influence the three constructs of SDT and promote autonomous motivation in patients.[4,9,15] Ultimately, the use of SDT-based intervention strategies in a clinical setting is linked to the prevention and management of chronic disease and the promotion of long-lasting behavior change.[4,16] Interventions that focused on enhancing how significant people – such as clinicians, family, and friends – supported an individual's basic psychological needs of autonomy, competence, and relatedness proved to increase perceptions of need satisfaction, and, more importantly, these improvements led to positive changes of health behaviors throughout the course of the intervention period.[15]

To date, most studies that implemented SDT-based interventions targeted physical activity, diet, sedentary behavior, and smoking cessation.[16] Interventions that utilized noncontrolling language positively impacted autonomy satisfaction while provision of a rationale increased autonomous motivation.[9] Similarly, identifying barriers was associated with increased autonomous motivation, while interventions that conveyed a person is valued were correlated with increases in autonomy satisfaction, reductions in amotivation, and even minor improvements in relatedness satisfaction.[15]

In addition, utilizing a community setting when delivering interventions can more effectively reduce amotivation and improve relatedness compared to mediations performed elsewhere.[15] Similarly, Sheeran et al.[16] determined that SDT-based interventions lead to significant changes in health behaviors; however, the degree of behavior change was small. When examining physical and psychological health outcomes, Ntoumanis et al.[15] found that SDT-based interventions had only a small benefit at follow-up and a nonsignificant effect at the end of the intervention period. Future research should focus on both the impact of SDT on health behaviors and on health outcomes as clinically significant data could further appeal to clinicians and policymakers.[15]

5.4.1 Practical Strategies for Fostering Autonomous Motivation

The way clinicians communicate with patients has an impact on facilitating change and supporting autonomous motivation. Presently, the predominant relational model in healthcare is more directive, in which clinicians focus on identifying problems, defining the visit agenda, and determining the lifestyle prescription, often with little to no input from the patient. This so-called "expert approach" is helpful and necessary in certain situations – such as conducting diagnostics and prescribing medications and procedures – yet it often yields limited success in encouraging the adoption of healthy behaviors, as knowledge of improved behaviors alone is not sufficient to foster lasting change.[18]

Conversely, the "coach approach" is a systematic, collaborative communication style that is geared toward supporting patients in adopting self-directed behavior changes.[19,20] While it is a systematic communication style in regards to how particular concepts and tools can be used, it is also fluid and experimental in how exactly the tools are used. The variety in which the systematic concepts and tools are used will vary depending on the patient and the unique nature of the clinical encounter. In evaluating the difference between the expert approach and coach approach, there are key differences in the roles of the clinician and patient, as well as the overall views and beliefs held by the clinician, as outlined in Table 5.1. This is similar to Table 13.2 provided in Chapter 13 on the differences between the COACH and the EXPERT in the materials and information regarding group interventions.

TABLE 5.1
Comparing an Expert Approach to a Coach Approach

Expert Approach	Coach Approach
Assumes ownership of patient's health	Empowers patient to take ownership of their health
Clinician as the expert	Patient as the expert in their own life
Patient told what to do	Patient is an active partner in creating action steps to accomplish the lifestyle prescription
Leads the process	Guides the process
Delivers the right answers	Asks the right questions
Motivates to comply	Uncovers motivation within

Source: Adapted fromMatthews, Jessica A., Margaret Moore, and Cate Collings. "A Coach Approach to Facilitating Behavior Change." *The Journal of Family Practice* 71, no. 1 Suppl Lifestyle (2022): eS93–eS99.

TABLE 5.2

Clinical Applications for a Coach Approach

Coach Approach	Values & Actions
Patient-centered	Create a trusting bond
	Have unconditional positive regard for the patient
Clinician elicits patient's agenda	Determine what is of value to the patient as well as what they want to focus on
	Evoke reason for change
Partners & collaborates	Respect for the patient as the expert of their life
	Find and mobilize their values and strengths
Patients are the ones talking the most, while the clinician listens with empathy	Mindful presence (listen, rather than thinking about what to say next)
	Tap into desire for connection
	Search for patient's capabilities
Clinician asks permission to give advice & asks open-ended questions	Ask for permission to offer expertise
	Be attentive and identify when support is needed
Patient determines goal	Co-create clear goals
	Clarify what the patient wants to achieve
	Focus on discrepancies between what they want and where they are presently
	Ensure SMART goal aligned with values
Brainstorms with patient & fosters possibilities; clinician and patient co-discover answers	Assess where the patient is presently in terms of readiness to change
	Can use questionnaires to determine motivation type
Use of self-discovery for patients to find their own answers	Inquire what value is behind the behavior
	When patients need help with creating steps, create opportunities for choice to honor autonomy
Clinician and patient co-create a plan based on the patient's values and intentions	Break down tasks into small, achievable steps
	Steps are in reach but provide just the right amount of stretch
Focuses on what is going right	Positive feedback--praise the mastering of an acquirable skill (rather than inherent talent)
	Celebrate accomplishments
	Emphasize consistent efforts that led to growth
Clinician learns from the patient's story	Respect & appreciate the patient's experience and perception of their experience
	Reframe the experience in positive terms (setbacks are part of the experience) rather than jumping to focusing on the problem and trying to fix it
Patient is responsible for their own choices; there is a shared responsibility of accountability	Acknowledge that patients have responsibility for choices in behavior

Source: Center for Self-determination Theory[35]; Liddy et al.[28]; Moore et al.[24]; Neuner-Jehle et al.[25]; and Proot et al.[36]

5.4.2 A COACH APPROACH TO FACILITATING BEHAVIOR CHANGE

Health coaching is a growth-promoting relationship designed to facilitate positive and sustainable lifestyle changes that support optimal health. Clinicians who utilize a coach approach can support patients in cultivating the knowledge, skills, tools, and confidence needed to become active participants in their care in order to reach self-determined behavioral goals and prevent or treat chronic diseases.[21,22]

5.4.2.1 Thrive

At the heart of a coach approach is the recognition that humans are wired to thrive.[23] Clinicians utilizing a coach approach view patients as not someone needing to be fixed but rather as someone who has the capacity and resourcefulness they need to make healthy behavior changes. Patients are more than their disease process or problem, as they have values and beliefs that empower them to engage in behaviors they feel are personally meaningful to them.[23,24] Patients have basic psychological needs surrounding their sense of competence in the behaviors they engage in, feeling connected and cared for by those around them, and having a sense of owning their life choices.[23,24] With this in mind, the clinician sees the patient as the expert of their life with valuable insights and significant potential to expand awareness and explore possibilities to move toward improved health and well-being. Tapping into the patient's values is where coaching can help elicit autonomous motivation for change.

5.4.2.2 Together

Second, there are key changes to the roles both the clinician and patient hold, as the patient holds the agenda and is the facilitator of the behavior change.[19] The patient determines where he or she wants to make a change and together, in collaboration with the clinician, devises a plan on how to get there. The clinician uses coaching communication skills to facilitate the patient toward their own self-discovery[19] and there is a shared responsibility between the clinician and patient for accountability.[23,25] By establishing positive relationships in which patients feel supported and empowered to recognize and leverage their strengths, they can begin to generate possibilities, initiate actions, and motivate the self-regulation needed to support meaningful, lasting changes.[24]

5.4.2.3 Communication

It is important to recognize that there is a continuum of communication styles that can be utilized to varying degrees within clinical visits. At one end of the continuum is a directing style, in which instructions, information, and advice are readily given yet with minimal input from the patient – more of an "expert approach." At the other end of the continuum is the following style, which employs good listening and trust in the patient's own wisdom while refraining from providing direct information or input. In the middle of this continuum, however, lies a guiding style, which skillfully blends active listening while also offering expertise where needed in the process.[26] This style of communication embodies a coach approach in a framework consistent with motivational interviewing (MI) to elucidate what information patients may want and need while also honoring their autonomy, making it particularly well suited for helping patients navigate health behavior changes.[27]

Within a clinical encounter clinicians can flow from an expert approach to coach approach through a transitional phrase, such as: "Until now, we have been discussing what I can do for you to help you with your condition. I am interested in what you would like to do for your own health. Is it okay with you if we talk about that?"[25, p. 6] In this example, the clinician is intentionally shifting the conversation to show interest and concern in what the patient views as most important to them, thereby honoring their autonomy. By eliciting the patient's agenda, the clinician can then utilize appreciative inquiry (AI) to facilitate patient self-discovery. AI comprises open-ended questions that invite patients to talk about their best accomplishments, what conditions generate their best moments, what strengths they feel proud of, and what they enjoy most. See Chapter 6 for more information on AI.

Conversely, when it is pertinent to share relevant information with patients, clinicians can maintain the spirit of a coach approach by utilizing the elicit-provide-elicit model from MI, as outlined in Chapter 4.

5.4.2.4 Further Evidence

A key determinant in chronic disease prevention and treatment is health-related behavior, yet many clinicians find addressing patients' health behaviors and their motivation to change unhealthy behaviors to be a challenge.[25] There is growing evidence supporting coaching as a valuable intervention for behavior change and chronic disease management.[19,28] Health coaching has been demonstrated to be an effective intervention even in brief encounters.[19,20,28] Studies have shown that using coaching communication practices, such as MI in brief clinical encounters within primary care settings can be more effective than usual care or information shared through didactic materials in helping patients achieve targeted outcomes, such as blood pressure reduction, weight loss, and smoking cessation.[29] However, the effects of MI on patient outcomes can vary greatly, particularly due to provider qualifications, training, and practice, higher levels of which have been shown to be more efficacious.

Despite some of the current limitations in the rapidly growing body of literature – such as consistent definitions and applications of coaching as well as lack of appropriate controls in study design to better examine coaching effect[30] – there is clear and promising evidence of the effectiveness of a coach approach in improving internal motivation and self-efficacy, supporting behavior change, and improving health outcomes and quality of life. Whether provided in person or via telehealth, health coaching has shown statistically significant improvements in physical and mental health status among adult patients with chronic diseases.[31] Improvements in health behaviors such as increased physical activity, dietary changes, self-care behaviors, medication adherence, tobacco and alcohol cessation and foot care in diabetes management have been documented, as well as an increase in patients' confidence in discussing their care plan with their provider.[31] With respect to patient populations and clinical outcomes, health coaching has been found to be particularly effective among patients with diabetes and obesity,[32] yielding clinically relevant improvements in hemoglobin A1c (HbA1c)[30,32,33] and reductions in weight and body mass index (BMI).[30–32] There is also promising emerging evidence of reductions in blood pressure and low-density lipoprotein cholesterol (LDL-C).[30,34]

5.5 CONSIDERATIONS FOR CLINICAL APPLICATION

The healthcare environment can positively or negatively influence a patient's sense of autonomy. As stated previously, a key aspect of the coach approach is that it is patient-centered and focused on self-management which are key to supporting patient autonomy.[22,25] With that in mind, the key beliefs associated with coaching must be at the forefront of the clinician's mind during brief clinical encounters. With the basic core beliefs in place, clinician can then use practical strategies associated with a coach approach, as highlighted in Table 5.2. Part of creating an environment that supports patient autonomy is through the use of open-ended questions and reflections (see Chapter 4), which necessitate listening with curiosity.[24]

Through the use of supportive, collaborative communication skills, clinicians can honor autonomy and cultivate the conditions for patients to find their own way and their own resources simply by being completely present and engaged, asking open-ended questions that open minds followed by offering reflections that deepen personal exploration and set the stage for intentional action.

5.5.1 ASSESSING AUTONOMY-SUPPORTING HEALTHCARE ENVIRONMENTS

The role of the clinician is to provide encouragement and support for more intrinsic and self-determined forms of patient motivation to better facilitate adoption and adherence to lifestyle prescriptions. To further guide application, there are a number of free tools and resources available at selfdeterminationtheory.org.[36] One such assessment tool is the Healthcare Climate Questionnaire (HCCQ) which evaluates from a patient's perspective to what degree the healthcare environment supports autonomous motivation. The items are scored using a 7-point Likert scale, with a score of 1 representing "strongly disagree" and 7 representing "strongly agree." Higher average scores reflect a higher degree of perceived autonomy support among patients.

Example questions from the HCCQ include:

- I feel that my healthcare professional has provided me choices and options about my health. (autonomy)
- My healthcare professional conveys confidence in my ability to make changes regarding my health. (competence)
- I feel a lot of trust in my healthcare professional. (relatedness)
- My healthcare professional has made sure I really understand my condition and what I need to do. (competence)
- My healthcare professional (HCP) encourages me to ask questions. (autonomy)
- I feel able to share my feelings with my healthcare professional. (relatedness)

5.6 SUMMARY

Behavior change is the foundation for effective lifestyle prescriptions, yet the journey toward health-promoting behaviors is an individualized and nonlinear experience influenced by a myriad of factors. In addition, the type and level of motivation will vary from patient to patient and also differ based on their individual readiness to change. Despite the personalized nature of the behavior change process, as illuminated in SDT, all patients share the same basic psychological needs to feel in control (autonomy), confident (competence) and connected (relatedness) in their lives.

By using the collaborative communication style of a "coach approach," clinicians can cultivate autonomy-supporting care environments that empower patients to foster more intrinsic and self-determined forms of motivation which, in turn, facilitates the adoption and sustainment of health-promoting behaviors.

5.7 KEY TAKEAWAYS

- Although motivation is often viewed broadly as a singular construct, it is the specific type of motivation a patient has that can best predict their future actions toward health behavior change.
- Motivation can be generally classified into two general types – intrinsic motivation and extrinsic motivation.
- Patients with autonomous motivation are more likely to initiate and sustain health-promoting behaviors.
- SDT posits that motivation is shaped by the fulfillment of three basic psychological needs – autonomy, competence, and relatedness.
- Clinicians can cultivate autonomy-supporting care environments by utilizing a "coach approach."

5.8 RESOURCES

- Deci, Edward L., and Richard M. Ryan. *The Handbook of Self-Determination*. Rochester, NY: University of Rochester Press, 2004.
- Deci, Edward L., and Richard M. Ryan. *Intrinsic Motivation and Self-Determination in Human Behavior*. New York: Springer Publishing Company, 1985.
- *The Handbook of Behavior Change*. Edited by Martin S. Hagger, Linda D. Cameron, Kyra Hamilton, Nelli Hankonen, and Taru Lintunen. Camberage, England: Cambridge University Press, 2020.
- Ryan, Richard M., and Edward L. Deci. *Self-Determination Theory: Basic Psychological Needs in Motivation, Development, and Wellness*. New York: Guilford Publications, 2018.
- Sheldon, Kennon, Geoffrey D. Williams, and Thomas Joiner. *Self-Determination Theory in the Clinic: Motivation Physical and Mental Health*. New Haven, CT: Yale University Press, 2003.
- Wade, Susan L. *Self-Determination Theory (SDT): Perspective, Applications and Impact*. Hauppauge, NY: Nova Publishers, 2017.

REFERENCES

1. Ryan, Richard M., and Edward L. Deci. *Self-determination Theory: Basic Psychological Needs in Motivation, Development, and Wellness*. New York: Guilford Publications Press, 2017.
2. Deci, Edward L., and Richard M. Ryan. "The General Causality Orientations Scale: Self-determination in Personality." *Journal of Research in Personality* 19, no. 2 (1985): 109–134.
3. Teixeira, Pedro J., Eliana V. Carraça, David Markland, Marlene N. Silva, and Richard M. Ryan. "Exercise, Physical Activity, and Self-determination Theory: A Systematic Review." *International Journal of Behavioral Nutrition and Physical Activity* 9, no. 1 (2012): 1–30.

4. Ng, Johan YY, Nikos Ntoumanis, Cecilie Thøgersen-Ntoumani, Edward L. Deci, Richard M. Ryan, Joan L. Duda, and Geoffrey C. Williams. "Self-Determination Theory Applied to Health Contexts: A Meta-analysis." *Perspectives on Psychological Science* 7, no. 4 (2012): 325–340.

5. Koponen, Anne M., Nina Simonsen, and Sakari Suominen. "Determinants of Physical Activity among Patients with Type 2 Diabetes: The Role of Perceived Autonomy Support, Autonomous Motivation and Self-Care Competence." *Psychology, Health & Medicine* 22, no. 3 (2017): 332–344.

6. Williams, Geoffrey C., Zachary R. Freedman, and Edward L. Deci. "Supporting Autonomy to Motivate Patients with Diabetes for Glucose Control." *Diabetes Care* 21, no. 10 (1998): 1644–1651.

7. Deci, Edward L., and Richard M. Ryan. *Intrinsic Motivation and Self-Determination in Human Behavior.* New York: Springer Science & Business Media, 2013.

8. Cook, David A., and Anthony R. Artino Jr. "Motivation to Learn: An Overview of Contemporary Theories." *Medical Education* 50, no. 10 (2016): 997–1014.

9. Gillison, Fiona B., Peter Rouse, Martyn Standage, Simon J. Sebire, and Richard M. Ryan. "A Meta-analysis of Techniques to Promote Motivation for Health Behaviour Change from a Self-Determination Theory Perspective." *Health Psychology Review* 13, no. 1 (2019): 110–130.

10. Ryan, Richard M., and Edward L. Deci. "Self-Determination Theory and the Facilitation of Intrinsic Motivation, Social Development, and Well-being." *American Psychologist* 55, no. 1 (2000): 68.

11. Pace, Emma J., Nicholas J. Somerville, Chineme Enyioha, Joseph P. Allen, Latrina C. Lemon, and Claudia W. Allen. "Effects of a Brief Psychosocial Intervention on Inpatient Satisfaction: An RCT." *Family Medicine* 49, no. 9 (2017): 675.

12. Kelley, John M., Gordon Kraft-Todd, Lidia Schapira, Joe Kossowsky, and Helen Riess. "The Influence of the Patient-Clinician Relationship on Healthcare Outcomes: A Systematic Review and Meta-analysis of Randomized Controlled Trials." *PLOS ONE* 9, no. 4 (2014): e94207.

13. Van Cappellen, Patty, Elise L. Rice, Lahnna I. Catalino, and Barbara L. Fredrickson. "Positive Affective Processes Underlie Positive Health Behaviour Change." *Psychology & Health* 33, no. 1 (2018): 77–97.

14. Deci, Edward L., and Richard M. Ryan. "The General Causality Orientations Scale: Self-Determination in Personality." *Journal of Research in Personality* 19, no. 2 (1985): 109–134.

15. Ntoumanis, Nikos, Johan YY Ng, Andrew Prestwich, Eleanor Quested, Jennie E. Hancox, Cecilie Thøgersen-Ntoumani, Edward L. Deci, Richard M. Ryan, Chris Lonsdale, and Geoffrey C. Williams. "A Meta-analysis of Self-Determination Theory-Informed Intervention Studies in the Health Domain: Effects on Motivation, Health Behavior, Physical, and Psychological Health." *Health Psychology Review* 15, no. 2 (2021): 214–244.

16. Sheeran, Paschal, Charles E. Wright, Aya Avishai, Megan E. Villegas, Jan Willem Lindemans, William MP Klein, Alexander J. Rothman, Eleanor Miles, and Nikos Ntoumanis. "Self-Determination Theory Interventions for Health Behavior Change: Meta-Analysis and Meta-analytic Structural Equation Modeling of Randomized Controlled Trials." *Journal of Consulting and Clinical Psychology* 88, no. 8 (2020): 726.

17. Ryan, Richard M., and Edward L. Deci. "Intrinsic and Extrinsic Motivation from a Self-Determination Theory Perspective: Definitions, Theory, Practices, and Future Directions." *Contemporary Educational Psychology* 61 (2020): 101860.

18. Phillips, Edward M., Elizabeth P. Frates, and David J. Park. "Lifestyle Medicine." *Physical Medicine and Rehabilitation Clinics* 31, no. 4 (2020): 515–526.

19. Boehmer, Kasey R., Suzette Barakat, Sangwoo Ahn, Larry J. Prokop, Patricia J. Erwin, and M. Hassan Murad. "Health Coaching Interventions for Persons with Chronic Conditions: A Systematic Review and Meta-analysis Protocol." *Systematic Reviews* 5, no. 1 (2016): 1–7.

20. Butterworth, Susan W., Ariel Linden, and Wende McClay. "Health Coaching as an Intervention in Health Management Programs." *Disease Management & Health Outcomes* 15, no. 5 (2007): 299–307.
21. Bennett, Heather D., Eric A. Coleman, Carla Parry, Thomas Bodenheimer, and Ellen H. Chen. "Health Coaching for Patients with Chronic Illness." *Family Practice Management* 17, no. 5 (2010): 24.
22. Wolever, Ruth Q., Leigh Ann Simmons, Gary A. Sforzo, Diana Dill, Miranda Kaye, Elizabeth M. Bechard, Mary Elaine Southard, Mary Kennedy, Justine Vosloo, and Nancy Yang. "A Systematic Review of the Literature on Health and Wellness Coaching: Defining a Key Behavioral Intervention in Healthcare." *Global Advances in Health and Medicine* 2, no. 4 (2013): 38–57.
23. Kimsey-House, Henry, Karen Kimsey-House, Phillip Sandahl, Laura Whitworth, and Alexis Phillips. *Co-Active Coaching: The Proven Framework for Transformative Conversations at Work and in Life.* Hachette, UK: Nicholas Brealey Publishing, 2018.
24. Moore, Margaret., Erika. Jackson, and Bob. Tschannen-Moran. "Design Thinking." In *Coaching Psychology Manual.* 2nd ed. Philadelphia, PA: Wolters Kluwer, 2016, pp. 125–140.
25. Neuner-Jehle, Stefan, Margareta Schmid, and Ueli Grüninger. "The 'Health Coaching' Programme: A New Patient-centered and Visually Supported Approach for Health Behaviour Change in Primary Care." *BMC Family Practice* 14, no. 1 (2013): 1–8.
26. Miller, William R., and Stephen Rollnick. *Motivational Interviewing: Helping People Change.* 3rd ed. New York: Guilford Press, 2013.
27. Rollnick, Stephen, William R. Miller, and Christopher Butler. *Motivational Interviewing in Health Care: Helping Patients Change Behavior.* New York: Guilford Press, 2008.
28. Liddy, Clare, Sharon Johnston, Kate Nash, Natalie Ward, and Hannah Irving. "Health Coaching in Primary Care: A Feasibility Model for Diabetes Care." *BMC Family Practice* 15, no. 1 (2014): 1–8.
29. VanBuskirk, Katherine A., and Julie Loebach Wetherell. "Motivational Interviewing with Primary Care Populations: A Systematic Review and Meta-analysis." *Journal of Behavioral Medicine* 37, no. 4 (2014): 768–780.
30. Dayan, Paula Helena, Gary Sforzo, Nathalie Boisseau, Luciana Oquendo Pereira-Lancha, and Antonio Herbert Lancha Jr. "A New Clinical Perspective: Treating Obesity with Nutritional Coaching versus Energy-restricted Diets." *Nutrition* 60 (2019): 147–151.
31. Kivelä, Kirsi, Satu Elo, Helvi Kyngäs, and Maria Kääriäinen. "The Effects of Health Coaching on Adult Patients with Chronic Diseases: A Systematic Review." *Patient Education and Counseling* 97, no. 2 (2014): 147–157.
32. Sforzo, Gary A., Miranda P. Kaye, Irina Todorova, Sebastian Harenberg, Kyle Costello, Laura Cobus-Kuo, Aubrey Faber, Elizabeth Frates, and Margaret Moore. "Compendium of the Health and Wellness Coaching Literature." *American Journal of Lifestyle Medicine* 12, no. 6 (2017): 436–447.
33. Wolever, Ruth Q., and Mark H. Dreusicke. "Integrative Health Coaching: A Behavior Skills Approach that Improves HbA1c and Pharmacy Claims-Derived Medication Adherence." *BMJ Open Diabetes Research & Care* 4, e00201 (2016): 1–7.
34. Sforzo, Gary A., Miranda P. Kaye, Sebastian Harenberg, Kyle Costello, Laura Cobus-Kuo, Erica Rauff, Joel S. Edman, Elizabeth Frates, and Margaret Moore. "Compendium of Health and Wellness Coaching: 2019 Addendum." *American Journal of Lifestyle Medicine* 14, no. 2 (2019): 155–168.
35. Center for Self-determination Theory. "Health-Care Self-Determination Theory Questionnaire (HCSDTQ)." Self-Determination Theory. Accessed August 14, 2022. https://selfdeterminationtheory.org/health-care-self-determination-theory-questionnaire/.
36. Proot, Ireen M., Huda Huijer Abu-Saad, Wilma P. de Esch-Janssen, Harry FJM Crebolder, and Ruud HJ ter Meulen. "Patient Autonomy during Rehabilitation: The Experiences of Stroke Patients in Nursing Homes." *International Journal of Nursing Studies* 37, no. 3 (2000): 267–276.

6 Appreciative Inquiry

Simon Matthews, MHlthSc

6.1 INTRODUCTION

Appreciation is a wonderful thing: It makes what is excellent in others belong to us as well.

Attributed to Voltaire

6.1.1 WHAT COULD BE?

There are times in medical and health care where quick assessment and evaluation of a problem, and a rapidly implemented solution, literally save a life. The skill set of problem solving is vital to develop and must form part of the toolkit for medical and health professionals. But not all medical and health concerns are critical or immediately life threatening and yet we often carry the "problem-solving" mindset into every clinical encounter.

The problem-solving approach is a mainstay of health assessment and treatment (and most other disciplines) and has been explained and conceptualized in different ways.[1] Its associated paradigm – Root Cause Analysis[2] – leads the inquirer deep inside the complexities of a problem to be addressed. There are frequently six steps identified in classical problem solving,[3] which can be summarized in Figure 6.1.

6.2 APPRECIATIVE INQUIRY

But is there more to healthcare than solving health problems and health crises? By contrast, Appreciative Inquiry (AI)[4] is described as a collaborative quest for what

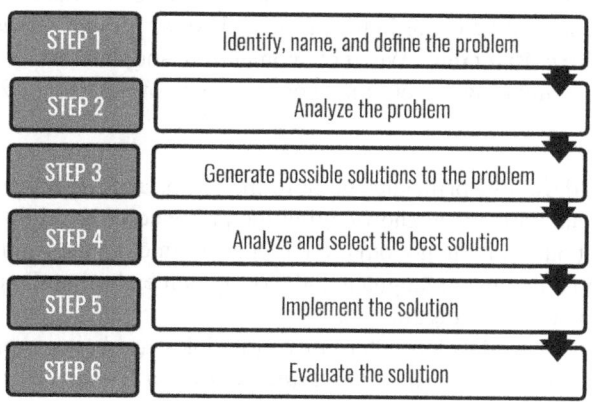

STEP 1	Identify, name, and define the problem
STEP 2	Analyze the problem
STEP 3	Generate possible solutions to the problem
STEP 4	Analyze and select the best solution
STEP 5	Implement the solution
STEP 6	Evaluate the solution

FIGURE 6.1 Steps to classical problem solving.

DOI: 10.1201/9781003161226-6

is best – in an individual and their environment – and the systematic uncovering of what leads to thriving. In this sense, it shares a great deal of commonality with the field of positive psychology, which seeks to understand the factors that lead to positive human functioning and flourishing.[5]

The AI approach invites the clinician to see the patient not as a person with a problem to be solved, or worse – as a problem to solve, but as a being with the capacity to imagine, act, and bring into reality a desired outcome in her life. In this way, it keeps us mindful that a person's health and well-being is an asset – a set of knowledge, skills, behaviors, and mindsets that enable the person to bring to life their own vision, purpose, dreams, and values.

Although AI, as a worldview and a set of skills, had its origin in the field of organizational development in the 1980s,[6] it has since been widely incorporated into the field of health care.[7-9] It has also been widely incorporated into the practice of health coaching.[10]

6.2.1 PRINCIPLES OF APPRECIATIVE INQUIRY

The principles guiding the practice of AI were not articulated until about 15 years after Cooperrider first began articulating the process of AI.[4] This was perhaps due to an absence of formal methodology early in the development of AI.[11]

The principles described by Cooperrider and Whitney[4] are as follows:

- **The Constructionist Principle**: Our subjective beliefs strongly influence what we do and the circumstances of our actions and choices. (*Words create worlds*)
- **The Simultaneity Principle**: The very act of making an inquiry serves as an intervention – it leads to the person reflecting, perhaps in ways they haven't before. (*Asking evokes Action*)
- **The Poetic Principle**: The language we use, the conversations we have, and the focus we choose to have all influence what and how we think – there are no neutral questions, comments, and reflections. (*Examine what's Excellent*)
- **The Anticipatory Principle**: The vision we have for ourselves and our future shapes our behavior in the present. (*Visions prompt Ventures*)
- **The Positive Principle**: We fuel momentum and interest in change by focusing on and drawing out the "positive core" of a person. (*Optimize the Outlook*)

Taken together, these five principles point to the importance of honoring the autonomy of clients and patients; acknowledging the presence of positivity in the person and seeking that out; looking not only to the present time but the future, to capture a compelling vision; and using language judiciously, remembering the power it has to shape belief and behavior (Figure 6.2).

As AI continues to develop, alternative principles are being proposed, including *wholeness, process of enactment, awareness, free choice, narrative,* and *synchronicity.*[12]

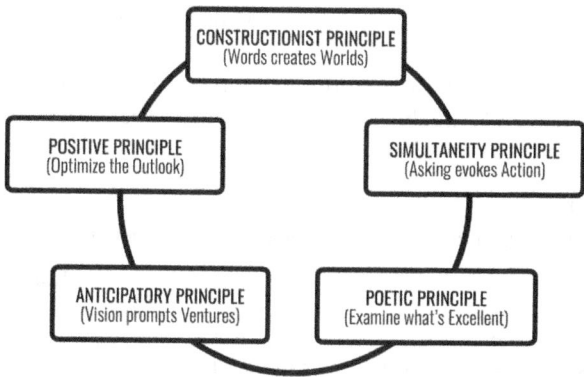

FIGURE 6.2 The Principles of Appreciative Inquiry. Adapted from Cooperrider and Whitney (2005).

6.2.2 THE PROCESS OF AI

The process is variously described either as the "4-D cycle"[4] or "5-D cycle." The 4-D cycle consists of four elements:

1. *Discover*
2. *Dream*
3. *Design*
4. *Destiny*

The earlier notion of an "affirmative topic" or "positive core" for discussion[6] was subsequently included in the process as the fifth "D" – *Define*, which established the 5-D cycle.[13] This cycle is explained in detail below. The 5-D cycle integrates the practice of honoring patient autonomy and is a desirable framework for health behavior change.

6.2.2.1 Define

The strongest principle of growth lies in the human choice.

(George Eliot, British author, 1819–1880)

In this first stage of the 5-D cycle, the clinician invites the patient to state the area of focus for behavioral change. In this way, the autonomy of the patient (addressed further in Chapter 5) is honored. Autonomy sits at the heart of Self-Determination Theory,[14,15] which seeks to explain what motivates individuals to action and is also central to the ethics of healthcare practice.[16]

The honoring of autonomy, by seeking to have the patient determine what should be the principal area of focus for health and well-being, is a powerful factor in behavioral change. In fact, a recent meta-analysis of factors specific to Self-Determination Theory showed that perceived autonomy support (the extent to which the treatment context is perceived by the patient as honoring their autonomy) produced the largest mean effect size for the examined studies ($g = 0.84$, 95%CI).[17] In health behavior change, autonomy is perhaps best captured by words attributed to Dr Peter Senge,

Senior Lecturer at the MIT Sloan School of Management – *"People don't resist change – they resist being changed."*

When autonomy is honored by inviting the patient to describe the area of focus that is most important and valuable to them at that time, the foundations are laid for compelling autonomous motivation.

6.2.2.2   Discover

Things don't turn up in this world until somebody turns them up.

James A Garfield
20th US President, 1831–1881

The primary task in this phase of the AI process is to uncover positive capacity or *"the best of what is"*.[18] It is an unabashed exploration of the positive. Research into human cognition has consistently pointed to what is known as the "negativity bias" or "negativity effect".[19] This is the notion that things of a perceived negative nature have a greater impact and influence on cognition and mental/emotional processes than equally intense things of a positive, or even neutral, nature. The negativity bias provides a good explanation for the observation that a neutrally expressed inquiry such as "How was your week?" is likely to evoke a "laundry list" response, frequently biased to the negative – *"Oh, it was okay I guess...busier than I would've liked and I felt like I didn't have much success improving my diet this week."* This bias is particularly the case in the realm of decision-making, where an individual is more likely to overvalue the perceived negative consequences of a decision than the perceived positive possibilities.[20] Thus a putative health behavior change may evoke fears about what will be lost rather than what will be gained. By contrast, the Discovery phase of AI is able to harness the "positivity offset"[21] in which neutrally weighted situations are more likely to be perceived as somewhat positive.

The Discovery phase of AI seeks to understand best experiences, best expressions of values, best use of strengths, best outcomes, proudest moments, and greatest achievements. Thus, an AI of this nature may be phrased: *"What was your best experience of managing your health this past week?"* or *"In what way did your determination to improve your health most show up this week?"*

6.2.2.3   Dream

What you can do, or dream you can, begin it. Boldness has genius, power, and magic in it.

Reflections of Irish poet John Anster, 1793–1825 on Faust – by German playwright Johann Wolfgang von Goethe, 1749–1832

The creation of a vision of a desired future (or a *dream*) fuels goal-directed behavior.[22,23] The converse is also true – that disappointment about dreams can lead to goal abandonment.[24] This is frequently the experience of patients who are engaging (yet again!) in an effort at behavioral change. They often describe a litany of past "failures" – attempts at dietary improvements, exercise and activity changes, and stress modulation strategies which have left them disappointed, dispirited, and with an internalized sense of low self-efficacy. Very often, these patients have created visions that weren't supported by well-crafted behavioral goals or sometimes they've stated impulsive goals for behavioral change not backed by a compelling vision or *"Why?"*

The Dream stage of the 5-D cycle represents an opportunity to support the patient to describe the future they wish for themselves – and to further cement the notion of working to the patient's agenda, not the treatment provider's agenda.

While working with a patient to articulate a vision or dream, it's vital that attention be paid to the creation of such a vision that is autonomously supported and represents the essence of what the individual really desires, not what they *think they should desire*. When people first consider behavioral change, it's often a result of prompting or urging by a significant other, or even by a physician or health care provider. This results in a reluctant and often guilt-laden approach to behavioral change.[25,26] Deeply rooted autonomous motivation remains at the heart of sustainable behavioral change.[27]

6.3   DESIGN

> You can't use up creativity. The more you use, the more you have.
>
> **Maya Angelou**
> *Author, poet, civil rights activist, 1928–2014*

This is the stage of the 5-D cycle of AI which most closely corresponds with the activity that many, or even most, clinicians immediately associate with behavioral change – goal setting; however, the entire AI cycle reminds us that goal setting is really a small component of long-term behavioral change and that many other elements, including a compelling vision and strong autonomous motivation must also be in place to support this process.

The Design process in AI is analogous to the process of planning a route between two cities on a world map, having first imagined traveling from one to another (the "Dream" process). In this example, it is immediately clear that there is no single way to do this, and not even a single "best" way. What is considered "best" will be informed by a number of factors relevant to the traveler including time available, level of comfort desired, the relative importance of the *experience* of traveling, the opportunity costs to be paid, and the perceived value of the journey. All of these factors differ from person to person, and a competent travel agent would not simply "prescribe" the same journey to different clients without first appreciating the clients' desires and needs.

Designing goals can be an intensively creative process, in which a patient who has been given permission to do so (from herself and the clinician) will often create ideas for goals and how to reach them that the health care provider alone would never have thought of. The Design phase leads to a "prototype" plan or an expression of "what should be." It is subject to modification and change, according to the outcomes of its implementation. Various factors, both internal to patients and external to their environment, may conspire to alter the imagined outcomes and necessitate a re-planning of goals.

6.4   DESTINY

> Que sera sera
>
> **Doris Day**
> *1922–2019*

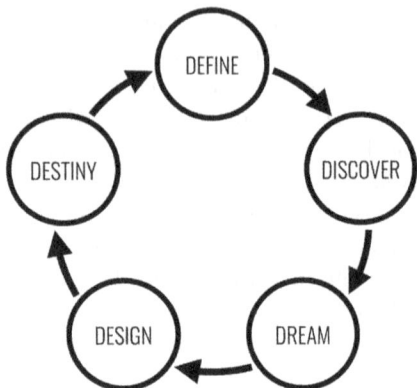

FIGURE 6.3   The 5D cycle of Appreciative Inquiry. Created from the work of Cooperrider and Whitney (2005).

You don't learn to walk by following rules; you learn by doing. And falling over. '

Sir Richard Branson
Business magnate, 1950–

The fifth stage of the AI process was originally named "Delivery." The authors reportedly thought that this notion did not sufficiently capture the liberation which may be experienced by the person who is in the process of experiencing long-desired behavioral change.[25] Some authors argue that the name "Destiny" suggests enabling a client to live his or her life fully and well[28]; however, the word also implies mindful acceptance of what is. In the Design phase a plan was developed and put into action. Now, what will be, will be. Perhaps the plan unfolded in the way the patient imagined and hoped. Perhaps it didn't. This is a stage of the AI process in which the health care provider supports the patient to accept what is; to continue to focus on the best experiences within that, even if they seem minor; to view errors or mistakes or failings as opportunities to learn more about oneself; to learn from what has emerged and continue to adapt this and other plans to work toward that long-desired vision.

During the "Destiny" phase, the health care provider works with the patient to recognize the elements of her vision which are beginning to emerge, even if the plan is not fully realized (*"in what ways have your efforts in the last week contributed to your overall vision?"*). The provider may also work with the client to manage the disappointment that almost always follows when a plan does not evolve and bear fruit as originally desired (*"What can you take from this experience to further boost your determination?"*). And importantly, when successes are experienced, they are celebrated (*"What makes you feel proud and capable? What would you most like to celebrate about yourself?"*) (Figure 6.3).

6.5   KEY PRACTICE POINTS

- The 5D cycle is intended as a recursive or iterative process, with each iteration building from the previous cycle. What is learned from one iteration can inform the focus for the following cycle. It is not a "one and done" approach to behavioral change.

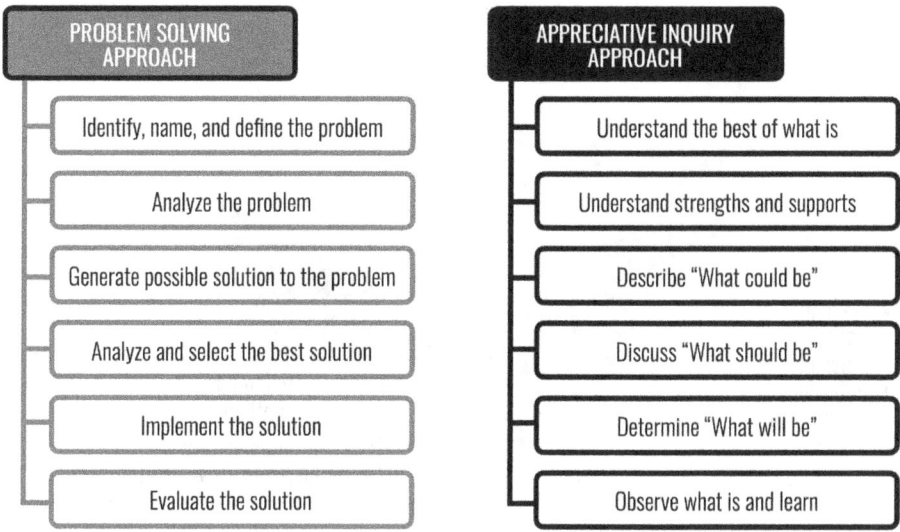

FIGURE 6.4   Problem-solving steps contrasted with Appreciative Inquiry steps.

- Powerful inquiries cannot be pre-determined precisely, any more than a builder can lay out tools at the beginning of a work day in the exact order in which he will use them. Each element of effective AI is built on the preceding response of the patient.
- The most powerful inquiries are not logistically focused – *"When will you begin this?"*, *"What will you do first?"*, *"Who will assist you?"*. Powerful inquiries are focused on values, strengths, purpose, and meaning – *"Which of your strengths will be most important here?"*, *"In what ways will this be an expression of your values?"*, *"What will be the significance of you accomplishing this?"*.

AI is not a replacement for all methods of engagement with patients. Problem-solving skills remain important. Problem-solving skills alone form only part of a useful tool-kit for supporting patients through the process of behavioral change. For comparison, the steps involved in a classical problem-solving approach are compared to the steps in the AI process below (Figure 6.4).

6.6   BRINGING AI TO LIFE

The basis of AI is, of course, inquiry. The skill of posing insightful and evocative inquiries is therefore key. Many clinicians have learnt about the difference between "open" and "closed" inquiry. This difference is frequently expressed in structural terms – an open inquiry is one that begins with "who, what, when, where or how" and a closed inquiry is one that evokes only a "yes or no" response. These inquiry types can also be understood more helpfully from a patient relationship perspective – a closed inquiry minimizes the data that a patient can provide in response and

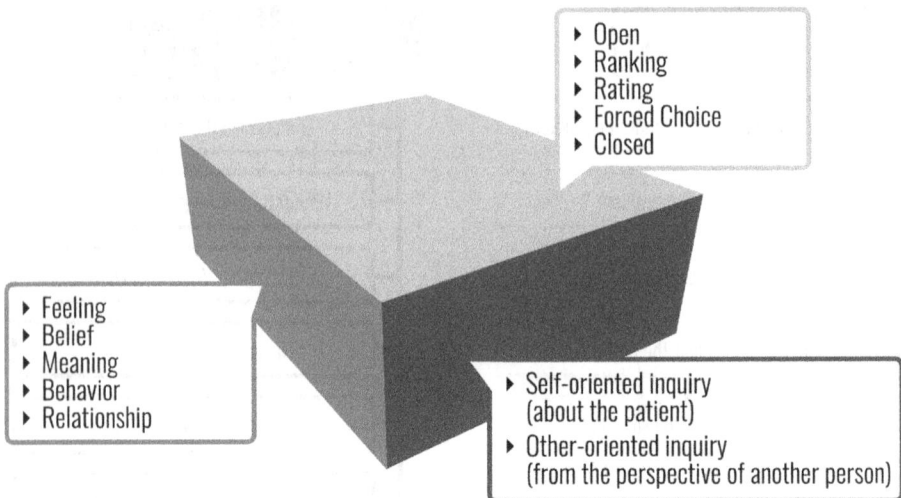

FIGURE 6.5   The Question Cube.[29]

an open inquiry maximizes that data flow. Clearly, to develop an understanding of anything, more open inquiry is desirable. One of the best methodologies for teaching inquiry is the "Question Cube".[29, 30] By understanding the elements of an inquiry, the process of forming useful and incisive open (and other) inquiries is made possible (see Figure 6.5).

As can be seen in Figure 6.5, any inquiry can be made by combining three elements – the type of inquiry (open, closed, forced choice, rating, and ranking), with a topic for discovery (feeling, belief, meaning, behavior, and relationship) and a focus (self, other).

Furthermore, the whole cube can be imagined to be sitting on rollers and able to move from the present, forward into the future and back into the past.

An example inquiry from the "Discovery" phase of AI, using the Question Cube approach might then be: ***What was a time (open) when your (self-oriented) values (topic) found their best expression in what you were doing? (appreciative focus).***

Although at first glance such an inquiry might seem to sit outside the domain of health care and well-being, we've already seen in Chapter 3 the roles that confidence and self-efficacy[31] play in generating and sustaining behavioral change. An inquiry such as this begins to invite the patient to access that part of their experience. A more comprehensive guide to examples of AI built on the Question Cube approach may be found in Table 6.1; however, the reader is reminded that genuine AI cannot be planned and fashioned outside of the context of the clinician/patient relationship. Powerful inquiries are built on genuine curiosity and deep listening, with the patient's response to an inquiry informing the next inquiry to be made.

Questioning alone does not adequately describe the skill set required to develop proficiency in the process of AI. Effective inquiry must also be supported by deep listening and a capacity for insightful and empathetic reflection. These are core skills of motivational interviewing[32] and addressed previously in Chapter 4 of this book.

TABLE 6.1
Examples of Appreciative Inquiry

Define   **What area of your health would you most like to focus on right now?**

What aspect of your well-being has your attention in this moment?

If something led to you experiencing a sense of achievement with your health a year from now, what would that be?

If you were advising your younger self, what would you suggest that you prioritize in your life?

Discover   Tell me about a time when your health and well-being were at their best for you

What's been your best experience of developing your own health and well-being?

What would your (husband/wife/partner/son/daughter) say is the best part of you being healthy and well? (note the "other" orientation)

Where in your body do you experience your best recollection of living life to the fullest?

Dream   What is the world calling you to be?

What's the inspiration for your health and well-being?

Imagine your best-self 1 year from now – what do you see?

If your strengths and values were on display for the world to see, what would that look like?

Design   What small gain in your health and well-being would lead you to feel like you were on the way to your vision?

Which past successes can you draw on to make a change to your health and well-being now?

What health behaviors would you be engaged in that would lead you to feel capable and proud?

Imagine that your dream (vision) for your health was true in this moment. What would you be doing?

Destiny   How would you most like to celebrate your achievements so far?

What has been your best learning about yourself so far?

What do you now feel strongly committed to as a result of what you've been doing?

Who would you most want to thank for the support they've provided you?

6.7   RESEARCH

Considerable use has been made of AI in the sphere of healthcare *system* analysis – using the approach to improve healthcare delivery and professional practice environments, for example Clossey et al. (2011) and Yoon et al. (2011).[33,34] A smaller body of work has focused on using AI as a tool to support individual patient health behavior change, although this work is growing. For example, McCarthy[35] provides a straightforward explanation for using AI to understand a patient's needs and avoid a behavioral management intervention. AI is typically deployed within the broader context of health coaching and this makes determining the specific outcomes attributable to AI more difficult. Nevertheless, some recent research, strongly featuring AI, is summarized below.

Scala and Costa[36] investigated the effectiveness of a coaching intervention, using AI, for chronic disease patients transitioning from hospital to home. While they encountered several challenges related to living conditions and readiness to change, the authors found AI to be an effective intervention for patients managing a transition to home, who are ready to make a behavioral change.

Purcell et al.[37] investigated the impact of the VA "Whole Health" program (which works with participants to develop personalized health plans based on values and needs) on health outcomes. Sixty-five veterans who participated in the program were interviewed prior to the start and following completion. In comparison with the intake survey, the completion surveys showed significant improvements and moderate effect sizes over baseline measures of mental health ($p = 0.006$; $d = 0.36$), stress ($p = 0.003$; $d = -0.38$), and perceived health competence ($p = 0.01$; $d = 0.35$). In addition, interviewees reported high levels of satisfaction with their coaching experience.

In a study conducted by Chen et al.,[38] 114 participants, with Type II Diabetes Mellitus and Hemoglobin A1c (HbA1c) levels of at least 7%, were assigned to a usual care (control) group or a coaching group (intervention). The aim of the study was to determine whether a coaching intervention, featuring AI, had a measurable impact on HbA1c levels. Overall, 67.2% of participants in the intervention group and 37.5% in the control group had a decrease in HbA1c levels within 6 months. Further, the coaching intervention was associated with a statistically significant decrease of 0.64% (CI = 0.45–0.83) in HbA1c level within 3 months ($p < 0.01$) and a decrease of 0.68% (CI = 0.40–0.96) within 6 months ($p < 0.01$).

While more research is indicated, two published compendia of health coaching outcomes[39,40] point reliably to the positive impact that a coaching intervention, often featuring the presence of AI, has on a number of chronic health conditions.

6.8 RECORDING PATIENT RESPONSES

A challenge in primary care settings is the expeditious and rapid recording of patient interactions. While it is not the intention of this chapter to provide guidance on when such recordings should be made, Table 6.2 provides a template for such notes, arising from an appreciative interaction with a patient. When used in conjunction with the style of inquiry featured in Table 6.1, the healthcare provider will be able to capture the essence and detail of what matters to the patient.

TABLE 6.2
Appreciative Inquiry Form

Patient Name   **Patient MRN**

Physician/AHP Name: **Date**:

Define (What does the patient want to focus on in this conversation? What area of their health currently has their strongest attention?)

Record patient responses to your inquiries here:

Discover (What is the patient's best experience of their health? Which of their values came to life at this time?)

Record patient responses to your inquiries here:

Dream (What does the patient's "best-self" look like with respect to their health? What would they love to be true about their health and well-being?)

Record patient responses to your inquiries here:

Design (Which health behaviors matter to the patient at this time? What small steps/achievable goals would they like to work on? What are they prepared to commit to?)

Record patient responses to your inquiries here:

Destiny (What was the patient's best experience of working on the goal? What challenges/obstacles did they overcome? What have they learnt along the way?)

Record patient responses to your inquiries here:

6.9   CASE STUDY

In the following case example, AI was used both to support the patient to engage in behavioral change and to review with her the changes she had made.

Ms P is a 53-year-old woman who has been managing Type II Diabetes since she was aged 25. In the ensuing years, her body weight increased from 130 to 230 lb. During this time, she also developed depression, as well as complications from diabetes, including peripheral neuropathy in her feet, and intense physical pain in her calves, ankles, and feet. She currently uses medication for diabetes, chronic pain, and depressed mood. She underwent a laparoscopic gastric band procedure at age 43. Her weight decreased initially from 230 to 160 lb, remaining stable there for 5–6 years, until steadily increasing again to 210 lb. She reported struggling with late-night snack foods and voluntarily staying awake through the night to complete hobby-related tasks. Ms P said that her treating physician and bariatric surgeon have both been urging her over a number of years to "quit the snacking" and do more exercise. She is married, with two adult children. She describes her husband as "alcoholic" and "depressed." She reports that she would not consider leaving their marriage and also reports that remaining in it exacts a high psychological toll on her. She also operated a successful consultancy for a number of years in her late 20s through early 40s. As her health declined, she was less able to work, and she is currently experiencing a great deal of financial strain. She presented for psychology and coaching support after deciding she was "sick of living like this," referring to her body weight, depressed mood, and apparent inability to effect any changes to her lifestyle.

Define – When asked, Ms P made clear that she wished to focus on being able to recapture the health she remembered having in her early 20s. She recalled being active and engaged in team sport and she spoke of the excitement she had for her life at that time. In particular, she said that she was tired of "chasing numbers" with respect to her body weight and wanted to focus on ways that she could reduce her use of medication.

Specific inquiries made during this stage included:

- *"What would you most like to focus on in our consultation today?"*
- *"What makes that important for you in this moment?"*
- *"How have you come to this point?"*

Discover – Ms P described her best experiences of her health as being part of her early adult life. In particular, she recalled being a teen and joining community running events, connecting with friends through team sport, discovering a love of food and cooking. She described the early days of her marriage and the weekend activities she and her husband would engage in such as bike riding and mountain hiking. This process evoked a spontaneous comment from her that she had forgotten how much she loved being outdoors (and how she had retreated further and further from that over recent years). This comment led to a discussion identifying these strengths and values that she saw emerging in herself at that time in addition to those that still had meaning and value for her and that she would like to recapture.

Specific inquiries made during this stage included:

- *"What is the best experience of your own health and wellbeing you recall?"*
- *"What emotions do you recall experiencing while you were engaged in those activities?"*
- *"What strengths and values came to life for you at that time?"*

[*Practice note – the point in an interaction where a client identifies something in their past that held value for them is often quickly followed by a problem-solving discussion on how that might be retrieved or re-discovered. In the practice of appreciative inquiry, it's important not to be diverted by this problem-solving or problem-focused approach. Rather – the focus remains on exploring the depth and complexity of those positive experiences for the person, so that they develop their own perspective on how they might wish to proceed.*]

Dream – Ms P described several "wished-for" elements of her health and well-being. Note that these are very different from short-term goals or strategies. She explained that she had always wanted to go on a walking holiday and imagined walking 10–15 miles per day for 2–3 weeks; however, the leg pain she experienced in addition to the discomfort of carrying excess body weight had always led her away from this dream. She said that she pictured herself spending 1 hour per day focused on maintaining her own physical fitness, adding that she had recently attended a spin class at the gym with her elder daughter and enjoyed this. She linked all of these behaviors to personal values of "living life to the full," "being the best I can with my family," and "living like my health is a resource to be looked after."

Specific inquiries made during this stage included:

- *"Picture yourself 5 years from now – what does your health and well-being look like?"*
- *"What else will your improved health allow you to do that aligns with your values?"*
- *"What will you be saying about your health behaviours in a year's time?"*

Design – As a result of reflecting on the best moments and experiences of her health and well-being (Discover), in addition to the "bold dreams" of how the future may look for her (Dream), Ms P was able to identify some specific activities she wished to engage in that would serve as short-term goals. She began by committing to continued participation in spin classes with her daughter, which she said gave her a physical fitness advantage and the opportunity to engage with her daughter in a shared interest. Ms P also set a goal of increasing her daily walking. She said she had withdrawn from this over the past few years due to leg pain and feared that she had become deconditioned. She therefore set a goal of walking for 20 minutes per day, in her neighborhood, for the next 2 weeks. Finally, Ms P said that on the advice of her endocrinologist, she had begun reducing the amount of added fat in her diet. She said she wanted to begin increasing the amount of fresh vegetables she consumed each day, as a means of feeling sated after eating, with a low caloric impact.

Specific inquiries made during this stage included:

- *"What would be a useful short-term goal for you to develop – something that you begin doing immediately and maintain for 1–2 weeks?"*
- *"Help me understand how you see this fitting with your vision of yourself 5 years from now"*
- *"What resources do you need to make this goal a reality for yourself?"*
- *"What obstacles do you see may inhibit you here? If you were to identify some strategies to manage those obstacles, what might that look like?"*

Destiny – In reviewing her first set of goals, (related to gym training, walking, and diet), Ms P reported that she had attended spin classes multiple times with her adult daughter and had not only noticed an increase in her aerobic capacity, but also a closer relationship with her daughter, which itself had encouraged her to remain committed to attendance at these classes. She also described having attempted to walk 20 minutes per day but had found she could only manage this on about 5 of 7 days due to the experience of pain in her legs. In exploring this outcome, Ms P said that she realized that "all or nothing is not the best approach" and had decided that having achieved her goal for 5 out of 7 days was still a satisfactory outcome for her. Even after only 10 days of goal-directed behavior, Ms P said that she felt like she had recaptured for herself a reason to want to keep developing and improving her health, which she had not expressly stated in earlier meetings. This was because she had regained a sense of control over her body, her decisions, and the direction in which she saw her life moving.

Specific inquiries made during this stage included:

- *"What has been your best experience of working on these goals?"*
- *"What strengths did you draw on to achieve what you did"*
- *"In what ways did you honor yourself and your values in what you did?"*
- *"What have you learned about yourself over these past 2 weeks that was not as clear to you before?"*

Over the course of 12 meetings, taking place across 7 months, Ms P reported the following outcomes:

- Adopting a whole food plant-based diet, exclusive of added fat
- An ongoing commitment to daily exercise, potentiated by the relational engagement with her daughter
- A reduction in the use of pain medication to nil
- A 75% reduction in the use of diabetes medication
- A reduction in the use of antidepressant medication to nil
- Increased stamina for physical exercise including the ability to walk for up to 2 hours daily
- Improvement in sleep and a consistent pattern of sleeping seven uninterrupted hours per night
- A decision to plan a walking vacation of 3 weeks, 6 months from the end of coaching consultations.

6.10 SUMMARY

The author Stephen Covey notes that "We must *look at the lens* through which we see the world... ...the *lens itself shapes* how we interpret the world" (italics added for emphasis). If we engage in problem-focused dialog, we will be inclined to interpret the elements of the story as "problem-laden." If we choose to engage in a solution-focused dialog, we will be more inclined to look at elements of the story as representing solutions (to problems). AI allows the health clinician to literally appreciate the patient's strengths, values, dreams, visions, and hopes and to explore with the patient all that sits within that. When used in an empathetically engaged manner, AI has the power to shape how our patients see their health and how we see our patients – as capable, competent, and hopeful people who want the best of health not for its own sake, but because of how it will lead them to thrive and flourish in life.

6.11 TAKEAWAYS

1. AI provides an effective interviewing framework to empower people to change.
2. The 5-D Cycle of AI includes Define, Discover, Dream, Design, and Destiny.
3. AI works to appreciate the positive and what is going well versus the general, standard interviewing process in healthcare during which the focus is often on what is not going well.
4. When working to appreciate the strengths, uniqueness, values, priorities, and hopes of an individual, the individual is better able to engage with their own potential and start harnessing to propel their own change process forward.
5. AI creates an opportunity for clinician and patient to explore how things can improve in an enjoyable, relaxed, growth-oriented, positive setting.

6.12 FURTHER READING AND RESOURCES

- The 5-D Cycle of AI: https://appreciativeinquiry.champlain.edu/learn/appreciative-inquiry-introduction/5-d-cycle-appreciative-inquiry/.
- Cooperrider, David L., and Diana Kaplin Whitney. 2005. *Appreciative Inquiry: A Positive Revolution in Change*. 1st ed. San Francisco, CA: Berrett-Koehler.
- Moore, Margaret, Jackson, Erika, and Tschannen-Moran, Bob. 2016. *Coaching Psychology Manual*. 2nd ed. Philadelphia, PA: Wolters-Kluwer.
- Orem, Sara L., Jacqueline Binkert, and Ann L. Clancy. *Appreciative Coaching: A Positive Process for Change*. John Wiley & Sons, 2007.

REFERENCES

1. Dunbar, Kevin. 1998. "Problem solving." *A Companion to Cognitive Science* 14:289–298.
2. Okes, Duke. 2019. *Root Cause Analysis: The Core of Problem Solving and Corrective Action*. Milwaukee WI: Quality Press.
3. De Mast, Jeroen. 2013. "Diagnostic quality problem solving: A conceptual framework and six strategies." *Quality Management Journal* 20 (4):21–36.

4. Cooperrider, David L, and Diana Kaplin Whitney. 2005. *Appreciative Inquiry: A Positive Revolution in Change*. 1st ed. San Francisco, CA: Berrett-Koehler.
5. Seligman, Martin EP, and Mihaly Csikszentmihalyi. 2014. "Positive psychology: An introduction." In M. Csikszentmihalyi (Ed.). *Flow and the Foundations of Positive Psychology*. New York: Springer, pp. 279–298.
6. Cooperrider, DL, and S Srivastva. 1987. Appreciative inquiry in organizational life In R. Woodman and W. Pasmore (Eds.). *Research in Organizational Change and Development*, Greenwich, CT: JAI Press, pp. 129–169.
7. Trajkovski, Suza, Virginia Schmied, Margaret Vickers, and Debra Jackson. 2013. "Using appreciative inquiry to transform health care." *Contemporary Nurse* 45 (1):95–100.
8. Moorer, Kerry, Schawan Kunupakaphun, Elilzabeth Delgado, Matthew Moody, Christina Wolf, Karen Moore, and Pracha Eamranond. 2017. "Using appreciative inquiry as a framework to enhance the patient experience." *Patient Experience Journal* 4 (3):128–135.
9. Moore, Shirley M, and Jacqueline Charvat. 2007. "Promoting health behavior change using appreciative inquiry: Moving from deficit models to affirmation models of care." *Family & Community Health* 30:S64–S74.
10. Moore, Margaret, Bob Tschannen-Moran, and Erika Jackson. 2016. *Coaching Psychology Manual*. 2nd ed. Wolters Kluwer Health/Lippincott, Williams & Wilkins, Philadelphia, PA.
11. Bushe, Gervase R. 2013. "Generative process, generative outcome: The transformational potential of appreciative inquiry." In D. Cooperrider, D. Zandee, L. Godwin, M. Avital, and B. Boland (Eds.). *Organizational Generativity: The Appreciative Inquiry Summit and a Scholarship of Transformation*. Bingley: Emerald Group Publishing Limited, pp. 89–113.
12. Whitney, Diana D, and Amanda Trosten-Bloom. 2010. *The Power of Appreciative Inquiry: A Practical Guide to Positive Change*. San Francisco, CA: Berrett-Koehler Publishers.
13. Magruder Watkins, Jane, Bernard J Mohr, and Ralph Kelly. 2011. *Appreciative Inquiry: Change at the Speed of Imagination*. San Francisco, CA: Wiley.
14. Deci, Edward L, and Richard M Ryan. 2010. "Self-determination." In E.W. Craighead and C. Nemeroff (Eds.). *The Corsini Encyclopedia of Psychology*. New Jersey: Wiley, pp. 1–2.
15. Ryan, Richard M, and Edward L Deci. 2000. "Self-determination theory and the facilitation of intrinsic motivation, social development, and well-being." *American Psychologist* 55 (1):68.
16. Beauchamp, Tom L, and James F Childress. 2001. *Principles of Biomedical Ethics*. New York: Oxford University Press.
17. Gillison, Fiona B, Peter Rouse, Martyn Standage, Simon J Sebire, and Richard M Ryan. 2019. "A meta-analysis of techniques to promote motivation for health behaviour change from a self-determination theory perspective." *Health Psychology Review* 13 (1):110–130.
18. Bushe, Gervase R. 1998. "Appreciative inquiry with teams." *Organization Development Journal* 16:41–50.
19. Jones, Edward E., David E. Kanouse, Harold H. Kelley, Richard E. Nisbett, Stuart Valins, and Bernard Weiner (Eds). 1972. *Attribution: Perceiving the Causes of Behavior*. Morristown, NJ: General Learning Press.
20. Kahneman, Daniel, and Amos Tversky. 1979. "Prospect theory: An analysis of decision under risk." *Econometrica* 47 (2):263. doi: 10.2307/1914185.
21. Norris, Catherine J, Jeff T. Larsen, L. Elizabeth Crawford, and John T. Cacioppo. 2011. "Better (or worse) for some than others: Individual differences in the positivity offset and negativity bias." *Journal of Research in Personality* 45 (1):100–111. doi: 10.1016/j.jrp.2010.12.001.
22. Locke, Edwin A, and Gary P Latham. 1990. *A Theory of Goal Setting & Task Performance*. New Jersey: Prentice-Hall, Inc.

23. Locke, Edwin A, and Gary P Latham. 2002. "Building a practically useful theory of goal setting and task motivation: A 35-year odyssey." *American Psychologist* 57 (9):705.

24. Bagozzi, Richard P, Hans Baumgartner, Rik Pieters, and Marcel Zeelenberg. 2000. "The role of emotions in goal-directed behavior." In S. Ratneshwar, D. Mick, and C. Huffman (Eds.). *The Why of Consumption: Contemporary Perspectives on Consumer Motives, Goals, and Desires*, New York: Routledge, pp. 36–58.

25. Cooperrider, David L, Diana Kaplin Whitney, and Jacqueline M Stavros. 2003. *Appreciative Inquiry Handbook: The First in a Series of AI Workbooks for Leaders of Change*, Vol. 1. San Francisco, CA: Berrett-Koehler Publishers.

26. Hurst, Megan, Helga Dittmar, Robin Banerjee, and Rod Bond. 2017. "'I just feel so guilty': The role of introjected regulation in linking appearance goals for exercise with women's body image." *Body Image* 20:120–129.

27. Deci, Edward L, and Richard M Ryan. 1985. Intrinsic Motivation and Self-Determination in Human Behavior. Berlin: Springer Science & Business Media.

28. Orem, Sara L, Jacqueline Binkert, and Ann L Clancy. 2007. *Appreciative Coaching: A Positive Process for Change*. San Francisco, CA: John Wiley & Sons.

29. Brown, Jacob Edward. 1997. "The question cube: A model for developing question repertoire in training couple and family therapists." *Journal of Marital and Family Therapy* 23 (1):27–40.

30. Matthews, SM. 2023. "The question cube re-imagined – A 5-dimensional model for cultivating coaches' capacity for curious inquiry in health behaviour change." *American Journal of Lifestyle Medicine*. doi:10.1177/15598276231172910

31. Bandura, Albert. 1986. *Social Foundations of Thought and Action*. Englewood Cliffs, NJ: Prentice-Hall, pp. 23–28.

32. Miller, William R, and Stephen Rollnick. 2012. *Motivational Interviewing: Helping People Change*. New York: Guilford Press.

33. Clossey, Laurene, Kevin Mehnert, and Sara Silva. 2011. "Using appreciative inquiry to facilitate implementation of the recovery model in mental health agencies." *Health & Social Work* 36 (4):259–266.

34. Yoon, Minn N, Mandy Lowe, Martha Budgell, and Catriona M Steele. 2011. "An exploratory investigation using appreciative inquiry to promote nursing oral care." *Geriatric Nursing* 32 (5):326–340.

35. McCarthy, Bernard. 2017. "Appreciative inquiry: An alternative to behaviour management." *Dementia* 16 (2):249–253.

36. Scala, Elizabeth, and Linda L Costa. 2014. "Using appreciative inquiry during care transitions: An exploratory study." *Journal of Nursing Care Quality* 29 (1):44–50.

37. Purcell, Natalie, Kara Zamora, Daniel Bertenthal, Linda Abadjian, Jennifer Tighe, and Karen H Seal. 2021. "How VA whole health coaching can impact veterans' health and quality of life: A Mixed-Methods Pilot Program Evaluation." *Global Advances in Health and Medicine* 10: 2164956121998283.

38. Chen, Ruey-Yu, Li-Chi Huang, Chien-Tien Su, Yao-Tsung Chang, Chia-Lin Chu, Chiao-Ling Chang, and Ching-Ling Lin. 2019. "Effectiveness of short-term health coaching on diabetes control and self-management efficacy: A quasi-experimental trial." *Frontiers in Public Health* 7:314.

39. Sforzo, Gary A, Miranda P Kaye, Irina Todorova, Sebastian Harenberg, Kyle Costello, Laura Cobus-Kuo, Aubrey Faber, Elizabeth Frates, and Margaret Moore. 2018. "Compendium of the health and wellness coaching literature." *American Journal of Lifestyle Medicine* 12 (6):436–447.

40. Sforzo, Gary A, Miranda P Kaye, Sebastian Harenberg, Kyle Costello, Laura Cobus-Kuo, Erica Rauff, Joel S Edman, Elizabeth Frates, and Margaret Moore. 2020. "Compendium of health and wellness coaching: 2019 addendum." *American Journal of Lifestyle Medicine* 14 (2):155–168.

7 Goal Setting and Planning

Marie Dacey, EdD

7.1 INTRODUCTION

Goals, goal setting, and *action planning* are behavior change techniques (BCTs). These three terms are used widely and sometimes interchangeably in various research and clinical settings. To offer consistency and clarity, we will use the following definitions in this chapter. *Goals* are mental representations of desired outcomes to which people are committed.[1] *Goal setting* is the BCT used to identify goals suitable for action planning.[2] *Action planning* identifies how one will specifically work to attain set goals.[3] Health behavior change coaching will optimally include collaboration and synergy between these three BCTs.

Goals encompass people's values, priorities, and hopes for the future. All goals represent some personal desired outcome. They are the principles, values, and desires behind any efforts to go forward. Goals lay the foundation for the health behavior change process, as they will inform the direction of general goal setting and then, more specifically, action planning. Goals may take many forms. Some key characteristics of goals are:

- Goals may be general and primarily address cognitive and emotional states (e.g., "I want to be healthier" or "I hope to have more energy"). Or they may be more specific (e.g., "I want to lose weight before my wedding in two months").
- Goals may be imposed by others, in that they are dictated by an authority figure and followed by the individual (e.g., "You need to stop smoking immediately"). Or they could be self-selected by the individual, alone or in collaboration with others. In these instances, the goals, goal setting, and action planning steps reflect a patient's preferences and independence throughout the process.
- Goals may be *approach*-oriented, focused on something positive to be gained (e.g., "I want to have a sense of calm more often"). Or, they may be *avoidance*-oriented, in that they target preventing or stopping something undesirable from occurring (e.g., "I want to argue less with my co-workers").

Goal setting is the process that helps to establish meaningful and suitable goals that have adequate motivation to invest thinking and behavior in order to achieve them (see Table 7.1 for the most recommended components and their level of research support). Goal setting is the most common behavior change technique among the 93 identified in the taxonomy of change strategies,[4] and it will optimally lay down the framework for developing and implementing an action plan.

Action planning[1] involves the detailed planning of specific behaviors to execute in order to accomplish set goals. Action planning sets the context, frequency, duration, and intensity of these behaviors.

DOI: 10.1201/9781003161226-7

TABLE 7.1
Research Support for Goal-Setting Components

Goal-Setting Component	Level of Support for Effectiveness
Meet individual's autonomy needs (i.e., choices should be based on one's own decisions and actions)	Good support[8]
Consider individual's values, needs, and preferences throughout goal-setting processes	Good support[2]
Tailor goal setting to individual's readiness to change	Good support[2]
Set goals that are challenging to the individual, yet attainable	Good support[7]
Establish sufficient commitment to a goal before proceeding to action planning (e.g., state strong intention along with personal importance of a goal)	Mixed support; value of commitment strongest with more difficult goals[7]
Set goals publicly (e.g., tell a friend or family member one's intention to establish and meet a goal)	Good support[7]
Establish goals that are not too complex, i.e., a low number of decisions and acts are required to accomplish a goal	Mixed support; complex goals can be suitable for certain individuals and/or circumstances[7]
Use other BCTs along with goal setting	Mixed support; highly dependent on the individual, which techniques, and type of goal[7]
Focus on outcome (results) or behavior (to-do) goals	Outcome and behavior goals are equally supported; one type of goal does not appear to be better than the other[7]
Work collaboratively with the patient to set goals in a clinical setting	Good support[2,9]
Set approach-oriented goals, and frame messaging to focus on gains	Good support, particularly for prevention behaviors. Both gain- and loss-framed messages are supported for detection behaviors[10]
Incorporate coping planning, i.e., formulate plans to overcome potential barriers to accomplishing goals	Good support[2,11,12]
Collaboratively reflect on patients' goals and progress in order to support ongoing self-regulation and persistence	Good support[13,14]

- *Context* is the situation in which someone will work toward a goal. Context may be physical (e.g., while exercising), social (e.g., when with other people), emotional (e.g., while feeling stressed), or cognitive (e.g., when automatic, negative thoughts intrude).
- *Frequency* establishes how often one will do the intended behavior (e.g., once weekly or twice daily).
- *Duration* sets the intention for how long a person will do the behavior (e.g., walk for 30 minutes, or meditate for 2 minutes).
- *Intensity* determines how much work or energy will be involved in doing the behavior (e.g., breathing heavily but still able to talk while running).

In this chapter, we will review the research evidence of the most recommended components of goal setting and action planning. Based on this review, we will offer practical suggestions for understanding goals, setting suitable and realistic goals, and establishing action plans most likely to be successful. A theoretical case study provides an application example in a health-coaching context.

7.2 EVIDENCE SUMMARY

An initial theory and the components of successful goal setting were originally proposed by Locke et al.[5] They described five elements of successful goal setting:

- *Clarity*: Set goals that are clear and precise
- *Challenge*: Optimal goals will not be too easy or too hard to achieve
- *Commitment*: Motivating goals will be consistent with personal aspirations
- *Feedback*: Set goals that can be monitored and adjusted if necessary
- *Complexity*: Break down overwhelming goals into smaller manageable units.

Locke and Latham's original work has led to considerable research on goal setting's role in health behavior change. Notable recent reviews include a systematic meta-review of meta-analyses conducted in the last 15 years,[6] which provides a synthesis of the evidence for multiple BCTs, including goal setting. Epton et al. (2017) conducted a robust systematic review and meta-analysis specific to goal setting's effectiveness.[7] These reports both note the range of study populations, settings, sample size, and quality of studies. They also state that goal setting is a complex process that inherently presents methodology challenges. It is difficult to isolate goal setting as an independent factor in the health behavior change process, and goal setting itself is comprised of many elements. Yet, some components of goal setting have been demonstrated to be more useful than others, particularly in certain circumstances. Table 7.1 outlines the most recommended components of goal setting, and the evidence for their effectiveness in accomplishing health behavior change goals.

7.3 PRACTICAL APPLICATION

The following tips are based on the evidence support cited above as well as previous reports of best practices. Providers should incorporate these application tips in a very patient-specific manner. Providers may also benefit from supplementing the information here with other recommendations offered in this book, as patients vary greatly in stage of change (Chapter 2), level of self-efficacy (Chapter 3), self-determination (Chapter 5), and perceived benefits and barriers to change (Chapter 9). Further, social and environmental circumstances, communication styles and skills, and life span developmental stage will all inform the goal setting/action planning segment of health behavior coaching. One size does not fit all. Thus, providers should flexibly incorporate these suggestions, in collaboration with each patient.

Faries (2016) proposed that goals and goal setting can be conceptualized as a hierarchical structure of gears that aid in the self-regulation of health behavior (Figure 7.1).[15] This structure encompasses Be, Do, and Act (or Action) Goals, and it offers a practical understanding to providers. This structure also syncs well with the terminology used in this chapter:

1. *BE Goals*: Who/what do you want to be? *(Goals)*
2. *DO Goals*: What do you think you could do to get there? *(Goal Setting)*
3. *ACT Goals*: Shall we set some specific behaviors to help get this done? *(Action Planning)*

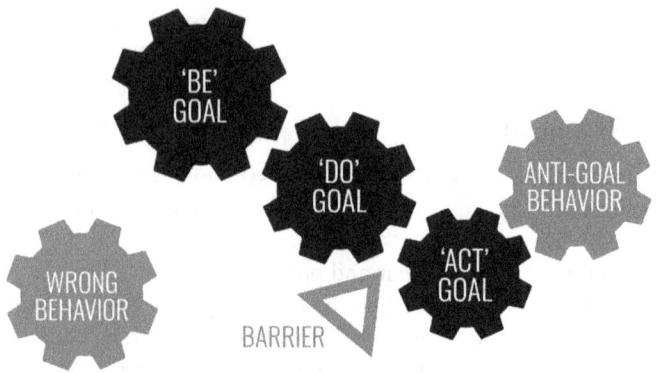

FIGURE 7.1 Hierarchical structure of goals (i.e., "Be" goals, "Do" goals, and "Act" or "Action" goals), depicted as gears. (Modified from Faries, 2016.[15])

7.3.1 PRACTICE TIPS: BE GOALS, AKA "GOALS"

- **Help patients establish reasons to change their behavior.** Explore with patients what matters most to them. Ask them about their values, desires for the future, and what their 'best self' is. Help patients acknowledge the discrepancy between their vision of a healthy life and their current life and lifestyle, using motivational interviewing (MI) tools as described in Chapter 4.
- **Acknowledge what is most relevant in the context of lifespan development.** Patients' age, social determinants, overall health, and function all need to be considered at the onset of establishing goals. For example, weight loss goals will present differently for a healthy overweight 10-year-old compared to a 65-year-old with multiple chronic conditions. It is important to note the context and adapt the coaching session, as warranted.
- **Cultivate a mindset of personal ownership in patients.** Goals belong to patients, not the provider. Allow time for self-disclosure and discovery. This allows patients' basic need for autonomy, as discussed in Chapter 5, to be met.
- **Encourage self-reflection and future-self visualization.** Reflection has been shown to be associated with an increased ability to focus, self-regulate one's actions, and be persistent.[13] Reflection also encourages realism in goal setting. Provider prompts might be to ask a patient to quietly consider what they would like from life, or what being satisfied would look like. Another possibility is to ask a patient if they might want to imagine and describe themselves living a life in the future that felt healthy and meaningful to them.
- **Use motivational interviewing (MI) skills**. Chapter 4 provides a thorough explanation of MI. Open-ended questions, Affirmations, Reflections, and Summary (OARS) are especially relevant during this initial stage of a Goals coaching session.
- **Be aware of contradictory anti-goals:** It is common for people to have goals that contradict their stated goal intentions. Patients may claim that they desire one thing, when they consciously or unconsciously regard other pursuits as equally important or more gratifying.[1] For example, a patient might say that it is important to feel physically strong. Thus, this is what

they would like to address in the goal-setting session. However, they also say they want to feel less tired. It is likely that the second goal (less fatigue) will take precedence over working toward the first (more strength), as simply resting has the potential to be immediately rewarded. Only if the provider takes the time to be aware of these seemingly contradictory goals, can they effectively address these throughout the coaching session.

- **Do not skip this first step!** Since goals, and people, are complex, providers should spend ample time with each patient to understand and establish individualized and valued 'Be' goals. Such goals will most likely result in success.

7.3.2 PRACTICE TIPS: DO GOALS, AKA "GOAL SETTING"

- **Guide patients in setting general goal(s), which could help achieve patients' BE goals.** Some examples of these general goal behaviors might be to improve nutrition, exercise more, stop smoking, sleep better, or practice stress management.
- **Explore patients' readiness to change.** As discussed in Chapter 2, understanding the five stages of change according to the transtheoretical model and where a client is on this continuum is key to relationship building, goal setting, and ultimate success.
- **Use a decisional balance matrix.** As discussed in Chapters 2 and 4, this activity helps patients clarify their perceived pros and cons of working on their general goals. This also serves to help verbalize contradictory anti-goals. This activity simply entails asking the patient what some advantages (pros) and disadvantages (cons) are of pursuing a particular goal. In response, a patient might state, for example, that they would like to eat a plant-based diet to order to improve their self-image (pro), but they believe it will take too much effort and time to alter their own and their family's cooking patterns (con). The 'con' also shows the anti-goal, i.e., to keep things simple and stay with the family's typical habits. As the perceived costs/cons of adopting new health behaviors are extremely powerful barriers to successful change, it is worthwhile to assess decisional balance during both the goal-setting and action planning stages of coaching.
- **Share with patients that goal setting is an intermediary step in the planning process.** It is important to continue to collaborate with patients on action planning after discussing and setting goals. Thus, patients should be aware that once they establish a goal, they still need to consider the specific steps necessary to accomplish the goal.

7.3.3 PRACTICE TIPS: ACT GOALS, AKA "ACTION PLANNING"

- Providers and patients should collaboratively set ACT Goals that are **SMART:**
  - *S – Specific*: Action items are specific and detailed. They leave little room for variable interpretation. Thus, rather than "Eat more fruits and vegetables," a specific ACT goal is "Eat five half-cup servings of fruit and/or vegetables each day this coming week."
  - *M – Measurable*: Action items are measurable and easily quantifiable behaviors. Thus, in the example above, the non-specific goal that states eat

"more" is not really measurable, as "more" is typically subject to interpretation. However, a goal of eating "five half-cup servings" daily is measurable.

- *A – Action-Oriented*: Action items are action-oriented, in that they involve performing a selected behavior. The behavior might or might not be directly obvious of observable. For example, if one sets a goal to run every day at 11 am, this action is observable. However, one might also set goals to meditate daily at 11 am or to note the number of automatic negative thoughts which occurred from 10 to 11 am. Such goals are still action-oriented, but the selected behavior (in these cases, meditation or mindfulness) is not observable.

- *R – Realistic*: Action items have a realistic level of difficulty, which is not boring but also not overwhelming. They can also readily fit into an individual's current life patterns. Providers need to be cautious of patients' tendencies to be unrealistically optimistic about what they can accomplish. Thus, a working parent might want to set an ACT goal to go the gym every day after work, but this is unrealistic as they need to pick up their child 2 days a week from childcare; so, a realistic action item may be to go to the gym three times weekly.

- *T – Time-sensitive*: Goals that are time-sensitive include a time period to commit to the ACT goal (e.g., a week or month). At the end of the period, one agrees to review progress and re-establish goals, which continue to be SMART. It is important to follow up at the end of the commitment time.

- **Establish ACT goals that are approach-focused rather than avoidance-focused.** As noted in Gallagher and Updegraff's robust review (2012), several studies have found that focusing on what one gains from doing a health behavior is often more effective than stating the negative consequences of not doing it.[10] Gain-framed messaging appears to be especially effective for prevention behaviors, such as when attempting to promote smoking cessation, skin cancer prevention, and physical activity. For detection behaviors, e.g., screenings, annual checkups, both gain- and loss-framed messages can be effective. For example, a provider would optimally ask a patient what they think they will gain from starting to walk for 30 minutes every day. The provider could also ask a patient what they are hoping to gain, or avoid, by getting an annual mammography.

- **Assess and support self-efficacy.** As discussed in Chapter 3, confidence in one's ability to accomplish a goal when faced with situational temptations is necessary to maintain motivation and achieve success. Self-efficacy assessment is especially important when establishing the specifics of action planning. Providers might use an MI tool, such as scaling, to assess and support self-efficacy. An example might be, "On a scale of 1–10, how confident are you that you will be able to eat 5 fruits and vegetables daily?" The response, e.g., "4," will demonstrate the level of self-efficacy. The provider can follow up with a question that will prompt a positive association and support increased self-efficacy, such as "What made you say 4 rather than 2 on the scale?"

- **Help patients become aware of and devise strategies to address conflicting, or anti-goals.** As stated above, dissonance is extremely common, and it is important to be aware of unstated contradictory goals and their potential to be strong deterrents to accomplishing stated goals. At any time during action planning, a provider may ask questions to illuminate anti-goals and then help the patient plan for how to cope when these goals present themselves. For example, a patient may want to commit to eating three healthy meals daily at consistent times. The provider could ask what other things the patient might want to do at mealtimes. When the patient responds, e.g., "keep working," or "watch TV," the provider could ask the patient how they could plan for these events. A patient might state, e.g., "I could make the meal ahead of time."

- **Establish implementation intentions, aka coping plans.** Similar to addressing anti-goals, providers should assist patients in establishing coping plans for other types of foreseeable barriers, e.g., a sick child, inclement weather, or increasing workload. It is useful for providers to recognize when patients present as strategic optimists or, in contrast, have unrealistic optimism when collaborating on coping plans.

  - Implementation intentions are most likely to be successful with strategic optimists.[11] Strategic optimists tend to have low levels of anxiety. They can acknowledge that challenges present possibility rather than automatic failure. And they can establish high expectations with simple planning for setbacks. They can note potential barriers when setting up an action plan and then independently devise plans to deal with the barriers when they occur. If a patient appears to have the overall qualities of a strategic optimist, it is recommended to support their view of challenges as opportunities to demonstrate one's self-identified strengths, e.g., persistence, personal organization, and commitment to what one values.
  - In contrast to strategic optimists, a more common presentation is unrealistic optimism. It is common for patients to think that they can set and accomplish difficult goals even with extraordinary barriers and minimal preparation to address these. This leads to setting goals that are not reached. MI (Chapter 4), which incorporates open-ended questions rather than confrontation, can be used to help patients understand discrepancies between stated goals and unrealistic action plans.

- **Include defensive pessimism strategies in patients with negative predictions for success.** Pessimism is another trait that hinders successful goal setting and outcomes. Individuals who are pessimists tend to focus solely on barriers and have low self-efficacy to overcome them. They doubt their ability to meet a goal. If a goal is important to one's health (e.g., cardiac rehab after a heart attack), anxiety is commonly present as well. Defensive pessimism strategies[12] can be useful in addressing patients' strong original negative predictions. Providers should prompt the pessimist to reflect on what it will feel like, in the future, if they are successful as well as if one fails. The patient is then typically able to more fully appreciate the positive aspects of successful change as well as proactively address the issues that may arise with failure. When pessimism is present, it is appropriate to encourage setting relatively easy goals and action plans, so success is highly probable.

- **Include process management.** Action planning is fluid and ongoing. After an initial plan is set in motion, process management involves monitoring the plan on a consistent basis, and flexibly changing it to maintain motivation (Chapter 8). A self-monitoring system that the client sets up, including phone apps can work well. Also, a provider or their clinical practice can monitor and provide feedback on progress. Overall, providers should encourage and support cognitive flexibility and adaptation so that the action plan can evolve as warranted. Positive reframing of setbacks will be important for all patients once action plans are set in motion. Optimally, self-efficacy remains high, and patients stay invested in the importance of their health behavior change goals.

7.4   THEORETICAL CASE STUDY

Martha, age 75, is meeting Dr. Yin for her annual physical exam. Martha is 5′6″ tall, weighs 180 lbs., has a BP of 158/92, and has a slight limp as she bruised her hip when she tripped two days ago in her new apartment at her senior retirement community. Martha's medical history is negative, except for hypertension, osteoporosis, and gastroesophageal reflux disease. Past surgeries include ureteroscopy for kidney stones, and knee replacement for osteoarthritis. She takes daily medication for hypertension, osteoporosis, and acid reflux. She has no history of any mental illnesses, and she has never considered herself particularly anxious or depressed. Her sleep is lighter than it was when she was younger, but she often takes an afternoon nap and then feels refreshed.

Martha is a retired elementary school teacher, who has lived alone since her husband passed away 6 years ago. She drives to see her nearby son and family 2–3 times weekly, where she visits and helps with chores as she is able. Other than these visits, she is sedentary. She eats most of her meals at the community dining room and admittedly enjoys the lavish desserts offered there.

Dr. Yin informs Martha that her BMI of 29 places her almost in the 'obese' range, and that her blood pressure has significantly risen in the last year. To assess Martha's overall readiness to adopt lifestyle changes, Dr. Yin asks Martha if she would like to discuss her health habits, in order to help address increasing risks from hypertension, weight gain, and falls. Martha says she would be willing to talk about her lifestyle, and Dr. Yin is encouraged that Martha is at least in the Contemplation stage of change.

Dr. Yin decides to help Martha clarify her "BE" goals, by asking her what is most important to her in her life. Martha states that her relationships with her family, and especially her son and grandchildren are most important to her. She wants to spend as much time as possible helping her son and daughter-in-law raise their children, and to be able to be a loving mentor to her grandchildren as they grow up. Dr. Yin sincerely affirms what Martha shares, by stating that he appreciates she is willing to talk about her lifestyle, and that the importance she places on her family relationships is admirable. He supports potential optimism and her self-efficacy, by stating that he will work with her to come up with some goals that she feels comfortable pursuing. Martha says she is willing to do this if it means she can continue to take care of herself for a long time and not be a burden to her family.

The coaching session continues toward the establishment of "DO" goals. Dr. Yin says it would be useful for Martha to talk more about what she wants to be able to do, before getting down to specifics. He asks Martha to describe some things that represent taking care of herself and not being a burden to her family. Martha says she wants to be adequately agile and alert so she can drive the grandchildren safely to school and sports, and she wants to have enough energy to "cook and clean some and keep up with the two youngest boys – they're only 5 and 7 now, and quite a handful!" Dr. Yin reflectively listens and summarizes that she would like to find a way to feel strong, agile, alert, and have more energy. Martha says he is correct.

Dr. Yin asks Martha what things come to mind as possible ways to feel more strong, agile, alert, and have more energy. She says she should probably exercise, and that there are classes offered at the retirement community's fitness center, and when she thinks about better health habits, exercise would be best for her. However, she really does not like to exercise. Dr. Yin affirms her belief that exercise would be good for her by sharing that physical activity, even moderately a few times a week, has been shown to have considerable health benefits. He also acknowledges that she does not like to exercise.

Dr. Yin stayed with setting a goal to exercise, since it was Martha's initial idea. He asks her if there was ever a time in her past when she did enjoy physical activity. She says when she was much younger, she liked to go to Zumba classes with her teacher friends after work. When Dr. Yin asked her what she liked about this, she said she liked the lively music, and laughing with friends. "Nobody took it too seriously – we just acted silly and enjoyed the music – it didn't feel like real exercise." Dr. Yin affirms what Martha shared, and then asks her if she would be interested in finding out if there were opportunities now to join classes that did not feel like serious exercise and had music and a fun group ambiance.

Martha says she would like to find an easy-going, fun class at the center, but she was skeptical that any were offered, and she feels self-conscious about her weight and potential clumsiness. Rather than immediately focus on her pessimistic concerns, Dr. Yin compliments Martha on being willing to explore if there is a class compatible with her preferences. He tells her it is great that she is open to some new ways to have fun and stay healthy. Martha says she will not commit to anything yet, but she could maybe at least check out the fitness center and find out more about their offerings. Dr. Yin says that sounds like a great idea, and suggests they talk a bit about how she will do this.

Dr. Yin and Martha continue to collaborate on a SMART ACT goal, i.e., a suitable action plan. Martha states she will go to the fitness center and speak to the fitness director about her desire to attend only classes that have music and have an easy-going, fun vibe (Specific). She will note when she completes this by telling a friend (Measurable). She needs to have a conversation (Action-oriented), which is easy to do (Realistic), and she will do this on Monday afternoon (Time-sensitive).

As Dr. Yin knows that there are obstacles that arise when patients make ACT goals, and Martha has already expressed some skepticism and self-consciousness, he asks Martha what may get in the way of her having this conversation with the fitness director. She says she feels awkward around fitness facilities, and she may feel too embarrassed on Monday to approach the fitness director. Dr. Yin again acknowledges he has heard and understands her, and he asks her what could make the conversation more comfortable for her. She said maybe she could talk to the fitness director at a place other than the fitness center, and maybe she could do it with a friend. Dr. Yin compliments her on these great ideas, and she says she feels confident that she and a friend can talk to the director together in the dining room. Dr. Yin reinforces that this is an excellent action plan. He also gave her some patient handouts with information on older adults and physical activity, which she can pursue if she wants. They set up a short virtual follow-up meeting for next week, and they conclude their meeting for today.

Note: This theoretical case study included setting a goal to exercise, yet the action plan is simply to explore fitness class options. It is a simple, single-step action plan that aligns with Martha's needs and stage of readiness. Dr. Yin always considered the importance of maintaining high self-efficacy and respecting Martha's autonomy. He recognized that goal setting is a complex process, and that Martha was not ready to commit to regular exercise. By conducting this short initial coaching session, he still utilized many of the evidence-based recommendations discussed in this chapter, which will help Martha become more positive about exercise. With small steps, Martha is likely to adopt and maintain a healthier lifestyle.

7.5   MEASUREMENT STRATEGIES

7.5.1   TRANSTHEORETICAL MODEL STAGE OF READINESS

Understanding a patient's readiness to change is key to goal setting and all other aspects of the behavior change process. There are several options offered by Drs. Prochaska in Chapter 2 for assessing the stage of change.

7.5.2   SELF-EFFICACY ASSESSMENT

To assess self-efficacy, practitioners can use the MI scaling question discussed earlier in this chapter. Additional useful information on the transtheoretical model, its assessment measures, and a goal-setting worksheet are available through the Preventive Cardiovascular Nurses Association https://pcna.net/wp-content/uploads/2018/12/16_ models_of_behavior.pdf

Finally, please see Chapter 3 of this book for more self-efficacy measurement strategies.

7.6   SUMMARY

Goal setting is an important part of the change process. There are BE Goals which include stating who or what you want to BE, and there are DO Goals which include the actions you do to get to who or what you want to BE. Then, there are ACT Goals or action planning. These are the SMART goals. Creating goals is an enjoyable process that a practitioner and patient can complete together as a team. The goal-setting process is ongoing. There are new stages of life and new obstacles that arise that require new goal setting for BE, DO, and ACT goals.

7.7   KEY TAKEAWAYS

- Goals, goal setting, and action planning are complex. It is important to allot adequate time to this component of health behavior coaching.
- Goal setting and action planning optimally is a collaboration between provider and patient.
- SMART ACT goals are determined in concert with 'BE' and 'DO' goals, so what is valued and important to patients is always acknowledged.

- Goal setting and action planning are matched with personal stage of readiness to change, decisional balance, and level of self-efficacy, so realistic goals are set and motivation remains high.
- Barriers to success, including conflicting anti-goals that are not always obvious or stated, may sabotage motivation in achieving stated goals. Coping planning, which involves implementation intentions is essential.
- Goal setting and action planning are not a one-and-done process. It is not linear, not a checklist. Rather it is fluid, sometimes circuitous and involves ongoing attention, feedback, and probably modification.

7.8 RESOURCES

7.8.1 Patient Resources

- The USDHHS Office for Disease Prevention and Health Promotion's 'Move Your Way' is an online resource to encourage physical activity, which includes interactive tools for goal setting and action planning: https://health.gov/moveyourway
- Several government agencies, e.g., CDC and NIH, offer free-of-charge videos, infographics, podcasts, and publications, which practitioners could use in their clinical settings or share with patients. These often provide general education regarding chronic disease and motivational messaging, which may be particularly useful for patients in the early stages of readiness to change. Some materials are available in Spanish. Resources are available at: https://www.cdc.gov/chronicdisease/resources/multimedia.htm or https://order.nia.nih.gov/
- This article from the Harvard Men's Health Watch offers a quick overview of SMART action planning and other key points from this chapter: https://www.health.harvard.edu/mens-health/an-easier-way-to-set-and-achieve-health-goals

7.8.2 Goal-Setting Apps

More than half of all mobile apps for behavior change incorporate goal setting.[16,17] Also, multiple goal-tracking apps to use once goals are set are readily available. However, most studies have found that using mobile apps does not provide significant behavioral change advantages over not using apps. Yet, participant feedback is generally positive,[16] in that people who choose to use them often state that they like them. Thus, apps may be desirable and ultimately useful for some patients. As the development and marketing of apps are in constant evolution, and highly personal in preference, it is recommended that providers and patients collaboratively explore available options when patients state they would like to use goal-setting or goal-tracking apps.

REFERENCES

1. Mann, Traci and de Ridder, Denise. 2013. "Self-Regulation of Health Behavior: Social Psychological Approaches to Goal Setting and Goal Striving. - PsycNET." *Health Psychology* 32 (5): 487–498. https://doi.org/10.1037/a0028533.
2. Lenzen, Stephanie Anna, Ramon Daniëls, Marloes Amantia van Bokhoven, Trudy van der Weijden, and Anna Beurskens. 2017. "Disentangling Self-Management Goal Setting and Action Planning: A Scoping Review." *PLoS One* 12 (11): e0188822. https://doi.org/10.1371/journal.pone.0188822.

3. Bailey, Ryan R. 2019. "Goal Setting and Action Planning for Health Behavior Change." *American Journal of Lifestyle Medicine* 13 (6): 615–618. https://doi.org/10.1177/1559827617729634.

4. Michie, Susan, Michelle Richardson, Marie Johnston, Charles Abraham, Jill Francis, Wendy Hardeman, Martin P. Eccles, James Cane, and Caroline E. Wood. 2013. "The Behavior Change Technique Taxonomy (v1) of 93 Hierarchically Clustered Techniques: Building an International Consensus for the Reporting of Behavior Change Interventions." *Annals of Behavioral Medicine: A Publication of the Society of Behavioral Medicine* 46 (1): 81–95. https://doi.org/10.1007/s12160-013-9486-6.

5. Locke, Edwin A., Gary P. Latham, Ken J. Smith, Robert E. Wood, and Albert Bandura. 1990. *A Theory of Goal Setting & Task Performance.* Englewood Cliffs, NJ: Pearson College Div.

6. Spring, Bonnie, Champion, Katrina, Acabchuk, Rebecca, and Hennessy, Emilie. 2021.021. "Self-Regulatory Behaviour Change Techniques in Interventions to Promote Healthy Eating, Physical Activity, or Weight Loss: A Meta-Review." *Health Psychology Review* 15 (4): 508–539. https://doi.org/10.1080/17437199.2020.1721310.

7. Epton, Tracy, Sinead Currie, and Christopher J. Armitage. 2017. "Unique Effects of Setting Goals on Behavior Change: Systematic Review and Meta-Analysis." *Journal of Consulting and Clinical Psychology* 85 (12): 1182–1198. https://doi.org/10.1037/ccp0000260.

8. Ryan, Richard, and Deci, Edward. 2000. "Self-Determination Theory and the Facilitation of Intrinsic Motivation, Social Development, and Well-Being." *American Psychologist* 55 (1): 68–78. https://doi.org/10.1037/0003-066X.55.1.68.

9. Grant, A. 2012. "An Integrated Model of Goal-Focused Coaching: An Evidence-Based Framework for Teaching and Practice." *International Coaching Psychology Review* 7 (2): 146–165.

10. Gallagher, Kristel M., and John A. Updegraff. 2012. "Health Message Framing Effects on Attitudes, Intentions, and Behavior: A Meta-Analytic Review." *Annals of Behavioral Medicine* 43 (1): 101–116. https://doi.org/10.1007/s12160-011-9308-7.

11. Spencer, Stacie M., and Julie K. Norem. 1996. "Reflection and Distraction Defensive Pessimism, Strategic Optimism, and Performance." *Personality and Social Psychology Bulletin* 22 (4): 354–365. https://doi.org/10.1177/0146167296224003.

12. Gasper, Karen, Regina H. Lozinski, and Lavonia Smith LeBeau. 2009. "If You Plan, Then You Can: How Reflection Helps Defensive Pessimists Pursue Their Goals." *Motivation and Emotion* 33 (2): 203–216. https://doi.org/10.1007/s11031-009-9125-5.

13. Martin, Andrew J., Herbert W. Marsh, and Raymond L. Debus. 2001. "A Quadripolar Need Achievement Representation of Self-Handicapping and Defensive Pessimism." *American Educational Research Journal* 38 (3): 583–610. https://doi.org/10.3102/00028312038003583.

14. Dineen-Griffin, Sarah, Victoria Garcia-Cardenas, Kylie Williams, and Shalom I. Benrimoj. 2019. "Helping Patients Help Themselves: A Systematic Review of Self-Management Support Strategies in Primary Health Care Practice." *PLoS One* 14 (8): e0220116. https://doi.org/10.1371/journal.pone.0220116.

15. Faries, Mark D. 2016. "Why We Don't 'Just Do It': Understanding the Intention-Behavior Gap in Lifestyle Medicine." *American Journal of Lifestyle Medicine* 10 (5): 322–329. https://doi.org/10.1177/1559827616638017.

16. Milne-Ives, Madison, Ching Lam, Caroline De Cock, Michelle Helena Van Velthoven, and Edward Meinert. 2020. "Mobile Apps for Health Behavior Change in Physical Activity, Diet, Drug and Alcohol Use, and Mental Health: Systematic Review." *JMIR MHealth and UHealth* 8 (3): 976–980. https://doi.org/10.2196/17046.

17. Payne, Hannah, Lister, Cameron, West, Joshua and Bernhardt, Jay. 2015. "Behavioral Functionality of Mobile Apps in Health Interventions: A Systematic Review of the Literature." *JMIR MHealth and UHealth* 3 (1): e20. https://doi.org/10.2196/mhealth.3335.

8 Maintaining Motivation

Lyra Heller MA, Monique Class MS, APRN,
BC, and Sandra Scheinbaum PhD

8.1 INTRODUCTION

Throughout this book, the reader has been introduced to a rich and multi-dimensional portfolio of evidence-based behavior change theories, research, results, tools, and assessment instruments written by the innovators and investigators in their respective fields. All highlight that changing a behavior or habit is challenging and complex. Each chapter offers a distinct and complementary perspective on ways to conceptualize change and sustain the motivation to change unhealthy lifestyle practices and acquire new ones.

Frates and Bonnet (2016) integrate and apply these theoretical constructs and communication skills in the "coach" approach – a flexible behavior change model that accommodates practitioner individuality, methodological preferences, self-expression, creativity, and the importance of therapeutic reciprocity between client and practitioner. The "coach" approach is a collaborative person-centered partnership described as, "…a purposeful interaction and a powerful connection between a lifestyle medicine practitioner and a patient that not only educates but also motivates and empowers the patient to participate in their own planning for a healthy lifestyle. It is this connection and empowerment that lead to sustained behavior change".[1] Chapter 1 reviews the COACH Approach (™).

While the significance of connection in relationship building is undeniable, the elements that contribute to a meaningful initial engagement and dynamic connection that build toward maintenance of motivation during behavioral change adoption are often elusive for the practitioner.[2-4] To help, this chapter presents *Let the client lead…*, a simple rubric that highlights the authors' clinical experiences, shared with Fifield and Suzuki (Chapter 4), attesting to the wisdom and veracity of how the quality and integrity of this connection can facilitate or undermine an individual's resolve to adhere to a change program. The avoidance of or inability to positively engage during each encounter can deflate drive and frustrate mutual trust, honest dialogue, and collaboration.[5-7]

Let the client lead… explores how to establish, strengthen, and maintain a powerful person-centered practitioner connection as a primary way to inspire and sustain the motivation to achieve healthy lifestyle habits. Here, we share our collective self-observations and reflections regarding prioritizing those core coaching behaviors that lead to deepening and regenerating the bond between client (or patient) and practitioner. The goal of *Let the client lead…* is cultivating the space for moments of *relational depth*, an interplay of three key actions: *being present, being authentic,* and *being in rapport* (Figure 8.1).

DOI: 10.1201/9781003161226-8

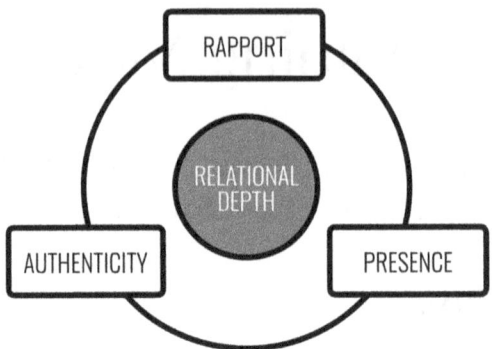

FIGURE 8.1   Let the Client Lead: Cultivating relational depth – the interplay of presence, authenticity, and rapport.

8.2   EVIDENCE REVIEW

8.2.1   RELATIONAL DEPTH

Relational depth (RD) can be described as those moments in a therapeutic relationship in which both the practitioner and the client have feelings of aliveness, satisfaction, and immersion.[8–11] Knox (2011) describes this experience as moments of identifiable and profound engagement and connectedness that can act as a positive catalyst supporting a prolonged sense of wellbeing post relationship.[11] Additionally, Knox's (2011) findings provide evidence that clients perceive a moment of relational depth as making a positive contribution to outcome, suggesting that practitioners should be prepared, ready, attuned, and willing to engage with their client at a level of relational depth should such a moment emerge.[11]

These awe-inspiring moments are akin to being "in flow" with another – a state that increases the satisfaction and enjoyment of both the practitioner and the client.[12–14] When viewed through the phenomenological lens, flow experiences draw us, "…willingly into interactions with the environment that call for full engagement and stretch our capacities."[15] The person-specific pre-conditions interacting to facilitate flow in a client encounter are *relatedness* where the practitioner demonstrates unconditional positive regard, common interests, and *commitment* to the coaching process and the client's agenda.[13]

Relational depth, the spontaneous experience of a powerful connection between client and practitioner, is theorized to assist in maintaining a client's motivation to change behavior by reinforcing trust and perceived authenticity that perpetuates the alliance. An awe-inspiring moment can organically generate self-reflection on both sides. For the client, *flow* can reveal fresh insights regarding personal strengths and obstacles, as well as a re-evaluation of rewards and goals, which can lead to a revised strategy and accountability. The practice of *presence* is assumed to facilitate *relational depth*.

8.2.2   PRESENCE

Being present involves the experience of being fully in the moment on multiple dimensions simultaneously – physical, emotional, cognitive, and relational.[16] The practitioner is fully aware of what is happening within themselves, with the client, and in the environment where the conversation is taking place.[16–18] Here, *flow* and *presence* might overlap, where both are characterized by a loss of self-consciousness, a distorted sense of time's passage, and the merging of action and awareness.[12]

Presence heightens awareness and sensitizes the practitioner to the nuanced verbal and non-verbal signals contributing to *relational depth*, identifying a client's stage of change,[19] asking appropriately synced *open-ended questions*, using *affirmations*, *reflections*, and *summaries*, readiness to talk change, work with ambivalence, and the need to address discrepancies between beliefs and action.[20] *Being present* increases practitioner "timing," and knowing when to invite the telling, the hearing, and the exploring of their client's story.[1,21]

From the client perspective, Geller and Porges (2014) theorize that when a practitioner attunes and is present to themselves, this facilitates attunement to the client which induces feelings of client calm and safety. From this space of safety, the client feels open to engage in self-reflective work contributing to the maintenance of a client's motivation to change unhealthy behavior.[22] Placing importance on staying connected from moment to moment not only reinforces a client's feeling safe but also supports their feeling accepted, being heard, and encourages the expression of feelings, thoughts, and desires.[16,17]

This level of engagement has the effect of decreasing the likelihood of resistance and "incongruent" dialogue between patient and practitioner.[23] Choosing to show up *present* enhances sensitivity to the ebb and flow of a practitioner's attention. Comfort with *being present* allows for a comfortable return to the moment when attention drifts, and the solicitation of client feedback if the client withdraws or is not engaged in response to the loss of connection. This builds coach and client confidence in each other by promoting openness in the exchange. Clients are motivated to stay in a relationship and work their plans when they feel cared for, accepted without judgment, heard, and free to question the practitioner without fear or anxiety.

Cultivating presence begins prior to a session.[17,23] Practitioners who practice being present report feeling *grounded* and *connected* to one's integrated and authentic (healthy) self and being open, receptive to, and *absorbed* in the moment.[24] There is a larger sense of spaciousness and *expansion* of awareness and perception that accompanies the intention, as Colosimo and Pos (2015) suggest, of being *with and for*, or *in communion with*, the client. From this expanded space, the client feels listened to, unconditionally accepted, and safe – prerequisites to experiencing a deeper relationship, relational depth, and positive outcomes.[16,17]

Psychologist Carl Rogers exemplifies the power of *presence* in maintaining both client and practitioner connection, facilitating *flow*, and providing the motivation to stay in relationship in a *A Way of Being* (1980) and *On Becoming a Person* (1961).[25,26]

When I am at my best, as a group facilitator or as a therapist, I discover another characteristic. I find that when I am closest to my inner, intuitive self, when I am somehow in touch with the unknown in me, when perhaps I am in a slightly altered state of consciousness, then whatever I do seems to be full of healing. Then, simply my presence is releasing and helpful to the other. There is nothing I can do to force this experience, but when I can relax and be close to the transcendental core of me, then I may behave in strange and impulsive ways in the relationship, ways in which I cannot justify rationally, which have nothing to do with my thought processes. But these strange behaviors turn out to be right, in some odd way: it seems that my inner spirit has reached out and touched the inner spirit of the other. Our relationship transcends itself and becomes a part of something larger. Profound growth and healing and energy are present.

Rogers, 1980, p. 129[25]

Colosimo and Pos (2015) offer a model for appreciating and practicing the nuance of presence in practice.[17] The researchers identify four interrelated dimensions of *being here*, *being now*, *being open*, and *being with and for the client* (*communion*) which are described below.

8.2.2.1   Being Here

Being Here is being "here and only here" in the immediate physical reality of the environment by anchoring attention in the place, whether inside or outside, where the conversation happens. This implies the practitioner is responsive to what is happening in their own bodily experience, to what the client embodies, as well to what occurs in the space. Distractions require noticing and getting back to the moment as swiftly as possible. Clinicians are subject to a wide variety of interfering factors, such as fatigue, mental chatter, distractibility, physical pain, emotional experiences (e.g., stress, anger, anxiety, boredom, self-doubt, and fear of the client), or hyper-intellectualization (i.e., feeling the need to lecture on a lifestyle-related topic like the best way to eat, exercise, or spend one's time), and preoccupation with the last client.[16,17] Returning to *being here* can be as simple as acknowledging the disconnect, such as asking the client, "Would you mind repeating what you just said? I lost my focus for a moment," or "I get excited when talking about food. If this is a topic that interests you, just let me know."

8.2.2.2   Being Now

Being Now reflects attunement to the immediate instant of time, not preoccupied by thoughts of what has just occurred (past) or might occur (future). Like *flow*, "now-ness" is a subjective state when the practitioner is completely involved to the point of forgetting time, fatigue, and everything else but the activity itself. To paraphase Wesson (2010), flow is what we feel when we get thoroughly absorbed in a well-crafted novel, our favorite sport or take part in a stimulating conversation. Flow is that intense experiential involvement in moment-to-moment activity where a person tends to function at their fullest capacity.[13]

> ...what we feel when we read a well-crafted novel, or play a good game of squash, or take part in a stimulating conversation. The defining feature of flow is intense experiential involvement in moment-to-moment activity. Attention is fully invested in the task at hand, and the person functions at his or her fullest capacity,

Wesson, 2010, p. 54

Being Now is an immersion in the moment, and it supports a developed sensitivity to *timing*. Poor timing in response to what a client says is evidenced by a sense of awkwardness in both counselor and client. The incongruence between being connected and disengaged becomes palpable. For example, non-verbal markers include the practitioner having a non-responsive, flat expression in face and body, or automatic head nodding that is unlinked to client tempo or narrative process.[16,17]

When conversations are frequently punctuated by poor timing, this signals practitioner boredom or disinterest in client welfare and frustrating connection. As stated previously, a powerful connection can maintain motivation and empower the client to participate in their own planning for a healthy lifestyle leading to sustained behavior change.[1] *Being Now* assists in adapting to the dynamism and volatility of staying connected, promoting excitement and energy.

8.2.2.3 Being Open

Being open, or "ready to receive," is having the capacity to maintain open readiness to perceive and receive what is in the here and now as well as the readiness to detect all relevant signals – the nuances.[16] This is the quality of a mind free from preconceptions, accompanied by a tone of unconditional positive regard and respect, refraining from interrupting, using empathic listening, and using open-ended questions and reflections to affirm client communication.[17] *Being open* involves *being present* to how a client's ethnicity, sexual orientation, economic and/or social standing, physical appearance, and other factors might inadvertently sabotage the clinician's capacity to form a therapeutic alliance. Practicing openness is an opportunity to observe when tightly held practitioner and client beliefs surface that may interfere with meaningful engagement.

Being "closed" permits personal prejudices and hindrances to presence discussed earlier (e.g., therapist preoccupation with thoughts, fear, boredom, fatigue) to increase the likelihood of the practitioner missing important client signals inviting collaboration.[16,17] As a result, the motivation for maintenance of behavior change is undermined by calling into question whether the practitioner is a trustworthy partner that truly understands and cares for their client's welfare.

8.2.2.4 Being with and for

Being with and for the client reflects *communion* with the intention of creating an emotionally safe space that promotes trust, self-discovery, and self-confidence.[17,20,26] Here, the quality of the interpersonal contact actively communicates, through words and body language, complete practitioner engagement congruent with the client's experience. For example, a practitioner's facial expression responds to a client in a manner that communicates a shared process, or the exchange embodies a flexible, relaxed, and spontaneous character. The nature of the dialogue supports collaboration and conveys an attitude of respect, compassion, and acknowledgment of client choice (i.e., autonomy). Conversely, the practitioner's response might not be in line with the client's experience, where there is a failure to notice or share the client's point of view.[17] In this instance, the client may feel uncomfortable, unsupported, and respond in several ways – argue, withdraw, and change the subject. This may require the practitioner to have the capacity to relinquish control. Intentionally choosing to be present nurtures a strong bond supporting partnership resiliency and acceptance of the volatile nature of staying connected. *Being with* and *for* leverages *being now* to invite client feedback, resolve misunderstandings, restore connection, and sustain the motivation to change.[26]

The four dimensions of presence coalesce and tap into the vibrancy and excitement of getting to know the client, hearing their story,[21] letting them lead, and giving them choice, which encourages autonomy (self-determination), self-confidence, and competence.[27] From the coaching perspective, choosing to be *here and now*, sit with uncertainty, strong emotions and *be open* and receptive to all possibilities, engenders a willingness to be vulnerable. The motivation to practice *being present* with clients is likely tethered to how the clinician answers larger phenomenological questions. For example, to what extent does the practitioner intrinsically believe that their clients[27,28]:

1. Are the experts in their own lives?
2. Have the desire and the freedom to choose?
3. With appropriately timed guidance, want to explore and discover their own solutions?

8.2.3 BEING AUTHENTIC

What does it mean to be *real, authentic, honest,* and *genuine* with a client? This is a complex question with many dimensions.[29,30] For the purposes of this discussion, *being authentic* is defined as the degree to which a particular behavior is congruent or consistent with a person's attitudes, beliefs, values, motives, and other dispositions.[31,32] This is referred to as *self-congruence.* Researchers conceptualize and operationalize *self-congruence* in different ways[31,33]:

1. Congruence with the *true self*
2. Congruence with beliefs, attitudes, or values
3. Congruence limited to specific contexts – cross-situational and cross-role consistency

The essence of authenticity, when associated with congruent behavior, is further demonstrated by the 3Cs – *consistency, conformity, connection,*[34] and *continuity* – the additional "C," contributed by Dammanns et al (2021) 4C-view adding a dynamic perspective.[35]

For example, if trust between friends is an assumed value, then exhibiting consistency in word and deed is crucial. The common expressions "saying what you're going to do and doing what you say" or "being your word" are high priority behaviors and measures of authenticity. Inconsistency undermines trust.

8.2.3.1   The Authentic Practitioner

Here, the person-centered therapeutic partnership is the context within which the practitioner commits to engage in congruent conversation and behavior with a client during each session.[23,26] Rogers (1961) said, when we are "real" with each other, this facilitates trust and communication. In turn, the alliance deepens and the client's confidence in their ability to achieve their goals continues. Congruence (being real), empathy, unconditional positive regard, and *presence* are inseparable practices[23] underlying a powerful client–practitioner connection that supports adherence to behavior change programs.

To be one's *authentic self,* within this person-centered model, depends on the practitioners' interest in knowing themselves.[31,32,36] By setting the intention to be present within the scope of this type of helping relationship, the practitioner commits to showing up "empty," "open" and suspending judgement. From this space, an honest exchange can evolve because openness begets openness, trust, acceptance and client-practitioner reciprocity.[17] There is a willingness to flow with the sense of vulnerability and uncertainty that accompanies not knowing. Both parties embark on an adventure of self-discovery through the exchange.

While the practice of *being present* increases the quality of all interactions, the expectations associated with authentic behavior, stated previously, can vary with the context. For example, what it means to be honest can fluctuate dramatically between the workplace, family, friends, clinician and coach. Here, where the clinical focus is a person's health and sustaining motivation, maintaining trust and connection is essential to partnering with a client on their change journey. In this situation, "being real" is synonymous with congruent behavior – "saying what you mean," "doing what you say," and "doing no harm with your words and actions."[37]

8.2.3.2 Congruent Dialogue and Action

For authenticity to occur, the practitioner must engage in congruent dialogue in practice. Congruent dialogue has two components[23,37]:

1. *Awareness* (the internal component)
2. *Transparency* (the external component)

Awareness refers to the ability to be aware of one's own internal experience, what might be happening to the client, and the influence of the physical environment in the moment – *to be here and now.*[17]

Transparency (openness and honesty) is the willingness to extend and share the practitioner's genuine inner experience with the client regarding what is going on *within* themselves during the immediate interaction. This includes calling attention to what they see might be going on within the client and/or checking in when transparency is helpful[23] – *being open* and *being with and here* for the client.[17] A transparent exchange between client and practitioner is reciprocal.[23]

In aligning *presence* with congruence and authenticity, the practitioner and client become aware of and present to an "incongruent" interaction. They recognize the discrepancy (inconsistency) between verbal and non-verbal behavior or changes in narratives (i.e., goals, story) within the current or past session. When fully present, incongruence is often experienced viscerally and is virtually impossible to ignore. In a collaborative person-centered atmosphere where the practitioner and client feel free to express what they hear and see in a respectful manner, dissonance, while usually uncomfortable and unpleasant, can be addressed openly and honestly. This reinforces a dynamic conversation of give and take where trust is continually renewed. Both practitioner and client are empowered to be themselves and practice unearthing conscious or unconscious agendas.[17,37,38]

Often, incongruent dialogue signals client ambivalence toward changing unhealthy behaviors or acquiring new ones.[20] Within the context of the motivational interview (MI), being present to client discrepancies during an exchange is viewed as a motivational accelerant.[20,39–41] Fifield and Suzuki in Chapter 4 describe specific MI communication skills that help transform a client's incongruent language into "arguing oneself into change,"[39] and ambivalence into self-discovery and profound insight.[42]

Presence and *authenticity* are our first two priorities. They are the path to achieving relational depth, flow, rapport and sustaining the client's motivation to stay in a relationship[16] leading to positive outcomes whether the agenda is changing behavior or personal growth. The practice of *being present* enables the practitioner to gain comfort with uncertainty, flexibility and experience the process of behavior change as an adventure. Choosing *to be in the moment* opens the opportunity to witness how physician behavior impacts the client, for better or worse, on the subtlest of levels, by increasing self-awareness, encouraging self-reflection, and suppressing the "righting reflex" – the tendency to want to "fix" a client's problems, impart clinician wisdom or insight, and offer unsolicited advice on how to get healthy as discussed by Frates in Chapter 1.

Showing up *present* and *real* with clients helps (1) demonstrate caring, genuine interest, empathy and compassion – the spirit of the motivational interview,[20,40,41] (2) engage in appreciative inquiry,[43,44] (3) use incongruent dialogue to explore intrinsic motivators.[27] (4) recognize a client's readiness to change within the transtheoretical model,[19] and (5) learn motivational interview communication skills such as open-ended questions, affirmations, reflective listening, summarizing (OARS), hear change talk cues, roll with resistance, and use ambivalence to inspire the motivation to adhere to programs.[20,40]

8.2.4   RAPPORT: BEING HERE, NOW AND OPEN

Rapport is often described as a close and harmonious relationship, frequently spontaneous, in which the people or groups concerned understand each other's feelings or ideas and communicate well.[4] Sometimes, this type of connection is referred to as "clicking," "being in sync," or "the right chemistry."[45] Tickely-degnan (1990) describes the nature of rapport as an experience of mutual attentiveness, positivity, balance, and harmony. There is consensus among researchers and clinicians across health domains that cultivating and sustaining rapport forms strong relational bonds that lead to patient satisfaction and treatment compliance.[2,4,6,27,46–49] Subsequently, motivation is reflected in the patient's willingness to stay involved. *Flow* and moments of *relational depth* are expressions of prioritizing rapport from session to session.

The inability to establish rapport within each encounter is widely recognized to contribute to any number of behaviors ranging from client resistance to stoicism, refusing to share, arguing, and being defensive. Frequent appointment cancellations are symptomatic of disinterest and declining motivation to comply. The quality of rapport influences the client's motivation to continue the relationship.[1,4,41]

8.2.4.1   How to Be in Rapport

How to be *in rapport* with the client is discussed in depth by Leach (2005) and Miller (2015).[4,20] This process includes the following and flows from the practice of *being present* and engaging authentically discussed previously[23,26]:

1. Disclosure, honesty, and respect
2. Recognizing the person/individual
3. Interacting socially without pretense
4. Caring and bonding

8.2.4.2   Honest Communication and Emotional Safety

Honest, congruent communication is the standard set by the practitioner. The practice of *being now and open* with the client[17] facilitates being real, creates *rapport*, and helps establish an emotional safe zone. A practitioner's willingness to choose *openness* supports the courage to participate in an aware and transparent discussion.[16,23]

Subsequently, a condition is set for meaningful exchanges that earn mutual respect and trust over successive encounters. Creating an emotionally safe space encourages the client to enter without fear of being judged, receiving unsolicited advice and unwanted instruction. This sense of "emotional safety" appears rooted in our neurophysiology where a variety of verbal and non-verbal communication styles have been postulated and demonstrated to influence limbic-hypothalamic-pituitary-adrenal (HPA) axis, promoting resilience and calming the nervous system.[17,23,27,50]

8.2.4.3 Rapport Is Dynamic

Rapport, like motivation, is dynamic and changing. You gain it, lose it, regain it, and sometimes it disappears for good.[45] The attached guide to sustaining rapport (Table 8.1) invites the practitioner to engage in a role-play where he or she meets a client for the first time and establishes connection by *being now* and *being open and receptive.*[17]

TABLE 8.1

Being Now and Being Open – A Guide to Sustaining Rapport from Moment to Moment and Session to Session

	Gaining Rapport
Warm greeting	• Open, inviting
	• Generous with eye contact
	• Smile
	• Share your name
	• Use their name frequently
	• Be yourself
Show genuine curiosity	…what interests you, what's your passion, how do you spend your free time, what do you think about, what is your current occupation?
Hear their story	• Ask Open-Ended Questions – How? When? Who? What? Where?
	• When really listening (being now), asking open-ended questions is connected to the content of what a person is saying
	• Advance questioning with "tell me more…"
	• Genuine inquiry promotes self-discovery and requires suppressing ego
	• Avoid "yes" and "no" questions – they are dead ends
	Sustaining Rapport
Five actions to reduce anxiety (yours and the clients) and build trust:	• Provide reassurance
	• Reaffirm it's okay to ask questions
	• Share any objective data, like lab results, and explain what they mean
	• Ask what they want and need from you
Listen empathically	• Stay present to what is being said – notice when you check out and drift to thinking about how you want to respond
	• Pause after the last word is spoken – notice the frequency with which you want to interrupt
	• Practice timing and acknowledgment – weave their story into your conversation when appropriate
	• Listen and/or feel for emotions as well as fact

(Continued)

TABLE 8.1 (*Continued*)

Being Now and Being Open – A Guide to Sustaining Rapport from Moment to Moment and Session to Session

	Losing Rapport
Feel, hear, and see a disconnect!	• Notice when you disappear from the talk and where you went… • Bring your attention back to the conversation with a simple statement like "do you remind repeating what you just said?" • Notice if the client "shuts down" and your reaction.

Common demotivating behaviors	• Giving unsolicited advice
	 • Expert trap:
	  • Using language and behaviors that are judgmental – how often do you rely on words like "good," "bad," "right," or "wrong" (or other versions of these words)? These types of words express that you have an opinion about what the other person is saying, rather than being open to their experience and listening to what they say.
	  • Lecturing and over-talking – too much information
	 • Lengthening gaze or inability to maintain eye contact
	 • Unintentional ambiguity – i.e., confusion regarding expectations
	 • Emotionally challenging "why" questions
	 • Violation of personal space – paremature "barely perceptible" touch
	 • Chaotic environment – background noise, front office disgruntlement, messy, etc.
	 • Poor hygiene
	 • Lack of professionalism – i.e., breach of confidentiality, unsafe setting like thin walls
	 • Failure to identify and acknowledge cultural differences when they arise

	Getting It Back
Acknowledge the disconnect	• If you are uncomfortable. Confirm if client fells disconnected too. • During a conversation, tuning in, listening without distraction, and paying attention to the current moment will reveal the questions to ask that help to address the disconnect and deepen understanding
What works	• A simple acknowledgment of the breakdown is usually sufficient and appreciated • If you disappear from the conversation and are lost when you return, apologize for missing what was said and ask them to repeat what was just said
Not so helpful	• There are no do-overs – whatever level of connection and closeness existed previously is over. Just move forward. • Trying to explain why you did what you did • Arguing your point • Correcting them • Saying their issue is somehow overblown or ill stated • Trying to discern "right from wrong"

The role-play: Choose to show up fully present and be yourself without an agenda other than what your partner chooses as their problem and meet them for the first time. This is an opportunity to let go of everything you have learned about the elements of coaching. Just enjoy the conversation, practice self-observation without self-judgment, simply listen and ask questions when it feels appropriate. If you feel like soliciting feedback, a simple question asking if they feel heard suffices, and then continue going where the exchange leads. Notice when you feel self-conscious, the frequency with which you use the "righting reflex" (offer unsolicited advice) or disappear from the conversation. Practice returning to *now* with simple statements of acknowledgment, such as, "Would you mind repeating what you just said. I got lost for a moment." Enjoy and laugh.[51] Be playful.[52] By experiencing the dynamic nature of rapport and staying in connection, the practitioner can glimpse the relationship between how being fully engaged in the moment and thoroughly immersed in getting to know the other can enhance a client's motivation to continuously renew his or her commitment to lifestyle change through dialogue.

8.3   PRACTICAL APPLICATION AND CASE STUDY

8.3.1   BEING WITH AND FOR THE CLIENT

To help the practitioner apply what has been learned, we re-emphasize the four modes of presence in practice and provide an opportunity for exploring their application. Specifically, Table 8.2 illustrates how the interrelationship between the four modes of presence sensitize the practitioner to hearing, seeing, and feeling the nuanced verbal and non-verbal signals associated with client satisfaction, the expression of ambivalence, and incongruent conversation. This attunement often leads to recognizing a client's stage of change (Chapter 2),[19] readiness to talk change (Chapter 4),[20] and the personalization of the integration of coaching methods (Chapters 1 and 12), tools and techniques covering the motivational interview (Chapter 4),[20] appreciative inquiry (Chapter 6), self-determination theory (Chapter 5), and goal setting (Chapter 7).

While Table 8.2 is not an exhaustive account of the nuances of the practitioner–patient experience, approaching each encounter with the intention of *being present* offers the benefit of dampening physician burnout, which Chipidza et al. (2015) describes as "…a state of detachment, emotional exhaustion, and lack of work-related fulfillment….".[53] The process of getting to know a client more deeply from session to session can inspire and refresh both the clinician and client by releasing the energy that supports their resolve to work together toward the client's successfully reaching their lifestyle goals.

8.3.2   INSIDE THE ENCOUNTER WITH JENNA

Jenna's story illustrates, through multiple practitioner–client encounters, analyses, and coach reflections, the seamless integration of *all aspects of presence, authenticity,* and *rapport* that forge a powerful and enduring connection sustaining Jenna's motivation to change an unhealthy behavior, discover and adopt a new one.

TABLE 8.2
Being With and For the Client

Being here Gather oneself	• Set the intention to be fully present, in this moment, suspending judgment of self and others • Prepare in advance – ground yourself in your body, prepare to immerse yourself in the encounter • Notice how what you see, hear, smell, taste, and touch influence your readiness to engage • Be mindful of the physical space – private, comfortable, free of distractions • Be mindful of appearance • Be mindful of your energy level • Know the client's name • Collect the appropriate tools for the session • Clear mind before engaging – take some deep breaths
Being now Greet warmly	• Be open, inviting, generous with eye contact, smile • Share your name • Use their name • Be yourself • Be kind • Notice how it feels to give 100% of your attention • Pay attention with all five senses to your client and the immediate surroundings

Being open
Establish rapport
	• Solicit the client's reason for the visit – capture their words
	• Practice "just listening" and be present to the opportunity for meaningful inquiry and dialogue
	  • Stay present to what is being said – notice when you check out and drift to thinking about how you want to respond
	  • Listen and/or feel for emotions as well as facts
	• Share reasons for the visit and discuss discrepancies between client and practitioner/coach understanding
	  • Be humble – if confronted, it's ok to admit you are distracted and return to the conversation
	  • Take a pause after the last word is spoken
	• Notice if and when you want to "fix" the client – be the expert in your field and let the client be the expert in their life
	  • Notice if and when you judge
	• Explain the person-centered relationship and conduct yourself accordingly
	• Be your word – say what you will do and do what you say: be on time, if you promise to provide resources in the form of article, books, recipes, follow through, etc.

Being with and for the client Meet the client where they are	• Understand the client's own motives for changing • Ask meaningful open-ended questions tethered to the immediate conversation • Listen for client cognitive, emotional, and spiritual strengths, skills and accomplishments

(*Continued*)

TABLE 8.2 (*Continued*)
Being With and For the Client

- Move the conversation forward by affirming, reflecting, and summarizing what you hear
- Trust your intuition when reflecting and summarizing – listen for and be open to client's possibilities
- Practice timing – notice the frequency with which you want to interrupt
- Discover "common ground" – weave client story into the conversation when appropriate
- Notice incongruency between client's expressed goals when it arises
- Notice if you experience the client's ambivalence as personally uncomfortable
- Notice how you handle internalizing the client's discomfort
- Speak the truth as it pertains to the exchange, find the courage to foster discrepancy, and heighten awareness of ambivalence by amplifying incongruences through questions and reflections
- Give a person the opportunity to vent – could be in the form of tears, frustration, anger…when finished, lightly and politely ask if they can access what is really going on
- Notice how it feels to sit with strong emotions
- Listen for the client to signal "it's time to act"
- Then, and only then, begin the process of exploring planning and goal setting

On display (Table 8.3), during each session, is the routine of (1) "gathering oneself" – *being here*, the process of preparing for the encounter, followed by (2) establishing rapport/connection – *being now* and *open* – those moments when connection is acknowledged, and transitioning to (3) meeting the client where they are – *being with and for the client*. By weaving the practitioner's session reflections throughout these exchanges, the clinician offers insights regarding Jenna's responses, and also shares moments in the conversation that signal unanticipated clinician personal challenges. In this context, every encounter can be compared to a journey, and every conversation a dance. Some encounters are exciting adventures punctuated with dramatic personal breakthroughs and breakdowns for both client and healthcare provider. Others milestones along the way are more subdued, dominated by quiet reflections, pauses and periods of silence leading to profound insights. Some conversations dance the tango and others a waltz. Between the words exchanged live the moments for *relational depth* and transforming insight.

8.3.2.1 Jenna's Story

The first time Jenna and I met was virtual. She immediately announced she was here for only "one" visit. That visit was to appease her mother who wanted me to give Jenna a food plan. Jenna is 23 y/o. Her mother was convinced that Jenna's anxiety, depression, eczema, and other health issues were related to what she ate. Jenna was angry and felt coerced.

TABLE 8.3
Jenna: Inside the Encounter

	1st Encounter
Coach reflections	Gathering myself – being here and now: • Preparation – tested audio and visual connections. • Reviewed reason for visit – mother made the appointment for me to create a personalized food plan to address Jenna's anxiety and depression. • Prejudgments: Jenna is in emotional pain, feeling continually discounted and needing to vent. Mother triggered feelings of anger. I anticipate either stoicism or anger. • My challenge – Silencing strong voice that prejudges mother as controlling. Resist discussing mom–daughter relationship with Jenna and "fixing" mom. • Choose to be present and now take a couple of deep breaths; notice how I am feeling in the moment. • Set intention to establish connection, build trust, let Jenna lead, and "fully" listen to who she is, her priorities, and what brings meaning to her life.
JENNA	Just so you know, I don't want to be here. My mom thought I needed to see a health coach. She's really into health. I'm only here so she would stop nagging me. But I'm only coming this one time.
Coach reflections	The moment Jenna sees my face on the screen she announces her protest. There is no opportunity to introduce myself. Initially, I could feel her anger. She makes little eye contact. She is glancing down. I assume her anger keeps her focused on staying true to her commitment to not yield. Feels uncomfortable for a moment. I breathe.
COACH	I appreciate you for being honest and telling me that you don't want to be here. Yet you showed up anyway.
JENNA	Just this one time. I'm not coming back.
Coach reflections	The affirmation is calming. Meeting Jenna where she's at, she acknowledges she wants nothing to do with advice and would like the opportunity to vent. Being with her anger is the theme of this encounter. I notice the pace of the conversation is fast, loud, and breathless. Being present to her voice, I slow the pace down by responding in a relaxed, normal cadence. I attempt eye contact and smile.
COACH	I respect whatever decision you make regarding continuing. Why do you think your mom wants you to work with me?
JENNA	She has a crazy idea that what I eat is making me anxious and depressed. And, also, that, because I don't exercise 10 hours a day like her, I'm depressed and angry. That's not the reason! She's upset because I was fired from my job. It wasn't my fault. Besides, I'm working on these things with my therapist. I don't need a health coach.
COACH	Ok, I hear you. You do not need a health coach. If you don't mind, would you share with me what you think a health coach does?
JENNA	Sure. You are supposed to tell me what to eat and give me information on everything food, like you do with my mom.

(Continued)

TABLE 8.3 (*Continued*)
Jenna: Inside the Encounter

COACH	Got it. Is it ok for me to share with you what I do?
JENNA	Yes
Coach reflections	Open-ended questions, selective summarizing, and reflective listening lead to a relaxation of Jenna's defensiveness.
COACH	My clients come to me and tell me what they want and need. My skills cover an array of health concerns ranging from everything food-special diets, cravings, as you said, to working with post-traumatic stress. My style is to be your advocate. Together we explore your interests related to lifestyle change if you have any. What would you like to work on?
Coach reflections	I took a chance and asked what she would like to work on rather than asking her if she was interested in working with me. Premature. However, this opened the opportunity for her to continue to vent and explain the types of suggestions she's been exposed to. I also demonstrated being with and for Jenna by my sustained willingness to be present to her anger and frustration over feeling bullied. I worked on withholding judgment and my desire to fix her – righting reflex.
JENNA	(Angry tone) I'm tired of people telling me what to do and making suggestions. My therapist told me to get this meditation app and I hate it. I don't like listening to meditations where people tell me how I should meditate. My mom is gluten free, dairy free, and has this freakish diet, which I don't want to follow or eat what she makes for me. It actually makes me mad. And really, I don't want to be here at all. I'm tired of going to different people
COACH	I appreciate you're being so honest and upfront with me. And I want you to know that I totally understand what you're going through. I don't like people telling me what to do either. I want you to know that as your coach, I'm not going to tell you what to do. I want to know what you want to do. You develop the plan for getting to where you want to be and how you want to feel. I heard that your mom wants you to work on your anxiety, but what do you want to work on? "What's the most important thing to you?"
JENNA	(Long pause) Well, I don't like how I look. I hate having such a fat stomach. It's really hard to buy jeans. Also, lately I've noticed tons of these tiny bumps on my arms and I try to hide them by wearing long sleeves. I don't care that I'm not skinny like my mom, but in college, there was a lot of body shaming from my so-called friends and that really hurt and made me feel bad about myself.
Coach reflections	The pace slows down. I take a few breaths and get comfortable with "fully listening." Lots of distracting thoughts come up making it hard to stay present. I resist "jumping in" and commiserating with her about school experiences. I notice how the word "shaming" triggers my early school experiences. Another breath. I want to "fix" mom. Then, I return to listening to what she needs and ask questions generated by our conversation. I continue to meet her where she is – honoring her demand for "no advice" – critical to staying connected and building trust. I support her autonomy, encouraging her to create her own plan.

(Continued)

TABLE 8.3 (*Continued*)
Jenna: Inside the Encounter

COACH	What have you worked on in the past that you've been successful with?
JENNA	Well, I could tell you what wasn't successful. I hated that meditation app, and all these imagery exercises that my therapist was trying to get me to do. They actually made me angrier and more anxious. Sometimes, I just like to drop into my body and go for walks at a forest preserve near my house.
Coach reflections	How ironic. My specialty, mind–body medicine, is a turn-off. I know that I can make imagery palatable. Again, I notice that I drift and quickly return.
COACH	That sounds like a fabulous idea. You've developed a great way to relax. Would you like to have some information on how deep breathing actually can help or change your nervous system?
JENNA	No, I don't want to hear any information. I really just don't want people telling me what to do or giving me information
Coach reflections	Trusted our connection. Tested my perception that Jenna may be open to hearing some mind–body information. Excited to share. I misjudged. Continued expressing appreciation for her honesty.
COACH	I'm good with that. I really appreciate your honesty and your feedback. I want you to know that you're in charge here. I'm just here to support your desires and help you create your plan. I'd like to hear more about how you drop into your body
JENNA	It's about moving. When I walk, my mind quiets. And when I.....
COACH	How many times a day would you like to do this to relax?
JENNA	I guess I could do this in the morning, maybe right before I go to bed. And in the middle of the day, maybe right after lunch? After I eat, I get bloated and feel disgusting, so that could be a good time.
Coach reflections	I validated that she was creating the protocols: "dropping into her body" which was calming to her nervous system rather than checking out of her body. Then we did a back and forth, where I had her expand upon her ritual of relaxation, including specifics as to frequency and what time of day. I also inquired about anything she could add to the current ritual. Questioning continues leveraging her digestive comments. I see this as an opportunity to tie into food.
COACH	This sounds like a great plan. What do you think is causing the bloating?
JENNA	I've been eating fast foods and a lot of carbs for lunch because that's when my mom isn't around. Maybe that's it.
COACH	You're on the right track. Foods could also be contributing to the bumps on your arms and your weight gain around the middle, which you said are your two main concerns. What would you say we explore these issues?
Coach reflections	I use reflective paraphrasing and summarizing to help her reflect on what she has shared as her concerns and to let her know I am listening and hearing her.
JENNA	(Thinks about it) ...yes, I would like to find out, because I'm embarrassed by these bumps and I hate how fat I look, like I'm pregnant. I'm not bothered by my anxiety; I'm not bothered by being depressed. I feel like if I don't have the bumps on my arms and the bloating gets better, I won't have as much anxiety. I won't feel so bad about myself, and I won't be so depressed.

(Continued)

TABLE 8.3 (*Continued*)
Jenna: Inside the Encounter

Coach reflections	The pace of our conversation flows now. It is punctuated with "ah hah" moments. By creating a safe space for her to be herself, express her anger without judgment, and share her plans, she begins to trust that I am there for her. The turning point arrived when she wants to find out how foods were impacting the bumps on her arm and the abdominal weight gain, because those are her two areas of concerns. She wants to look a particular way to fit in with her peer group. Although this is an external motivator, she is also internally driven to make her own decisions and not be told what to do. At the conclusion of the session, for the first time in the conversation, she was open to receiving information from me.
COACH	How do you want to change your food plan?
JENNA	Definitely don't want to eat the way my mom eats. I could add more fruits and vegetables, stop eating so much fast food. I've been thinking about becoming a vegetarian. I think I'm going to give up meat for a month.
COACH	How about recipes and meal plans? I could share some with you if you're interested.
JENNA	Sure, that would be great.

2nd Encounter

Coach reflections	Just prior to our second visit, my mind was cluttered with other client distractions. I gathered myself and chose to be present by breathing for 3 minutes and then, reviewing my previous visit with Jenna. When we meet, she reported that she had implemented all the changes that she designed. She was walking and "dropping into her body."
	She had changed her food plan and become a vegetarian. She reported that the bloating after lunch was resolved, but the bumps on her arms were still present. I then inquired about what else she would like to work on. She wanted to refine her food plan and learn more about breathwork. We discussed diaphragmatic breathing and how engaging in "micro meditations" throughout the day could change her nervous system as much as longer practices.
	She decided that when she was transitioning from one online class to the next, she would practice deep breathing and walk around her house, as she didn't particularly like to sit still. She described her food plan as going well. She noticed more energy, her stomach was flatter, and she was having more bowel movements. She made the decision to continue with the plan and reduce consumption of gluten.
	Within a three week period, by this second meeting, Jenna created her own plan and made her own decisions.

3rd Encounter

Coach reflections	I was excited to meet Jenna. She returned for the third meeting feeling, a month later, encouraged. The bumps on her arms had started to improve, which was very encouraging to her. Consequently, she was even more motivated to keep her food plan clean and continue to practice the relaxation techniques that she had designed. She was engaging in the coaching process and smiling during our conversation. We celebrated her success by reviewing her journey.

(Continued)

TABLE 8.3 (*Continued*)
Jenna: Inside the Encounter

<table>
<tr><td></td><td align="center">**4th Encounter**</td></tr>
<tr><td>Coach reflections</td><td>During this final visit, a month later, she reported that because she felt better about her stomach being flatter and the bumps on her arms were receding, she was engaged more with her friends.

The client continued to create her own plan and make her own decisions. We terminated our formal visits with Jenna knowing that she could call or text me if she wanted to talk, needed support, and share how well she was doing any time.</td></tr>
</table>

The first encounter was spirited and dominated by venting. The energy generated by the expression of strong emotions was a powerful and potential motivating force for change and self-discovery because Jenna was engaged. The challenge was to establish rapport and gain enough trust during our first meeting so Jenna could envision the benefits of continuing our relationship.

This coach–client dialogue illustrates how choosing *to be present*, in the moment, influences the capacity to fully listen and handle distractions. During each exchange, disturbed concentration shows up in many forms – from background noise to internal conversations that shift attention away from the client. As we talked, Jenna's life experience triggered my memories. I aligned with her emotional pain and frustration. Empathy became sympathy. Interfering thoughts vacillated between fixing mom and fixing Jenna. I struggled with refraining from giving unsolicited advice about the connection between food and mood. By setting the intention, at the outset of each encounter, to notice interruptions and immediately return to fully listening, I was able to sustain connection. By the end of the first session, Jenna genuinely believed that I was motivated solely by her desires and not those of her mother.

The first encounter rolled into four despite her predetermined decision to not cooperate on any level. This coaching relationship was the first relationship where someone asked her what she wanted and fully listened. In terms of stages of change, Jenna began in precontemplation and during the first visit transitioned to being in action with minimal setbacks as she progressed. Jenna developed a fluid, self-directed care plan adjusting the details based on observed tangible, positive results, From the initial encounter, she had the power. For Jenna, control over decision making was intrinsically motivating. As a result, she engaged fully in the change process. Previously, she resisted because "everyone was telling her what to do." I chose to not interfere with her decision-making at any level and respect her desire for complete autonomy. Our relationship based on mutual respect and reciprocity had a ripple effect that impacted all facets of her life. My great challenge was to silence my "righting reflex" that surfaced continuously within each session.[1]

8.3.3 Closing Remarks

An inspired and motivated client reflects an engaged practitioner "who lets their client lead." This relationship is bi-directional, dynamic, and fluid. Honoring this reciprocity, the give and take between practitioner and patient, generates the power and durability of the connection that generates the motivation to stay motivated throughout the behavior change process.

Our clinical experiences mirror the passionate statement of Siminovitch and Van Eron (2008) – "Coaches need to be guided by a knowledge base, emotional intelligence and a resonance with their clients. The coach's 'presence' and developmental journey is important, for it is how a coach is present or how the coach is 'being' that offers a catalyzing force in the client's learning. Presence is a far more potent variable than tools and techniques, allowing the coach to respond to the moments of uncertainty with distinctive impact and transparency that inspires others" (p. 90).[18]

8.4 KEY TAKEAWAYS

1. Establishing, strengthening, and maintaining a powerful person-centered practitioner connection is a primary way to inspire and sustain the motivation to achieve healthy lifestyle habits.
2. The specific elements that contribute to a meaningful initial engagement and dynamic connection are sometimes elusive for the practitioner.
3. *Let the Client Lead…* is a practical approach that identifies the interplay of those specific elements – *being present, authentic,* and *in rapport* that contribute to powerful engagement, *flow* and transformational moments of *relational depth.*
4. *Presence* is the experience of being fully in the moment and fully aware of what is happening within the practitioner, with the client, and in the environment where the conversation is taking place.
5. *Authenticity* or *being your real self* is the degree to which a particular behavior, verbal and non-verbal, is congruent or consistent with the expressed attitudes, beliefs, values, motives, and other dispositions of the practitioner within the context of a coaching conversation.
6. *Rapport* is a close and harmonious relationship, often spontaneous, where people or groups understand each other's feelings or ideas and communicate well – being "in sync" and "clicking." Within the context of a coaching conversation, rapport's effortless quality becomes dynamic and fluid through each successive encounter. Initiation and maintenance requires presence and authenticity.
7. Choosing to "show up" fully present and engage in authentic (aware and transparent) dialogue is intentional and the predicate to a dynamic connection/rapport where trust, mutual respect, collaboration, empathic listening, creativity, courage, joy, and motivation flourish.

8.5 RESOURCES

- Functional Medicine Coaching Academy. https://functionalmedicinecoaching.org
- Motivational Interviewing: https://motivationalinterviewing.org. Motivational Interviewing Network of Trainers (MINT), Training for New Trainers (TNT), Resources for Trainers.
- Houston E. 2020. 12 Best Compassion Training Activities and Exercises. https://positivepsychology.com/compassion-training/ Accessed January 19, 2022.

REFERENCES

1. Frates, E.P., and J. Bonnet. 2016. Collaboration and negotiation: the key to therapeutic lifestyle change. *American Journal of Lifestyle Medicine* 10(5):302–312.
2. Dang, B.N., R.A. Westbrook, S.M. Njue, and T.P. Giordano. 2017. Building trust and rapport early in the new doctor-patient relationship: a longitudinal qualitative study. *BMC Medical Education* 17(1):1–10.
3. Harkey, J., C. Sortedahl, M.M. Crook, and P.V. Sminkey. 2017. Meeting people "where they are". *Professional Case Management* 22(1):3–9.
4. Leach, J. 2005. Rapport: a key to treatment success. *Complementary Therapies in Clinical Practice* 11(4):262–265.
5. Flückiger, C., A.C. Del Re, B.E. Wampold and A.O. Horvath. 2018. The alliance in adult psychotherapy: A meta-analytic synthesis. Psychotherapy, 55(4), p.316.
6. Hamovitch, E.K., M. Choy-Brown, and V. Stanhope. 2018. Person-centered care and the therapeutic alliance. *Community Mental Health Journal* 54(7):951–958.
7. Pinto, R.Z, M.L. Ferreira, V.C. Oliveira et al. 2012. Patient-centred communication is associated with positive therapeutic alliance: a systematic review. *Journal of Physiotherapy* 58(2):77–87.
8. Cooper, M. 2005. Therapists' experiences of relational depth: a qualitative interview study. *Counselling and Psychotherapy Research* 5(2):87–95.
9. Knox, R., and M. Cooper. 2011. A state of readiness: an exploration of the client's role in meeting at relational depth. *Journal of Humanistic Psychology* 51(1):61–81.
10. Kim, J., S. Joseph, and S. Price. 2020. The positive psychology of relational depth and its association with unconditional positive self-regard and authenticity. *Person-Centered & Experiential Psychotherapies*, 19(1):12–21.
11. Knox, R. 2011. Clients' Experiences of Relational Depth, PhD diss., University of Strathclyde, Glasgow Scotland.
12. Csikszentmihalyi, M., and J. Nakamura. 2018. Flow, altered states of consciousness, and human evolution. *Journal of Consciousness Studies* 25(11–12):102–114.
13. Wesson, K.J. 2010. Flow in coaching conversation. *International Journal of Evidence Based Coaching & Mentoring* 4:53. http://www.business.brookes.ac.uk/research/areas/coaching&mentoring/.
14. Nakamura, J., and M. Csikszentmihalyi. 2002. The concept of flow. In *The Handbook of Positive Psychology*, ed. C.R. Snyder and S.J. Lopez, 89–105. England: Oxford University Press.
15. Tse, D.C.K., J. Nakamura, and M. Csikszentmihalyi. 2022. Flow experiences across adulthood: preliminary findings on the continuity hypothesis. *Journal of Happiness Studies*, 23(6), pp.2517-2540.

16. Geller, S.M., and L.S. Greenberg. 2012. The experience of therapeutic presence. In *Therapeutic Presence: A Mindful Approach to Effective Therapy*, ed. S.M. Geller and L.S. Greenberg, 109–131. American Psychological Association. https://www.apa.org/pubs/books/4317278

17. Colosimo, K.A., and A.E. Pos. 2015. A rational model of expressed therapeutic presence. *Journal of Psychotherapy Integration.* 25(2):100. https://doi.org/10.1037/a0038879.pdf.

18. Siminovitch, D., and A. Van Eron. 2008. The power of presence and intentional use of self: coaching for awareness, choice and change. *International Journal of Coaching in Organizations* 3:90–111.

19. Prochaska, J.O. 2008. Decision making in the transtheoretical model of behavior change. *Medical Decision Making* 28(6):845–849.

20. Miller, WR. 2015. Enhancing motivation for change in substance abuse treatment: treatment improvement protocol (TIP) series 35. Motivation for Change in Substance Abuse - Treatment Improvement Protocols (TIPS). HHS Publication No. (SMA) 12-4212.

21. Spencer, A.C. 2016. Stories as gift: patient narratives and the development of empathy. *Journal of Genetic Counseling* 25(4):687–690.

22. Geller, S.M., and S.W. Porges. 2014. Therapeutic presence: neurophysiological mechanisms mediating feeling safe in therapeutic relationships. *Journal of Psychotherapy Integration* 24(3):178.

23. Greenberg, L.S., and S. Geller. 2001. Congruence and therapeutic presence. *Rogers' Therapeutic Conditions: Evolution, Theory and Practice* 1:131–149.

24. Abravanel, M. 2018. Coaching Presence: A Grounded Theory from the Coach's Perspective. PhD diss., Concordia University, Montreal, Quebec, Canada.

25. Rogers, C.R. 1980. *A Way of Being*. Boston, MA: Houghton Mifflin.

26. Rogers, C.R. 1961. *On Becoming a Person*. Oxford, England: Houghton Mifflin.

27. Deci, E.L, and R.M. Ryan. 2012. Motivation, personality, and development within embedded social contexts: an overview of self-determination theory. In *Oxford Handbook of Human Motivation*, ed. R.M. Ryan, 85–107. Oxford, UK: Oxford University Press.

28. Ntoumanis, N., J.Y.Y. Ng, A. Prestwich et al. 2021. A meta-analysis of self-determination theory-informed intervention studies in the health domain: effects on motivation, health behavior, physical, and psychological health. *Health Psychology Review* 15(2):214–244.

29. Sutton, A. 2020. Living the good life: a meta-analysis of authenticity, well-being and engagement. *Personality and Individual Differences* https://doi.org/10.1016/j.paid.2019.109645.

30. Kernis, M.H., and B.M. Goldman. 2006. A multicomponent conceptualization of authenticity: theory and research. *Advances in Experimental Social Psychology* 38:283–357.

31. Jongman-Sereno, K.P., and M.R. Leary. 2019. The enigma of being yourself: a critical examination of the concept of authenticity. *Review of General Psychology* 23(1):133–142.

32. Sutton, A. 2018. Distinguishing between authenticity and personality consistency in predicting well-being: a mixed method approach. *European Review of Applied Psychology* 68(3):117–130.

33. Chen, S. 2019. Authenticity in context: being true to working selves. *Review of General Psychology* 23(1):60–72.

34. Lehman, D.W., K. O'Connor, B. Kovács, and G.E. Newman. 2019. Authenticity. *Academy of Management Annals* 13(1):1–42.

35. Dammann, O., K.M. Friederichs, S. Lebedinski, and K.M. Liesenfeld. 2021. The essence of authenticity. *Frontiers in Psychology* 11:4021.

36. Butt, M.F. 2021. Approaches to building rapport with patients. *Clinical Medicine* 21(6):e662–e663.

37. Greenberg, L.S. 2014. The therapeutic relationship in emotion-focused therapy. *Psychotherapy* 51(3):350.
38. Leleko, M. 2020. Exploring Coaches' Perceptions of Authenticity in Their Coaching Practice: An Interpretative Phenomenological Analysis, 1–34. London: School of Psychology, University of East London.
39. Dobber, J., M. Snaterse, C. Latour, R. Peters, G. Ter Riet, W. Scholte op Reimer, L. De Haan, and B. van Meijel. 2021. Active ingredients and mechanisms of change in motivational interviewing for smoking cessation in patients with coronary artery disease: a mixed methods study. *Frontiers in Psychology* 11:78.
40. Cook, P.F., S. Manzouri, L. Aagaard, L. O'Connell, M. Corwin, and B. Gance-Cleveland. 2017. Results from 10 years of interprofessional training on motivational interviewing. *Evaluation & the Health Professions* 40(2):159–179.
41. Widder, R. 2017. Learning to use motivational interviewing effectively: modules. *The Journal of Continuing Education in Nursing* 48(7):312–319.
42. Apodaca, T.R., K.M. Jackson, B. Borsari, M. Magill, R. Longabaugh, N.R. Mastroleo, and N.P. Barnett. 2016. Which individual therapist behaviors elicit client change talk and sustain talk in motivational interviewing? *Journal of Substance Abuse Treatment* 61:60–65.
43. Hung, L., A. Phinney, H. Chaudhury, P. Rodney, J. Tabamo, and D. Bohl. 2020. "Appreciative inquiry: bridging research and practice in a hospital setting." *International Journal of Qualitative Methods* 17(1):1–10.
44. Naude, L., T.J. van den Bergh, and I.S. Kruger. 2014. "Learning to like learning": an appreciative inquiry into emotions in education. *Social Psychology of Education* 17(2):211–228.
45. Tickle-Degnen, L., and R. Rosenthal. 1990. The nature of rapport and its nonverbal correlates. *Psychological Inquiry* 1(4):285–293.
46. Abendroth, K.J., and J.E. Whited. 2021. Motivation, rapport, and resilience: three pillars of adolescent therapy to shift the focus to adulthood. *Perspectives of the ASHA Special Interest Groups* 6(5):1254–1262.
47. Ackerman, S.J., and M.J. Hilsenroth. 2003. A review of therapist characteristics and techniques positively impacting the therapeutic alliance. *Clinical Psychology Review* 23(1):1–33.
48. Baier, A.L., A.C. Kline, and N.C. Feeny. 2020. Therapeutic alliance as a mediator of change: a systematic review and evaluation of research. *Clinical Psychology Review* 82:10:1921.
49. Tahan, H.A., and P.V. Sminkey. 2012. Motivational interviewing: building rapport with clients to encourage desirable behavioral and lifestyle changes. *Professional Case Management* 17(4):164–172.
50. Williamson, J.B., E.C. Porges, D.G. Lamb, and S.W. Porges. 2015. Maladaptive autonomic regulation in PTSD accelerates physiological aging. *Frontiers in Psychology* 5:Article 1571. https://doi.org/10.3389/fpsyg.2014.01571.pdf.
51. Yim, J.E. 2016. Therapeutic benefits of laughter in mental health: a theoretical review. *The Tohoku Journal of Experimental Medicine* 239(3):243–249
52. Wheeler, S. 2020. An exploration of playfulness in coaching. *International Coaching Psychology Review* 15(1):45.
53. Chipidza, F.E., R.S. Wallwork, and T.A. Stern. 2015. Impact of the doctor-patient relationship. *The Primary Care Companion for CNS Disorders* 17(5):27354.

9 Overcoming Obstacles

Mark D. Faries, PhD and Sofia Chandler, MS

9.1 INTRODUCTION

An obstacle is something that blocks one's way, hinders, or even prevents progress – an apt description of the barriers encountered in the initiation or adoption of healthy lifestyle prescriptions. Barriers are a key factor in common theoretical approaches to behavior change, such as the Health Belief Model, Social Cognitive Theory, Social-Ecological Theories, and the Transtheoretical Model. In addition, almost all theoretical models are embedded factors that, while not specifically defined as a barrier, can hinder or prevent progress in health behavior change (e.g., attitudes, behavioral beliefs, outcome expectations, temptations, attributions, social norms or pressures, or lack of autonomy).

Barriers span dimensions of influence within a person's life, including personal, social, environmental, economic, and spiritual/religious factors. The question this chapter aims to answer is how does the practitioner help the patient overcome obstacles (barriers) to initiating and maintaining healthy lifestyle prescriptions? For simplicity, this chapter will focus on a literature review that highlights two key lifestyle factors in adults: physical activity and healthy eating, both of which are instrumental in the prevention, treatment, and reversal of chronic disease.

9.2 EVIDENCE SUMMARY

9.2.1 OBSTACLES ARE COMMON

Overall, the most common self-reported barriers to healthy eating and physical activity are[1–6]:

1. Lack of Motivation
2. Lack of Time
3. Lack of Interest/Enjoyment
3. Lack of Energy/Willpower
4. High Cost

Large, national-level studies have provided a consensus of common barriers, which span across age, sex, socio-economic status, and geography. To highlight a few examples:

9.2.1.1 Healthy Eating

A nationwide cross-sectional study in Switzerland found that the leading barriers to healthy eating (≈ 30%–40% self-reporting) were *price, fondness of good food, time constraint*, and *daily habits/constraints*, while *lack of willpower* was reported in

DOI: 10.1201/9781003161226-9

approximately 20% of adults.[1] In a subsequent longitudinal nationwide study, the researchers discovered that over 15 years, barriers to healthy eating remained prevalent (≥20%) and tended to change in similar patterns across sex, age, education, and income.[7]

In a Spanish national sample, the main barriers to healthy eating were *irregular work hours* (30%), *willpower* (30%), and *unappealing food* (21%). For healthy eating with fruit and vegetable (FV) consumption, the Scottish Health Survey ($N = 8,319$) found that the leading barriers for both women and men, respectively, were *lack of willpower* (35%, 29%), *too expensive* (17%, 15%), *hedonics* (i.e., *healthy foods are too boring*, or *do not like taste/do not enjoy healthy foods; 10%, 16%*), *availability* (11%, 11%), and *preparation time* (7%, 7%).[3]

Across these examples, the most commonly reported barriers to healthy eating are:

- High Cost
- Lack of Time
- Lack of Willpower
- Taste/Enjoyment (displeasure with healthy food, pleasure with unhealthy food)

When examining recent literature reviews, the most common self-reported barriers to healthy eating are[2,8]:

- High Cost
- Lack of Time (planning, shopping, preparing food)
- Lack of Motivation, Apathy
- Lack of Knowledge
- Lack of Confidence/Competence (shopping, cooking, preparing food)
- Unhealthy Food Availability/Access (cheap, convenient, widely available)
- Healthy Food Availability/Access (expensive, supermarket access, healthy food deserts)
- Social Environments (eating socially, unhealthy diets of friends/family)

9.2.1.2 Physical Activity

A sample of over 2,000 adults in Portugal revealed that 55% cited *lack of time* as a barrier, followed by costs (20%), the *desire to do other things* (15%), *failure to consider themselves as athletes* (15%), and *lack of infrastructures* near where they live (Sequeira et al., 2011). It should also be noted that only 31% of individuals in this sample were meeting physical activity recommendations. Similarly, 50% of Australian adults aged 25–54 years cited *lack of time* as a leading obstacle to physical activity, followed by *lack of enjoyment* (44%), *prefer to do other things* (43%), *lack of confidence* (21%), *nobody to exercise with* (19%), and *lack of money* (16%).[9] Across these examples, the most commonly reported barriers to physical activity are:

- Lack of Time
- Lack of Enjoyment
- Prefer Other Activities
- Lack of Confidence
- Availability/Access Issues

When examining the more recent literature reviews, the most common self-reported barriers to physical activity are[2,10,11]:

- High Cost
- Lack of Time
- Lack of Motivation, Intention; Tired
- Lack of Knowledge
- Lack of Confidence/Competence
- Appearance Concerns (social physique anxiety, self-consciousness, social concerns)
- Health and Physical Condition Concerns (physical/chronic conditions, injury fear)
- Safety (neighborhood), Weather
- Access (Places, Facilities, Transport)
- Life/Work/Family Obligations
- Lack of Social Support/Role Models

9.2.2 Obstacles Are Perceived

Barriers are most often defined as *perceived*, such as an individual's own estimation of the level of challenge they experience when adopting a specific lifestyle behavior. For example, over 200 women were asked to keep 7 days of diary data of all activities lasting at least 10 minutes. Interestingly, most women, even those perceiving time as a barrier, had approximately 28 hours of leisure-time available per week, which was spent doing sedentary activities (e.g., watching television, reading, napping, or sitting quietly).[12]

Another study among young adults illustrated that as hours of work per week increased (particularly when hitting >40 hours/week), so did the perception of various time-related barriers to healthy eating, such as being too busy to eat healthy, being too rushed in the morning to eat a healthy breakfast, and eating healthy meals takes too much time.[13] However, difference in dietary intake (i.e., fast food, FV) between those working less than versus those working greater than 40 hours did not differ. Such findings emphasize the difficulty with perceived barriers as their potential effect on behavior appears to be individualized, where the same barrier might hinder and prevent progress toward healthy lifestyle adoption in one patient but not in another.

9.2.3 Obstacles Are Difficult

"The primary distinguishing feature of a perceived barrier is that it is a judgment of the *degree of difficulty* of a set of diverse factors (barriers) that can interfere with accomplishment of a specified health behavior" (emphasis added).[14] The type and degree of difficulty (or intensity) of obstacles determines the level of interference on behavior change – from a manageable pest to a stalwart impediment.

In a cross-national study, psychological barriers (*eating habits* and *willpower*) had as strong an effect on healthy eating behavior ($\beta = -0.39$), albeit negative, as common motives ($\beta = 0.41$; lose/control weight, look attractive, prevent disease, staying healthy, feel better, quality of life, control an existing problem, like oneself better).[15] On the other hand, physical barriers (*time, food preparation, cost, availability, amount and quality of information about healthy eating, nutritional information*) were not a statistically significant predictor of behavior across both national samples.

A study of Australian men illustrated how self-reporting "key barriers" differed between those who either meet or do not meet FV or physical activity recommendations.[16] A *higher* frequency of those eating ≤3 servings of FV/day self-reported *dislike taste of healthy foods* as a key barrier (34%) than those eating >3 servings of FV/day (12%), but a *lower* frequency of the key barrier *social influence (partner, family, friends do not eat healthy)* (8%) than those eating >3 servings/day (28%). For those *not meeting* physical activity recommendations, a *higher* frequency of the following barriers was noted than those meeting recommendations, respectively: *lack of motivation to exercise* (77% vs. 60%), *intimidation/embarrassment* (36% vs. 19%), and *lack of skills/knowledge* (23% vs. 9%). These findings suggest that certain barriers might be perceived as stronger in those who are not currently meeting healthy recommendations, and they also illustrate the reciprocal impact that adopting health behaviors can have on reducing the perception of barriers. Also, in all cases, those meeting recommendations were still reporting barriers, most particularly *lack of motivation to exercise*. These findings emphasize the need to encourage barrier plans and train barrier management skills.

For interventions, a study of the impact of perceived barriers to healthy eating on weight loss over 24 months illustrated that as mean fat intake, energy intake, or body weight decreased or increased, perceived barriers to healthy eating fluctuated with mirror-like precision.[17] Barriers can also influence health interventions. For example, specific obstacles have been found to moderate the effect of an educational intervention on physical activity behavior, including *general health, depressive symptoms, neighborhood crime rate,* and other *personal,* perceived barriers.[18] Also, there can be a dose–response association between the number of perceived barriers and the level of physical activity or healthy eating.[4,19,20] Such findings re-emphasize the perceived intensity of barriers, when unabated, can have on adoption of healthy lifestyle prescriptions. Of course, the perceived intensity or influence each obstacle might have on one's behavior will vary from patient to patient, stressing that obstacles could be most effectively assessed and accommodated at the individual level (see Section 9.3).

9.2.4 OBSTACLES CHANGE OVER TIME

Differences in perceived barriers across age categories have been reported for both physical activity and healthy eating. For example, de Mestral and colleagues (2016) noted other significant differences in perceived barriers to healthy eating between age groups for *time constraints, daily habit constraints, fondness of good food, fondness of abundant food,* and *lack of willpower.*[1] Generally, perceived barriers declined slightly with age, except *fondness of good food,* which increased in women from 18 to 35 years of age (35%) to >65 years (54%) and in men from 45% to 65%, respectively.

Transitions in life, obligations, careers, needs, motivations, environments, and social influences bring with them new challenges and obstacles, strengthening some and weakening others. For example, in a sample of over 7,000 adult women across the lifespan, physical activity commonly decreased with *marriage* and *childbirth* in young women, or with *declining health* in older women, but increased with *retirement* or *death of a spouse* in middle-aged women.[21] In contrast, a study of young, midlife, and older Korean-American adults revealed no differences in barriers to physical activity across the lifespan, with *takes too much of my time* and *tires me* as the leading barrier.[22] Ultimately, it is to the practitioner's benefit to be aware that perceived barriers can change over time and be more prominent following transitions that occur during life.

9.2.5 OBSTACLES ARE INDIVIDUALIZED

9.2.5.1 Sex

Individual differences in perceived barriers have been expressed between men and women. For physical activity, women have more often self-reported the barrier of *costs* (12%, 25%), while men more often self-reported the *lack of infrastructures* in the neighborhood (14%, 9%, $p < 0.001$).[23] However, Hoare and colleagues (2017) found no statistically significant difference in the common self-reported barriers to physical activity between men (M) and women (W) within Australian adults ($N = 894$).[9]

- Lack of Time: 47% (M), 54% (W)
- Lack of Enjoyment: 39% (M), 49% (W)
- Prefer Other Things: 39% (M), 48% (W)
- Lack of Confidence: 22% (M), 19% (W)
- Nobody to Exercise With: 17% (M), 21% (W)
- Lack of Money: 15% (M), 18% (W)

For healthy eating, a nationwide cross-sectional study in Switzerland found that 43% of women and 36% of men, respectively, self-reported *price of food*, as their most prevalent barrier to healthy eating, followed by *fondness of good food* (39%, 16%), *time constraints* (35%, 29%), and *lack of willpower* (22%, 21%).[1]

9.2.5.2 Body Mass Index

Excess body weight (or body fat) can be a commonly reported barrier, particularly in women, and those classified as "obese" (OB) by body mass index (BMI).[24] In a sample of over 700 women in West Virginia, specific differences in self-reported barriers to physical activity were found between those classified as "normal weight" (NW) and OB.[25]

- Lack of Time: 40% (NW), 26% (OB)
- Lack of Willpower: 43% (NW), 55% (OB)
- Don't Need More: 15% (NW), 5% (OB)

Notice that women classified as OB self-reported *higher* frequency of *lack of willpower*, but *lower* frequency of *lack of time* and *don't need more physical activity* than NW. In the aforementioned nationwide Swiss Health Survey, statistically significant differences were found between women and men classified as either "under/normal weight" (NW) or "obese" (OB) by BMI for healthy eating barriers.[1]

Women

- Fondness of Good Food: 34% (NW), 50% (OB)
- Lack of Willpower: 22% (NW), 28% (OB)
- Time Constraints: 36% (NW), 30% (OB)
- Daily Constraints: 41% (NW), 37% (OB)

Men

- Fondness of Good Food: 44% (NW), 63% (OB)
- Time Constraints: 31% (NW), 25% (OB)
- Daily Constraints: 40% (NW), 35% (OB)

Notice that *fondness of good food* and *lack of willpower* were *more* frequently reported in those classified as OB than NW, while *time constraints* and *daily constraints* were *less* frequently reported. These findings emphasize caution by the practitioner in assuming that those with higher BMI will automatically have more barriers than their lower BMI counterparts, or that all barriers that are perceived hinder progress toward a healthy body weight.

To note, logistic regression revealed that in women, being OB increased odds of self-reporting *fondness of abundant food* (OR = 1.86), *daily habit constraints* (OR = 1.78), *fondness of good food* (OR = 1.63), and *no social support* (OR = 1.62). The only two barriers that increased odds in men were *fondness of good food* (OR = 2.02) and *fondness of abundant food* (OR = 1.64). Such analyses are helpful because they visualize the strength of the hedonistic aspects of unhealthy food consumption (i.e., pursue what is pleasurable), which are theoretically intrinsically motivating and rewarding and act as a barrier against healthy eating. They also stress that simply prescribing healthy food, especially if not perceived as highly pleasant and rewarding, might not be strong enough to overcome the pleasure and reward experienced with unhealthy foods.

9.2.5.3   Socio-demographic Factors

Individual differences of perceived barriers across social-economic class have also been observed, as in a large European Union study ($N = 9,829$) that found differences between high, middle, and low social classes.[26] Approximately 55% of inactive women in low or middle social class perceived *feeling discriminated* as a barrier, compared to 90% in the high social class. The opposite was found with physical activity being *too expensive*, with 50%–60% of low and middle social class reporting this as a barrier compared to less than 10% of high social class. This study also highlighted gender differences across multiple barriers, except for *time*, which was about 50%–60% across men and women, and across all three social classes.

A large cross-sectional study with more than 2,000 adults clarified how socio-demographic variables can influence the perception of barriers to physical.[26] The authors found that marital status and educational level were the strongest predictors for several perceived barriers – those with partners and with a higher education

TABLE 9.1

Odds of Perceiving Barriers to Physical Activity by Marital Status and Education

Barrier	Marital Status *Married or with partner compared to single or no partner (OR)*	Educational Level *Primary/secondary compared to higher education (OR)*
Lack of motivation	0.54	1.76
Fear of injury	0.44	2.70
Lack of resources	0.38	2.78
Lack of energy	0.37	2.56
Lack of skill	0.35	3.27
Lack of social support	0.29	3.81

Source: Data from Herazo-Beltrán et al. (2017).[27]
OR, odds ratio.

perceiving fewer barriers, respectively. As shown in Table 9.1, marital status most prominently *reduced* odds, whereas educational level *improved* odds of perceiving particular barriers.

9.2.5.4 Geographical Location

Perceived barriers can differ by geographical location. In rural areas, for example, a majority of adults have been found to experience more specific barriers to physical activity, such as *fear of stray dogs, no safe place to exercise, access to free or low-cost facilities, discouragement from others,* or *caregiving duties/no childcare.*[4,28,29] Compared to those performing 30 minutes per day of physical activity in rural areas, those not achieving 30 minutes self-reported *feeling less safe walking in their neighborhood* (day or night) and *heavier traffic.*[30] Compared to those meeting FV recommendations, those not meeting FV recommendations noted *less affordable healthy food in neighborhood,* while being similar across other accessibility and affordability barriers.

Compared to those performing 30 minutes per day of physical activity in urban areas, those not achieving 30 minutes self-reported similar barriers of *accessibility* and *availability.*[30] Yet, compared to those meeting FV recommendations, those not meeting FV recommendations noted *less selection of fresh FV, less opportunities to purchase a healthy meal,* and a trend toward *lack of public transportation limiting food store choices.*

Interestingly, the interaction of geography and income reveals that urban, low-income adults ($0–$29,900) self-report higher frequency of *low enjoyment* as a barrier than rural adults.[28] However, both rural and urban adults have overlapping barriers, such as those aforementioned "common" obstacles. In direct comparisons, both groups had similar frequencies of *being self-conscious about appearance, lack of time, too tired, bad weather, not in good health, lack of energy, safety,* and *preference for or confidence in physical activity.*[28,30,31]

9.2.5.5   Experience and Behavior

Finally, there appears to be variation in perceived barriers, based on where the individual is in the behavior adoption process, including their current/past experience with the behavior. For example, in the U.S. Physical Activity Study, Eyler (2003) found that perceived barriers can vary between current walking level groups. A higher frequency of Never Walkers (NeW) reported specific barriers, compared to Regular Walkers (ReW)[32]:

- No Sidewalks: 43% (NeW) vs. 34% (ReW)
- No Time: 26% (NeW) vs. 10% (ReW)
- Too Tired: 23% (NeW) vs. 15% (ReW)
- No Energy: 22% (NeW) vs. 6% (ReW)
- No Motivation: 21% (NeW) vs. 11% (ReW)
- Afraid of Injury: 12% (NeW) vs. 6% (ReW)

The most frequent barriers across all walkers were *no walk/jog trails* (56%–66%), *do not see people exercising* (52%–64%), and *unattended dogs* (40%–45%). Interestingly, one particular reported barrier in Regular Walkers (28%) was not only higher than Never Walkers (16%), but also a barrier resulting from *getting enough exercise at work*.

A few studies have examined how perceived barriers can differ across the stages of change. For example, Rye and colleagues (2009) highlight the uniqueness of the interaction between specific barriers and stages of change for physical activity (Figure 9.1).[25]

While the barrier *don't need more physical activity* did not differ much between the stages, *lack of time* increased with individuals in Action and Maintenance stages. On the other hand, *lack of willpower* is a higher perceived barrier during the early Precontemplation, Contemplation, Preparation stages but drops upon engagement of physical activity (Action and Maintenance).

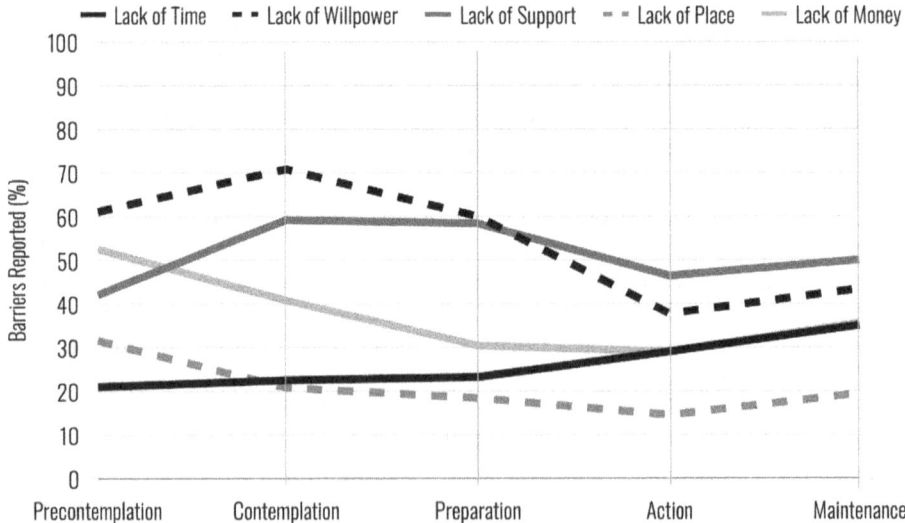

FIGURE 9.1   Perceived barriers to physical activity according to stage of change. (Re-created from data presented in Rye et al., 2009.[25])

In a national study from Norway, Sørensen and Gill (2008) examined how four different groupings of barriers differed across the stage of change in relation to exercise behavior.[33]

- Health Barriers: health problems, need more rest/relaxation, bothered by dizziness
- Practical Barriers: lack of opportunity, nobody to do it with, lack of transport, too expensive
- Affective/Cognitive Barriers: do not think will get anything out of it, not of importance to my health, do not like to be physically active, do not see myself as a physically active person
- Priority Barriers: feel like doing other things, do not have time and energy

Generally, they found, as perhaps would be expected, that the overall perceived mean of barriers was lower across stages, from precontemplation ($\approx$4.5 barriers) to maintenance ($\approx$3 barriers). However, the overall mean difference in various types of barriers between stages was not very pronounced, approximating to about 2 barriers each, with slightly greater variation in differences depending on the age group. Interestingly, perceived barriers in both men and women spiked during the Action stage, highlighting that implementing the lifestyle prescription can bring about an awareness of new barriers that were perhaps not perceived before the behavior change process was initiated.

9.2.5 SUMMARY

These findings reiterate both the individualized nature of barriers and the complexity of factors that can influence one's perception of obstacles to performing healthy lifestyle behaviors. Common barriers are not mutually exclusive, rather they often conglomerate into a mixed effect on perceptions and behavior. They also challenge the assumption that patients or clients must be hindered by the same traditional barriers or obstacles in the same way, and worse, they subsequently dismiss efforts to provide lifestyle prescriptions. Thus, while having a general understanding of barriers can be helpful, the evidence emphasizes the need to assess individual-level barriers with patients and clients, so that individualized applications and adaptations of lifestyle prescriptions can be made in practice.

9.3 PRACTICAL APPLICATION AND CASE STUDIES

Overcoming obstacles is very likely an iterative process, with no single method that works for everyone. Below, we provide brief key steps to consider in practice.

9.3.1 STEP 1: IDENTIFY INDIVIDUAL BARRIERS

9.3.1.1 Identification

The first step is to help the patient or client identify their leading barriers. You can use existing measures[1] for specific behaviors (e.g., barriers for healthy eating, barriers for physical activity), you can create your own (see Section 9.4), or simply have the patient or client list their barriers to specific lifestyle prescriptions (e.g., completed online or in waiting room).

- In the waiting room, patient Karen completes the physical activity barrier scale in Table 9.2, rating *lack of time* as her leading barrier to participating in physical activity. She has also chosen *walking* as her preferred activity.

TABLE 9.2
Example Barrier Assessment for Physical Activity and Healthy Eating

Physical Activity

Directions: Below are common barriers to physical activity. Rate how important of a problem each barrier is against your own physical activity behavior.

Barrier	Not at All a Problem	A Slightly Important Problem	A Moderately Important Problem	A Very Important Problem	An Extremely Important Problem
Lack of time	0	1	2	3	4
Lack of motivation	0	1	2	3	4
Lack of interest/ enjoyment	0	1	2	3	4
Lack of confidence	0	1	2	3	4
Lack of knowledge	0	1	2	3	4
Lack of support	0	1	2	3	4
Lack of options	0	1	2	3	4
Availability/access issues	0	1	2	3	4
Appearance concerns	0	1	2	3	4
Safety concerns	0	1	2	3	4
High cost	0	1	2	3	4
Health/pain/discomfort	0	1	2	3	4
Life/work obligations	0	1	2	3	4
Bad weather	0	1	2	3	4

Do you have any barriers to physical activity that are not listed above? If so, list and rate each one in the spaces below.

Barrier	Not at All a Problem	A Slightly Important Problem	A Moderately Important Problem	A Very Important Problem	An Extremely Important Problem
	0	1	2	3	4
	0	1	2	3	4
	0	1	2	3	4

Healthy Eating

Directions: Below are common barriers to healthy eating. Rate how important of a problem each barrier is against your own physical activity behavior.

Barrier	Not at All a Problem	A Slightly Important Problem	A Moderately Important Problem	A Very Important Problem	An Extremely Important Problem
Lack of time	0	1	2	3	4
Lack of motivation	0	1	2	3	4
Lack of interest/enjoyment	0	1	2	3	4

(Continued)

TABLE 9.2 (*Continued*)
Example Barrier Assessment for Physical Activity and Healthy Eating

Lack of confidence	0	1	2	3	4
Lack of knowledge	0	1	2	3	4
Lack of support	0	1	2	3	4
Lack of options	0	1	2	3	4
Availability/access issues	0	1	2	3	4
High cost	0	1	2	3	4
Preparation time	0	1	2	3	4
Don't like taste of healthy food	0	1	2	3	4
Like taste of unhealthy food	0	1	2	3	4
Family/friends eat unhealthily	0	1	2	3	4

Do you have any barriers to physical activity that are not listed above? If so, list and rate each one in the spaces below.

Barrier	Not at All a Problem	A Slightly Important Problem	A Moderately Important Problem	A Very Important Problem	An Extremely Important Problem
	0	1	2	3	4
	0	1	2	3	4
	0	1	2	3	4

9.3.1.2 Intensity

Identification of each barrier is commonly paired with its *intensity*, which elucidates the potential strength of the barrier to hinder progress. For example, if *lack of time* is the identified barrier, a follow-up question would assess how big/not big, strong/weak, or impactful/not impactful the barrier is to the individual. Most barrier scales include intensity, including our example scale in the Section 9.4.

- Using the scale in Table 9.2, Karen rates *lack of time* at the maximum intensity as an "extremely important problem" to her physical activity behavior.

9.3.1.3 Causes

The specific root causes of barriers can also be assessed. For example, an individual might first report a general *lack of time*, which can then be further explored.

Fixed causes represent those key factors that are commonly embedded in one's life, making them more stable and less flexible to change; so, to better navigate these difficult barriers (having to work long hours, getting kids ready for school, care of aging parent), the fixed causes need to be recognized and autonomy and self-regulatory abilities should be supported.

Flexible causes represent those key factors that are either more transient or specific in their occurrence in one's life, thus having a higher potential for early modification (e.g., when work is busy, during certain times of year, during holidays, or when traveling).

Note: As previously noted, perceived barriers might very likely spike during the Action stage of change. Thus, a baseline perception of barriers might not be indicative of the barriers experienced once the patient or client enacts behavioral efforts. Re-assessing barriers at various times during behavior change could be advantageous to recognize an increase, addition, or change in perceived barriers.

- Noting Karen's leading, *lack of time* barrier, the practitioner asks, "Why is time such a barrier?" Karen shares that she has been having to work late, and then her afternoons are consumed with getting children to extracurricular activities, feeding family, and getting children ready for bed.

9.3.2   Step 2: Make a Plan

Individualizing the lifestyle prescription can help in identifying an appropriate plan of action to overcome the obstacles, beginning with those that are perceived to be most personally meaningful, malleable to change, and that the patient is most confident to change.

- Karen could make a general plan to walk in the mornings before work, 3 days each week for 15–30 minutes. She also notes that getting up early might be an obstacle too, so a plan is also made to walk each Saturday mornings and Sunday afternoons, for now.

9.3.2.1   Action and Coping Plan

Action and coping plans can be beneficial here (see Chapter 7). Coping planning, in particular, helps anticipate barriers that might hinder the patient's implementation of the lifestyle prescription.

- Karen's *action plan* for the upcoming week:
  "*When* I wake up at 6:00 am Thursday morning, *then* I will get ready and immediately go for a 15-minute walk in the neighborhood."
- To help anticipate this key barrier of waking up earlier, Karen's *coping plan* could be:
  "If I sleep too late Thursday morning, then I will go for a 15-minute walk this Saturday in the neighborhood."

9.3.2.2   Help Sheet

Volitional help sheets have been promoted to help in the planning stage by providing patients with various situations (e.g., temptations, barriers) and then choices for solutions (appropriate responses). Such help sheets have been found to be beneficial in improving physical activity, having participants identify situations, and stressing the importance of self-selecting solutions.[34]

- For Karen's *Situation*: "If I'm tempted not to be physically active, because I feel I don't have the time…"
- Her chosen *Solutions*: (full volitional help sheet provided by Armitage and Arden, 2010[34])
  - "…then I will remember how warnings about the health hazards of inactivity move me emotionally."
  - "…then I will think about how my inactivity affects those people who are close to me."
  - "…then I will tell myself that being more physically active would make me a healthier, happier person to be around."
  - "…then I will tell myself that I am being good to myself by taking care of my body in this way."
  - "…then I will make myself do some physical activity anyway, because I know I will feel better afterward."
  - "…then I will make myself do something, because some physical activity is better than none at all."

Also, de Mestral and colleagues (2016) provide other tips for health practitioners to help patients plan to overcome common barriers to healthy eating[1]:

- Provide healthier products and cheaper alternatives with similar nutritional value.
- Cover medical nutrition therapy as part of treatment and prevention.
- Provide healthy ready-to-eat meals.
- Promote time spent preparing meals.
- Create time slots for cooking and eating, especially for patients.
- Increase number of healthy and tasty meal options.
- Promote healthy foods as tasty foods.
- Promote cooking methods to improve taste.
- Provide counsel and advice on methods of behavior change at healthcare facilities.
- Advertise and promote different options of healthy foods and ways to eat them.
- Promote behavior change as part of healthier, more enjoyable lifestyle.
- Work closely with patients to increase self-confidence and empower them to eat healthier foods.

9.3.3   STEP 3: PROVIDE FEEDBACK

Providing informative feedback to patients can help diagnose if specific plans were successful or not in overcoming obstacles. This allows for problem solving and building of confidence (self-efficacy) in one's ability to continue in or modify a lifestyle prescription in the face of obstacles.

9.3.4 STEP 4: REFER TO COMMUNITY PARTNERS

Helping patients and clients overcome obstacles to initiate and maintain lifestyle prescriptions is not a simple task, this requires time and assistance from a lifestyle medicine team, including in practice when available (e.g., medical assistants, health coaches, exercise physiologists), as well as community resources, such as healthy lifestyle programs offered by the local Extension service and other community, or public health programs aimed at teaching barrier management.

9.4 MEASUREMENT STRATEGIES

There are numerous ways to measure barriers to healthy lifestyle. When reading the research, it is important to remember that the authors of separate studies operationalize and assess barriers in different ways. Thus, when taking a research-based approach, knowing how and which barriers were measured will better elucidate the application of the findings in a clinical population as well as give healthcare practitioners a source of a measurement to use in their practice.

There are also several validated scales of perceived barriers (and benefits) to both physical activity and healthy eating, or more specifically, FV intake. While these can be a good start, all will be limited in the number and type of barriers assessed. Thus, it can be beneficial to include the barriers that are most pertinent to your practice. We provide in Table 9.2 an example barrier assessment that includes the most common barriers reviewed here, but this tool can be easily tailored to any practice.

- Barriers to Healthy Eating Scale[35]
- Exercise Benefits/Barriers Scale[36]
- Exercise Barriers Self-Efficacy Scale [www.epl.illinois.edu/barse][37,38]

9.5 SUMMARY

To fully understand behavior change, one must honor, address, and become comfortable with obstacles and barriers to change. Everyone has their own behavior change journey with varying obstacles and barriers. As someone who is working to empower individuals to adopt and sustain healthy lifestyles, it is important to be comfortable discussing obstacles. Research findings guide effective ways to counsel individuals about barriers and provide scales to assess barriers in practice. Identifying barriers is critical and helping to find strategies around the barriers is equally important. Knowing the intensity and the cause of a barrier can help in developing a plan around a given barrier. To empower people to change, the practitioner needs to be comfortable with conversations about both the details of barriers and the many options that can be employed to overcome them. The following Key Takeaways are provided to help guide practitioners.

9.6 KEY TAKEAWAYS

- Remain mindful that perceived barriers are dependent on several factors including (but not limited to) age, sex, marital status, and education level.
- Identify individual barriers and their intensity.
- Formulate an action plan that addresses perceived barriers within the lifestyle prescription, and then provide constructive feedback to help build barrier self-efficacy.
- Remember to check in with patients/clients when they begin managing perceived barriers, as obstacles can completely change or vary in intensity throughout the behavior change process.

9.7 RESOURCES

We were unable to review all of the research on specific obstacles (barriers) for every subgroup. However, the research has largely moved beyond general barriers to specific groups of people and can be helpful in understanding individual, condition-specific barriers encountered in healthcare practice. As a resource, Table 9.3 provides a recent list of such studies.

TABLE 9.3

Evidence Review List for Physical Activity and Healthy Eating Barriers of Specific Subgroups within Healthcare

Physical Activity

Arthritis

Rheumatoid	Veldhuijzen et al. (2015)[39]
Knee/hip osteoarthritis	Kanavaki et al. (2017)[40]

Autism Healy et al. (2021)[41]

Autoimmune Disease Sharif et al. (2018)[42]

Cancer

With breast cancer (in treatment)	Lavallée et al. (2019)[43]
With ovarian cancer	Morrison et al. (2020)[44]
With prostate cancer	Fox et al. (2019)[45]
History of breast/endometrial	Burse et al. (2020)[46]
Of cancer practitioners discussing	Keogh et al. (2017)[47]

Children/Youth

Young children	Hesketh et al. (2017)[48]
Disabilities	Mckenzie et al. (2021)[49]
Cystic fibrosis	Denford et al. (2020)[50]
Intellectual disabilities	McGarty and Mellville (2018)[51]

Dementia van Alphen et al. (2016)[52]

Diabetes

Type 1 diabetes	Brennan et al. (2021)[53]

(Continued)

TABLE 9.3 (*Continued*)
Evidence Review List for Physical Activity and Healthy Eating Barriers of Specific Subgroups within Healthcare

Pregnancy	
During	Harrison et al. (2018),[54]
	Coll et al. (2017)[55]
Postpartum	Ryan et al. (2021)[56]
Pulmonary Rehabilitation	Robinson et al. (2018)[57]
Healthy Eating	
Children/youth	Shepherd et al. (2006)[58]
Pregnancy – postpartum	Ryan et al. (2021)[56]
Physical challenges	Wetherill et al. (2021)[59]

NOTE

1 Some measures are copyright protected and require permission to use or reproduce.

REFERENCES

1. de Mestral, Carlos, Silvia Stringhini, and Pedro Marques-Vidal. "Barriers to Healthy Eating in Switzerland: A Nationwide Study." *Clinical Nutrition*, 35, no. 6 (2016): 1490–1498.
2. Kelly, Sarah, Steven Martin, Isla Kuhn, Andy Cowan, Carol Brayne, and Louise Lafortune. "Barriers and Facilitators to the Uptake and Maintenance of Healthy Behaviours by People at Mid-life: A Rapid Systematic Review." *PLoS One*, 11, no. 1 (2016).
3. McMorrow, Liam, Anne Ludbrook, Jennie I. Macdiarmid, and Damilola Olajide. "Perceived Barriers towards Healthy Eating and Their Association with Fruit and Vegetable Consumption." *Journal of Public Health*, 39, no. 2 (2017): 330–338.
4. Osuji, Thearis, Sarah Lovegreen, Michael Elliott, and Ross C. Brownson. "Barriers to Physical Activity among Women in the Rural Midwest." *Women & Health*, 44, no. 1 (2016): 41–55.
5. de Pinho, Maria Gabriela Matias, Joreintje Mackenbach, Hélène Charreire, Jean-Michel Oppert, Helga Bárdos, Ketevan Glonti, Harry Rutter, Sofie Compernolle, Ilse De Bourdeaudhuij, Joline W.J. Beulens, Johannes Burg, Jeroen Lakerveld. "Exploring the Relationship between Perceived Barriers to Healthy Eating and Dietary Behaviours in European Adults." *European Journal of Nutrition*, 57, no. 5 (2018): 1761–1770.
6. Sogari, Giovanni, Catalina Velez-Argumedo, Miguel I. Gómez, and Cristina Mora. "College Students and Eating Habits: A Study Using an Ecological Model for Healthy Behavior." *Nutrients*, 10, no. 12 (2018): 1823.
7. de Mestral, Carlos, Saman Khalatbari-Soltani, Silvia Stringhini, and Pedro Marques-Vidal. "Fifteen-year Trends in the Prevalence of Barriers to Healthy Eating in a High-income Country." *The American Journal of Clinical Nutrition*, 105, no. 3 (2017): 660–668.
8. Munt, Alex E., Stephanie R. Partridge, and M. Allman-Farinelli. "The Barriers and Enablers of Healthy Eating Among Young Adults: A Missing Piece of the Obesity Puzzle: A Scoping Review." *Obesity Reviews*, 18, no. 1 (2017): 1–17.

9. Hoare, Erin, Bill Stavreski, Garry L. Jennings, and Bronwyn A. Kingwell. "Exploring Motivation and Barriers to Physical Activity among Active and Inactive Australian Adults." *Sports*, 5, no. 3 (2017): 47.

10. Joseph, Rodney P., Barbara E. Ainsworth, Colleen Keller, and Joan E. Dodgson. "Barriers to Physical Activity among African American Women: An Integrative Review of the Literature." *Women & Health*, 55, no. 6 (2015): 679–699.

11. Spiteri, Karl, David Broom, Amira Hassan Bekhet, John Xerri de Caro, Bob Laventure, and Kate Grafton. "Barriers and Motivators of Physical Activity Participation in Middle-aged and Older Adults—A Systematic Review." *Journal of Aging and Physical Activity*, 27, no. 6 (2019): 929–944.

12. Heesch, Kristiann C., and Louise C. Mâsse. "Lack of Time for Physical Activity: Perception or Reality for African American and Hispanic Women?" *Women & Health*, 39, no. 3 (2004): 45–62.

13. Escoto, Kamisha Hamilton, Melissa Nelson Laska, Nicole Larson, Dianne Neumark-Sztainer, and Peter J. Hannan. "Work Hours and Perceived Time Barriers to Healthful Eating Among Young Adults." *American Journal of Health Behavior*, 36, no. 6 (2012): 786–796.

14. Glasgow, Russell E. *Perceived Barriers to Self-management and Preventive Behaviors*. National Cancer Institute, Bethesda, MD. (2008). Retrieved from: https://cancercontrol. cancer.gov/sites/default/files/2020-06/barriers.pdf.

15. Michaelidou, Nina, George Christodoulides, and Katerina Torova. "Determinants of healthy eating: A cross-national study on motives and barriers." *International Journal of Consumer Studies*, 36, no. 1 (2012): 17–22.

16. Ashton, Lee M., Melinda J. Hutchesson, Megan E. Rollo, Philip J. Morgan, and Clare E. Collins. "Motivators and Barriers to Engaging in Healthy Eating and Physical Activity: A Cross-sectional Survey in Young Adult Men." *American Journal of Men's Health*, 11, no. 2 (2017): 330–343.

17. Wang, Jing, Lei Ye, Yaguang Zheng, and Lora E. Burke. "Impact of Perceived Barriers to Healthy Eating on Diet and Weight in a 24-month Behavioral Weight Loss Trial." *Journal of Nutrition Education and Behavior*, 47, no. 5 (2015): 432–436.

18. Schoeny, Michael E., Louis Fogg, Susan W. Buchholz, Arlene Miller, and JoEllen Wilbur. "Barriers to Physical Activity as Moderators of Intervention Effects." *Preventive Medicine Reports*, 5 (2017): 57–64.

19. Reichert, Felipe F., Aluísio JD Barros, Marlos R. Domingues, and Pedro C. Hallal. "The Role of Perceived Personal Barriers to Engagement in Leisure-time Physical Activity." *American Journal of Public Health*, 97, no. 3 (2007): 515–519.

20. Ross, Anna M., and Trish Melzer. "Beliefs as Barriers to Healthy Eating and Physical Activity." *Australian Journal of Psychology*, 68, no. 4 (2016): 251–260.

21. Brown, Wendy J., Kristiann C. Heesch, and Yvette D. Miller. "Life Events and Changing Physical Activity Patterns in Women at Different Life Stages." *Annals of Behavioral Medicine*, 37, no. 3 (2009): 294–305.

22. Shin, Cha-Nam, Young-Shin Lee, and Michael Belyea. "Physical Activity, Benefits, and Barriers across the Aging Continuum." *Applied Nursing Research*, 44 (2018): 107–112.

23. Sequeira, Sebastião, Cristina Cruz, Diogo Pinto, Luís Santos, and Adilson Marques. "Prevalence of Barriers for Physical Activity in Adults According to Gender and Socioeconomic Status." *British Journal of Sports Medicine*, 45, no. 15 (2011): A18–A19.

24. Ball, Kylie, David Crawford, and Neville Owen. "Obesity as a Barrier to Physical Activity." *Australian and New Zealand Journal of Public Health*, 24, no. 3 (2000): 331–333.

25. Rye, James A., Sheila L. Rye, Irene Tessaro, and Jay Coffindaffer. "Perceived Barriers to Physical Activity According to Stage of Change and Body Mass Index in the West Virginia Wisewoman Population." *Women's Health Issues: Official Publication of the Jacobs Institute of Women's Health*, 19, no. 2 (2009): 126–134.

26. Moreno-Llamas, Antonio, Jesús García-Mayor, and De la Cruz-Sánchez. "Physical Activity Barriers According to Social Stratification in Europe." *International Journal of Public Health*, 65, no. 8 (2020): 1477–1484.

27. Herazo-Beltrán, Yaneth, Yisel Pinillos, José Vidarte, Estela Crissien, Damaris Suarez, and Rafael García. "Predictors of Perceived Barriers to Physical Activity in the General Adult Population: A Cross-sectional Study." *Brazilian Journal of Physical Therapy*, 21, no. 1 (2017): 44–50.

28. Pelletier, Chelsea A., Nicole White, Annie Duchesne, and Larine Sluggett. "Barriers to Physical Activity for Adults in Rural and Urban Canada: A Cross-sectional Comparison." *SSM-Population Health*, 16 (2021).

29. Reed, Jill R., Bernice C. Yates, Julia Houfek, Wayne Briner, Kendra K. Schmid, and Carol Pullen. "A Review of Barriers to Healthy Eating in Rural and Urban Adults." *Online Journal of Rural Nursing and Health Care*, 16, no. 1 (2016): 122–153.

30. Becker, Tyler Brian, Dawn Contreras, and Olivia Porth. "Differences in Eating and Physical Activity Behaviors, and Perceived Accessibility and Availability Barriers between Midwestern Rural and Urban Adults." *Journal of Hunger & Environmental Nutrition*, (2021): 1–16.

31. Wilcox, Sara, Cynthia Castro, Abby C. King, Robyn Housemann, and Ross C. Brownson. "Determinants of Leisure Time Physical Activity in Rural Compared with Urban Older and Ethnically Diverse Women in the United States." *Journal of Epidemiology & Community Health*, 54, no. 9 (2000): 667–672.

32. Eyler, Amy A. "Personal, Social, and Environmental Correlates of Physical Activity in Rural Midwestern White Women." *American Journal of Preventive Medicine*, 25, no. 3 (2003): 86–92.

33. Sørensen, Marit, and Diane L. Gill. "Perceived Barriers to Physical Activity across Norwegian Adult Age Groups, Gender and Stages of Change." *Scandinavian Journal of Medicine & Science in Sports*, 18, no. 5 (2008): 651–663.

34. Armitage, Christopher J., and Madelynne A. Arden. "A Volitional Help Sheet to Increase Physical Activity in People with Low Socioeconomic Status: A Randomised Exploratory Trial." *Psychology and Health*, 25, no. 10 (2010): 1129–1145.

35. Sun, Ran, Jeffrey M. Rohay, Susan M. Sereika, Yaguang Zheng, Yang Yu, and Lora E. Burke. "Psychometric Evaluation of the Barriers to Healthy Eating Scale: Results from Four Independent Weight Loss Studies." *Obesity*, 27, no. 5 (2019): 700–706.

36. Sechrist, Karen R., Susan Noble Walker, and Nola J. Pender. "Development and Psychometric Evaluation of the Exercise Benefits/Barriers Scale." *Research in Nursing & Health*, 10, no. 6 (1987): 357–365.

37. McAuley, Edward. "The Role of Efficacy Cognitions in the Prediction of Exercise Behavior in Middle-Aged Adults." *Journal of Behavioral Medicine*, 15, no. 1 (1992): 65–88.

38. Rogers, Laura Q., Kerry S. Courneya, Steve Verhulst, Steve Markwell, Victor Lanzotti, and Prabodh Shah. "Exercise Barrier and Task Self-Efficacy in Breast Cancer Patients during Treatment." *Supportive Care in Cancer*, 14, no. 1 (2006): 84–90.

39. Veldhuijzen, van Zanten, J. C. S. Jet, Peter C. Rouse, Elizabeth D. Hale, Nikos Ntoumanis, George S. Metsios, Joan L. Duda, and George D. Kitas. "Perceived Barriers, Facilitators and Benefits for Regular Physical Activity and Exercise in Patients with Rheumatoid Arthritis: A Review of the Literature." *Sports Medicine*, 45, no. 10 (2015): 1401–1412.

40. Kanavaki, Archontissa M., Alison Rushton, Nikolaos Efstathiou, Asma Alrushud, Rainer Klocke, Abhishek, and Joan L. Duda. "Barriers and Facilitators of Physical Activity in Knee and Hip Osteoarthritis: A Systematic Review of Qualitative Evidence." *BMJ Open*, 7, no. 12 (2017): e017042.

41. Healy, Sean, Benjamin Brewer, Paige Laxton, Brittany Powers, Julie Daly, Joseph McGuire, and Freda Patterson. "Brief Report: Perceived Barriers to Physical Activity among a National Sample of Autistic Adults." *Journal of Autism and Developmental Disorders*, (2021): 1–9.

42. Sharif, K., A. Watad, N. L. Bragazzi, M. Lichtbroun, H. Amital, and Y. Shoenfeld. "Physical Activity and Autoimmune Diseases: Get Moving and Manage the Disease." *Autoimmunity Reviews*, 17, no. 1 (2018): 53–72.

43. Lavallée, Jacqueline F., Shanara Abdin, James Faulkner, and Margaret Husted. "Barriers and Facilitators to Participating in Physical Activity for Adults with Breast Cancer Receiving Adjuvant Treatment: A Qualitative Metasynthesis." *Psycho-Oncology*, 28, no. 3 (2019): 468–476.

44. Morrison, Kittani S., Catherine Paterson, Celeste E. Coltman, and Kellie Toohey. "What Are the Barriers and Enablers to Physical Activity Participation in Women with Ovarian Cancer? A Rapid Review of the Literature." *Seminars in Oncology Nursing*, 36, no. 5 (2020): 151069.

45. Fox, Louis, Theresa Wiseman, Declan Cahill, Katharina Beyer, Nicola Peat, Elke Rammant, and Mieke Van Hemelrijck. "Barriers and Facilitators to Physical Activity in Men with Prostate Cancer: A Qualitative and Quantitative Systematic Review." *Psycho-Oncology*, 28, no. 12 (2019): 2270–2285.

46. Burse, Natasha R., Nishat Bhuiyan, Scherezade K. Mama, and Kathryn H. Schmitz. "Physical Activity Barriers and Resources among Black Women with a History of Breast and Endometrial Cancer: A Systematic Review." *Journal of Cancer Survivorship*, 14, no. 4 (2020): 556–577.

47. Keogh, Justin WL., Alicia Olsen, Michael Climstein, Sally Sargeant, and Lynnette Jones. "Benefits and Barriers of Cancer Practitioners Discussing Physical Activity with Their Cancer Patients." *Journal of Cancer Education*, 32, no. 1 (2017): 11–15.

48. Hesketh, Kathryn R., Rajalakshmi Lakshman, and Esther MF van Sluijs. "Barriers and Facilitators to Young Children's Physical Activity and Sedentary Behaviour: A Systematic Review and Synthesis of Qualitative Literature." *Obesity Reviews*, 18, no. 9 (2017): 987–1017.

49. Mckenzie, Georgia, Claire Willis, and Nora Shields. "Barriers and Facilitators of Physical Activity Participation for Young People and Adults with Childhood-Onset Physical Disability: A Mixed Methods Systematic Review." *Developmental Medicine & Child Neurology*, 63, no. 8 (2021): 914–924.

50. Denford, Sarah, Samantha van Beurden, Paul O'Halloran, and Craig Anthony Williams. "Barriers and Facilitators to Physical Activity among Children, Adolescents, and Young Adults with Cystic Fibrosis: A Systematic Review and Thematic Synthesis of Qualitative Research." *BMJ Open*, 10, no. 2 (2020): e035261.

51. McGarty, Arlene M., and Craig A. Melville. "Parental Perceptions of Facilitators and Barriers to Physical Activity for Children with Intellectual Disabilities: A Mixed Methods Systematic Review." *Research in Developmental Disabilities*, 73 (2018): 40–57.

52. van Alphen, Helena J.M., Tibor Hortobagyi, and Marieke JG van Heuvelen. "Barriers, Motivators, and Facilitators of Physical Activity in Dementia Patients: A Systematic Review." *Archives of Gerontology and Geriatrics*, 66 (2016): 109–118.

53. Brennan, Marian C., Janie A. Brown, Nikos Ntoumanis, and Gavin D. Leslie. "Barriers and Facilitators of Physical Activity Participation in Adults Living with Type 1 Diabetes: A Systematic Scoping Review." *Applied Physiology, Nutrition, and Metabolism*, 46, no. 2 (2021): 95–107.

54. Harrison, Anne L., Nicholas F. Taylor, Nora Shields, and Helena C. Frawley. "Attitudes, Barriers and Enablers to Physical Activity in Pregnant Women: A Systematic Review." *Journal of Physiotherapy*, 64, no. 1 (2018): 24–32.

55. Coll, Carolina VN, Marlos R. Domingues, Helen Gonçalves, and Andréa D. Bertoldi. "Perceived Barriers to Leisure-Time Physical Activity during Pregnancy: A Literature Review of Quantitative and Qualitative Evidence." *Journal of Science and Medicine in Sport*, 20, no. 1 (2017): 17–25.

56. Ryan, Rachel A., Hope Lappen, and Jessica Dauz Bihuniak. "Barriers and Facilitators to Healthy Eating and Physical Activity Postpartum: A Qualitative Systematic Review." *Journal of the Academy of Nutrition and Dietetics*, 122, no. 3 (2021): 602–613.

57. Robinson, Hayley, Veronika Williams, Ffion Curtis, Christopher Bridle, and Arwel W. Jones. "Facilitators and Barriers to Physical Activity Following Pulmonary Rehabilitation in COPD: A Systematic Review of Qualitative Studies." *NPJ Primary Care Respiratory Medicine*, 28, no. 1 (2018): 1–12.

58. Shepherd, Jonathan, Angela Harden, Rebecca Rees, Ginny Brunton, Jo Garcia, Sandy Oliver, and Ann Oakley. "Young People and Healthy Eating: A Systematic Review of Research on Barriers and Facilitators." *Health Education Research*, 21, no. 2 (2006): 239–257.

59. Wetherill, Marianna S., Ashten R. Duncan, Hartley Bowman, Reagan Collins, Natalie Santa-Pinter, Morgan Jackson, Catherine M. Lynn, Katherine Prentice, and Mary Isaacson. "Promoting Nutrition Equity for Individuals with Physical Challenges: A Systematic Review of Barriers and Facilitators to Healthy Eating." *Preventive Medicine*, 153 (2021): 106723.

10 Using Strengths

Mark D. Faries, PhD, Marcus W. Kilpatrick,
PhD, and Miquela G. Smith, MPH

10.1 INTRODUCTION

In its simplest form, self-regulation is a process of monitoring and changing behavior to stay in line with a goal, such as a lifestyle prescription. In its more complex form, "Self-regulation is the ability to flexibly activate, monitor, inhibit, persevere and/or adapt one's behavior, attention, emotions and cognitive strategies in response to direction from internal cues, environmental stimuli and feedback from others, in an attempt to attain personally-relevant goals" (p. 835).[1] Self-regulation can also be visualized as a system of gears, which represent the self-regulatory abilities or skills that must be acquired, activated, and maintained by the patient, such as self-monitoring, goal setting/reviewing, implementation intentions, action and coping planning, barrier and problem solving, time management, receiving personalized feedback, inhibitory control, emotional control and regulation, self-talk, and cognitive/positive reframing.

Ideally, the practitioner and the lifestyle medicine team would work to add, develop, and "oil" these abilities in their patients. However, time is limited. Also, two recent meta-reviews of meta-analyses aggregating the results of interventions to improve health behavior, including diet and physical activity, only to find the effectiveness of self-regulatory behavior change techniques was low to moderate and inconsistent.[2,3] While some inconsistencies are attributable to methodological issues of the limited research, such findings also highlight that successfully self-regulating health behavior is fraught with challenges, and wanting for new solutions. In this chapter, we highlight two simplified opportunities for the practitioner to improve successful self-regulation of lifestyle prescriptions when little time is available for the patient–practitioner interaction: *the trigger* and *the response*.

10.2 EVIDENCE SUMMARY

10.2.1 THE TRIGGER

Considering self-regulation as a process of monitoring and changing behavior *when normalcy is interrupted* – the patient–provider interaction, screenings, and/or clinical or behavioral diagnoses can interrupt the normalcy by providing awareness of a personal discrepancy. According to the feedback processing model of self-regulation, a desire to change is proposed to be initiated with a perceived discrepancy about oneself in relation to a standard[4] – such as not meeting a clinical standard in blood work, dietary intake, or physical activity behavior, or a diagnosis of overweight,

DOI: 10.1201/9781003161226-10

hypertension, or diabetes. The discrepancy is thought to act as a spark or *trigger* for subsequent efforts to reduce the discrepancy and/or any associated negative feelings (or restore positive feelings). Other common approaches, such as those based on Dissonance Theory or Self-Determination Theory (e.g., motivational interviewing), also emphasize the importance of developing discrepancies to hopefully spark behavior change.

Medical triggers are those sparks for change that are related to a diagnosis of risk and health concerns. Triggering events for weight loss have been cited in successful losers and maintainers of at least 10% of initial body weight for greater than one year.[5] Similar findings have been found in smoking cessation literature, with medically related triggering events (e.g., myocardial infarction) substantially increasing one's odds of quitting.[6] However, not all perceived discrepancies become a trigger for positive change. Two patients can be presented with an identical discrepancy for high blood sugar at 110 mg/dL and a diagnosis of prediabetes, of which are then linked to their unhealthy eating behavior. *Patient A* is motivated to change, but *Patient B* is not. We might ask,

Why are certain discrepancies perceived triggers for change, but others are not?

The discrepancies that trigger positive behavior change and self-regulation of behavior are those that likely have connection to personal meaning, values, and beliefs. In support of this, medical triggers are theorized to be more effective if they transcend into a deeper meaning or reason for that specific patient.[7] For example, the most common triggering events for control behaviors are those related to diagnosis of personal health concerns, improving appearance, and emotional or ongoing discontent.[5,8,9]

The next challenge for the practitioner is determining if a health concern or discrepancy is *personally meaningful* to the patient, which is a precursor to transforming a discrepancy or health concern into a medical trigger for healthy behavior change. We might ask,

Why are certain discrepancies perceived as meaningful, but not others are not?

There are numerous proposed answers to this question. However, there are far fewer solutions that translate to clinical applications when there is limited time for patient–practitioner interaction. We propose three considerations: needs, values, and past experiences.

10.2.1.1   Needs

Maslow's hierarchy of needs proposes that people seek and self-regulate behavior to satisfy progressively higher human needs, from *physiological* to *self-actualization*. "I should then say simply that a healthy man is primarily motivated by his needs to develop and actualize his fullest potentialities and capacities" (p. 394).[10] Progression through needs gratification is holistic, where a person, at a given time, has a certain percentage of needs met at each level.

- *Physiological Needs*: Homeostasis (e.g., water content in blood, nutrition, body temperature); physiological drives, particularly for sex and survival, such as food and drink, shelter, and clothing.
- *Safety Needs*: Safety concerns for oneself and family; protection from danger (e.g., elements, crime, fear); financial concerns; emergency concerns (e.g., war, disease, natural catastrophes).
- *Love Needs*: Give and receive love (not synonymous with sex), affection, and a sense of belongingness and relatedness.
- *Esteem Needs*: Desire for stable, high evaluation of self, respect, worth, and self-esteem; confidence, achievement, adequacy; reputation, prestige.
- *Self-Actualization Needs*: Self-fulfillment, to become actualized in one's potential, capable of being; doing what one is fitted for; "what a man *can* be, he *must* be."

Unfortunately, there is limited research on utilizing the hierarchy of needs in clinical or health coaching practice, with the noted exception of hospice care,[11] hemodialysis care,[12] type 1 diabetes,[13] a model for pharmacy,[14] healthcare employees,[15] medical resident wellness,[16] and an intervention for coronary heart disease surgery.[17] In summary, lifestyle prescriptions are not limited to lower-level need gratification rather can be modified to help fulfill and progress to higher-level needs. For example:

Physiological and/or *Safety Needs*. Lifestyle prescriptions can help gratify such needs through improving disease risk factors and financial concerns (e.g., lower medication costs, healthy eating on a budget), yet are challenged by gratification of physiological needs in other ways, such as craving for high fat, high sugar food or conserving energy, will likely challenge exchanging routine behaviors of unhealthy foods and physical inactivity with healthy foods (lower in fat and sugar) and physical activity (does not conserve energy).

Love Needs. Lifestyle prescriptions can help gratify love and belonging needs (e.g., group activity or cooking sessions, walking groups, social activities, cooking with family, actively serving the community). There are also benefits of prescribing meaningful social interactions, such as community groups or events and religious participation[18–20] – especially when considering that the effect sizes of church service attendance on all-cause mortality can be similar to those from other important preventative lifestyle prescriptions, including physical activity, tobacco smoking cessation, and consumption of fruits and vegetables.[21]

Self-Esteem and Self-Actualization Needs: Lifestyle prescriptions can help gratify such needs when they are modified to meet patients where they are, and they can also build confidence and hope in face of challenges as well as provide connection to and opportunities for improving self-worth, value, and personal strengths to achieve their highest personally meaningful purpose in life. To note, this view of self-esteem need not be consistent with the ancient, *negative* view of self-esteem (i.e., vainglory, self-love; *philautos* in Greek), which is more of a mindless, impassioned love for one's own self and body – begetting pride, and expressing domination and control by pleasures and passions. Similarly, self-esteem in this context is not necessarily encompassing a spiritual reality (e.g., self-glory to please man rather than God), although it can include such a perspective in those who see the process toward self-actualization as one of growth – as an acorn with freedom to grow toward its full potential as an oak tree.

10.2.1.2 Values

Like the hierarchy of needs, the perceived view of oneself (self-concept), evaluation of oneself (self-esteem), and value of oneself (self-worth) are conceptualized to exist atop a hierarchy of lower-level domains. For example, global or overall self-esteem is made up of several **domains**, such as *professional competence, social competence,* and *physical self-worth.*[22] For the domain of *physical self-worth,* the **subdomains** are commonly *physical condition, sport competence, attractiveness* of one's body, *physical strength,* and *perceived health.* The hierarchy can even extend further into the patient's attitude of the subdomain, how they compare to others or their ideal self, and how important they perceive the subdomain.[23]

Generally, our overall view and evaluation of self is contingent on meeting certain standards within valued subdomains. As summarized by Crocker and colleagues (2006), "Contingencies of self-worth can facilitate self-regulation because people are highly motivated to succeed and avoid failure in domains of contingency. However, because boosts in self-esteem are pleasurable and drops in self-esteem are painful, protection, maintenance, and enhancement of self-esteem can become the overriding goal. Several pitfalls for self-regulation can result, especially when tasks are difficult and failure is likely" (p. 1749).[24]

Common screenings, health concerns, and diagnoses can activate contingencies if they are perceived to threaten *a valued (personally meaningful)* subdomain of the hierarchy. Theories of social self-preservation suggest that when threatened in this way, behavior is self-regulated in order to restore the perceived integrity and view of self.[25,26] From this perspective, the role of the practitioner can be to help this restoration process, positively impacting the patient's past, present, and future view of self. "Our drive to make meaning from our experiences shapes and is shaped by our self-concept," (p. 300).[27]

One way to do this is by helping connect the discrepancy and a healthy restoration process to valued subdomains. For example, if a patient is told by her practitioner that she is 15 pounds over ideal body weight – (1) is this diagnosis a threat to any one of these subdomains? and (2) if so, which one(s)? If the practitioner emphasizes the threat to her *health,* but that is not the primary subdomain of value, then she might not be as motivated to follow the lifestyle prescription. However, if she values *body attractiveness* and *physical conditioning* (or *professional, social, spiritual,* and so on) and this excess weight diagnosis is a perceived threat to one or both subdomains, then she might choose to self-regulate behavior as a means of restoring view of self – albeit, not always with the healthiest choices, of which the practitioner should be attentive.[7,28]

In summary, within routine care, medical triggers can threaten subdomains of self that connect to a patient's overall value and self-worth. The practitioner can benefit self-regulation by knowing what (sub)domains of self-worth are most valued by the patient, so that lifestyle prescriptions can be made in supportive, compatible fashion, and counter any unhealthy behaviors chosen by the patient to restore self-worth. Also, engagement in lifestyle prescriptions can positively alter perceived value at the lower levels of the hierarchy, as has been shown with physical activity participation improving physical self-worth, and subsequently overall self-esteem in adults and adolescents.[29–31]

10.2.1.3 Past Experiences

Patients will interpret their response to medical triggers and lifestyle prescriptions through the lens of their past experiences. Has the patient had this diagnosis before? Has the patient attempted to change before, and if so, was it believed to be successful? Is the patient confident he or she can change? What is his or her attitude of a healthy lifestyle or specific behavior: boring-enjoyable, difficult-easy, not helpful-helpful?

Past experiences can be *hedonic*, informing each patient if enacting the lifestyle prescription will be pleasurable or painful, of which they might then approach or avoid, respectively. Past experiences can also be *reflective*, incorporating values, attitudes, feelings, and fears. Past socio-cultural and environmental factors are also incorporated into interpretation, such as effects of experiencing famine/poverty, lack of childhood consumption of fruit and vegetables, and culture/tradition on current healthy eating behavior.[32] As shown in the next section, both hedonic and reflective interpretations of past experiences and responses to physical activity are powerful shapers of current and future behavior.[33] Adverse childhood experiences (ACEs) can have adverse effects on numerous lifestyle behaviors, as well as an independent predictor of health outcomes (see Box 10.1).

BOX 10.1   ADVERSE CHILDHOOD EXPERIENCES (ACES) AND LIFESTYLE PRESCRIPTION CONSIDERATIONS

We have noted that patients bring their current and past experiences with them to the patient–practitioner interaction, which can impact their response to health concerns or discrepancies, as well as their experience of engagement with a lifestyle prescription. Adverse Childhood Experiences (ACEs) have recently been highlighted for consideration in lifestyle medicine, particularly as an important downstream cause of unhealthy lifestyles and disease risk.[35,38,39] For example:

Patient C has had "inconsistent" past experiences with healthy eating, although she enjoys fruits and vegetables. She lives in a supportive environment with moderate access to healthy foods, but has experienced adverse trauma in childhood (distal causes). She now has high levels of stress, learned helplessness from failed past attempts to lose weight, and is in a dissociative state (medial causes). She uses junk food to cope and extended periods of caloric restriction, resulting in binge eating and weight cycling (proximal causes).

ACEs provide a complex and delicate situation for lifestyle prescriptions, which require a more careful and nuanced response to use the strengths of the patient or client. ACEs have been associated with a propensity to adverse health behaviors and treatment non-compliance.[38] Primary care interventions to improve health in adults survivors of ACEs have been reviewed,[40] with the authors concluding that the most consistent positive outcomes were seen with cognitive behavioral therapy (CBT), especially those developed specifically for ACEs. In general, CBT seeks to identify and modify maladaptive thoughts and behaviors to improve overall psychological health, and in turn, physical health through lifestyle changes.

While ACEs-specific CBT and more advanced care is beyond the scope of this chapter, we use this opportunity to: (1) highlight the need for more research of ACEs and expansion of strength-based approaches in lifestyle medicine practice. Below, as a starting point, we highlight six basic principles for healthcare practitioners to consider when engaging patients and/or clients where trauma could be a contributing factor for lifestyle-related disease(s).

Trauma-Informed Approach	Medical Health Providers (e.g., MDs, DOs, RNs, FNP)	Other Health Professionals (e.g., PTs, RD/LDs, fitness)
Safety	The environment promotes a sense of safety and calm. Staff and clients feel physically and psychologically safe. Providers ask permission before touching a patient/client.	
Trustworthiness and transparency	Decisions about the patient's care are conducted with transparency and with the goal of building and maintaining trust.	
Collaboration and mutuality	Power dynamics are minimized, and patient/client is asked about concerns and to provide input during treatment planning and goal setting.	
Empowerment, voice, and choice	Individuals' strengths and experiences are built upon. Providers view patients as partners in designing lifestyle behavior modifications plans, with their own contributing voice, and not as "subjects of care." Patients are provided with choices and autonomy support in making those choices (for example, see the brief *health care climate questionnaire*).[a]	
Past experiences and individual differences	Awareness and recognition of adverse past experiences, biases, stereotypes, and trauma related to individual differences (e.g., age, religion, culture, geography, economic status, race/ethnicity, sex/gender, sexual orientation). Incorporate policies, protocols, and processes that are responsive to related concerns and needs.	
Peer support	Refer patients to relevant peer support groups offered at your healthcare office or with partner mental and behavioral health providers.	Encourage clients to discuss peer support options with their medical provider if specific concerns or experiences are disclosed.

[a] Czajkowska et al. (2017).[41]

Thus, when lifestyle medicine aims to "treat the true cause" of disease, the meaning expands beyond treating *risk factors* (e.g., blood pressure, high blood sugar or cholesterol), and even the more *proximal* causes of lifestyle behaviors that increase risk (e.g., smoking, poor diet, physical inactivity, sleep). Rather, there is a hierarchy of current and past factors, including *medial* causes (e.g., past experiences, psychological factors, stress), as well as *distal* causes (e.g., environment, technology, financial situation, other social determinants) – all of which patients are bringing with them to practitioner interactions.[34–37]

As an example, Patients A and B are told by their practitioner (you) that they have high cholesterol (risk factor), which is mainly as a result of their unhealthy eating (proximal cause).

- *Patient A* has had "terrible" past experiences with healthy eating, resulting in an *unpleasant attitude* of the taste of vegetables (medial cause), but lives in a supportive, suburban environment with *good access* to healthy foods (distal cause).
- *Patient B* has had "difficult" past experiences with healthy eating, resulting in *low confidence* in abilities (medial cause), and also lives in a challenging, rural environment of *poor access* to healthy foods, such as fruits and vegetables (distal cause).

How might you adjust your healthy eating prescription for both patients? Perhaps:

- *Patient A*: The patient shares that the "terrible" experiences were likely a result of being forced to eat the same three, unpleasant vegetables as a kid. The patient now thinks all vegetables taste bad, "like cardboard and grass." So, you connect the patient to a few restaurants and several simple recipes of your favorite (and tasty) vegetable dishes to try and rank order from most favorite to least favorite, with a plan to discuss at the next visit.
- *Patient B*: The patient shares that the "difficult" experiences are likely a result of lack of confidence in abilities. So, to help build self-efficacy, you (1) co-decide upon a "challenging, yet attainable" task of trying one new recipe the coming week for breakfast, lunch, snack, and/or dinner (to foster *mastery experience*), (2) connect the patient to another patient who faces similar concerns of access, but is successfully navigating the rural environment to eat healthfully (to foster *vicarious experience*), and (3) spend a bit more time in the follow-up discussion to provide support and feedback on why some strategies have worked and others have not (to foster *verbal persuasion*).

10.2.2 THE RESPONSE

If the medical trigger experience goes well, the patient will likely be motivated to receive and implement the lifestyle medicine prescription within the complexities of their own life. However, another layer of challenges can hinder patients' progress when they begin to put the lifestyle prescription into practice, as they "take their medicine." By analogy, some medicines taste good, while others do not. There are big pills and small pills. The directions that go along with the prescription are sometimes simple, other times complex; sometimes clear, other times confusing.

Lifestyle prescriptions have the advantage of being modifiable to leverage preferences and strengths of the patient, meeting them where they are, and maximize potential of medication adherence, when lifestyle is the medicine.

10.2.2.1 Two Minds

A prominent consideration in health behavior practice and research is determination of what factors influence and control behaviors. A longstanding approach to these kinds of issues has been the application of theories that rely on the basic presumption that behaviors are the byproduct of cognition, defined here as the mental processes associated with thought and experience. This perspective has produced a number of theories based on this cognitive behavior tradition, and although they can vary greatly with respect to individual factors (e.g., motivation, self-efficacy, decisional balance, social contexts), each is based on the presumption that cognition is a primary force in behavior. So, while the importance of these theories and concepts is clear, it is also the case that by relying on cognition, each assumes that human decision-making is mainly driven by a rational evaluation of information. The core idea that humans will dependably act in ways that are rational is challenged by the long list of healthy behaviors that are not completed despite a clear reason for doing so.

This is also true for lifestyle prescriptions. We know that recognition of guidelines does not signify patients' understanding, and neither does the perceived credibility of the source (the practitioner) guarantee use of guidelines.[42] There is also recognition of the elusive problem of the intention-behavior gap, where intention, alone, is an unreliable predictor of physical activity and dietary behavior.[43]

Mostly lacking within these approaches is the importance of affective and automatic processes, and consideration of these variables is important in understanding adoption of lifestyle prescriptions. The response has been the development of so-called dual-process theories. The primary tenet of these theoretical approaches is that humans have "two minds" that inform our behavior through two different processes.[44] *Type-1 processes* are thought to be fast, automatic, impulsive, effortless, unconscious, and emotional. In contrast, *type-2 processes* are slow, reflective, conscious, effortful, deliberate, and sober. While type-1 processes are generally believed to be outside of our awareness, type-2 processes are evaluative and full of cognition. These important principles have been nicely summarized by the concept of "thinking fast and slow",[44] which implies that behaviors are more than the sum and outcome of fully elaborated rational thought.

Physical activity behavior provides an excellent example and model for how this might be realized in practice. Suppose that a healthcare practitioner engages a patient or client and makes the determination that participation in regular exercise would be beneficial. This interaction takes on elements of a counseling or coaching session, and the details of the conversation and communication could be critical in determining whether exercise is initiated. For example, it is clear that interactions supporting autonomy and providing support are more likely to result in behavior change when compared to interactions whereby the professional is instructing and dictating the terms of an exercise prescription.[45,46] This very useful process is thoughtful and represents the type-2 process that was described earlier.

A logical conclusion would be that individuals who have autonomously determined the value of exercise would initiate and maintain a physically active lifestyle,
but as previously stated, human behavior is not entirely built around rational thought
and goals, but is instead also impacted by other forces. As such, what would objectively be described as a positive patient–practitioner interaction may lead to great
behavior change success but could also fail to produce a positive outcome. To help
explain this phenomenon from a dual-process perspective, a better understanding is
required of how patients respond to participation in the lifestyle prescription (i.e.,
taking their medicine), and subsequently, how the practitioner can modify lifestyle
prescription to increase probability of adherence. While the research is limited in
healthy eating, the research from the exercise literature can help us better understand
the complex response.

10.2.2.2   Feelings after Exercise

One especially important factor within the exercise domain is the influence of psychological considerations such as affect and emotion, which are referred to here as
mood. It has become increasingly clear that mood responses to exercise are important
considerations. A longstanding truth for most everyone is that mood after completing
exercise tends to be more positive than the mood that existed before exercise.[47] This
response is almost always the case, though it is possible that something uniquely
unpleasant or painful can worsen mood after exercise. The simple reality is that exercise tends to make people feel good, and with this outcome, the expectation would be
that human beings would be inclined to repeat those things which produce pleasure
and satisfaction and this is the case, but a focus exclusively on how one feels after the
completion of exercise does not tell the full story.

10.2.2.3   Feelings during Exercise

Another critical element about the exercise experience is not just how we feel *after*
exercise, but also how we feel *during* exercise. While feeling good after exercise is
a nearly universal phenomenon, perceptions during the exercise session is varied
and depends on many factors. Perhaps the most important factor about the experience is exercise intensity, which could be linked to simple perceptions of effort or
could link to cardiovascular or metabolic workloads. Easy and moderate exercise
reliably produce positive moods, while somewhat more intense exercise produces
mood responses that are more mixed, and very high intensities produce reliably negative responses.[48] Relatively easy exercise feels good while we are doing it, because
it is comfortable, and we know that we are doing a very healthy thing for our body.
In contrast, very intense exercise tends to feel more negative, because the height-
ened physiological response is associated with some very noxious symptoms, such
as hyperventilation and the accumulation of metabolic byproducts (e.g., lactic acid).

Perhaps the most interesting exercise intensity to consider is the intensity that
lies somewhere in between easy and very intense. The mood responses associated
with this middle intensity, which is proximal to what is known as the anaerobic or
lactate threshold, are highly dependent on the thoughts and perceptions of the exerciser.[48] Specifically, individuals who tend to be more confident in their abilities to
manage the exercise and are highly motivated to engage in exercise are more likely

to appraise the exercise as *positive*, while low confidence and motivation are more likely to yield *negative* responses. One example study compared moderate exercise against exercise that was slightly above the anaerobic threshold and results indicated that moderate exercise produced pleasure, while intense exercise created a mood state that was on average neutral but also varied significantly.[49] Truly negative mood responses are also possible during intense or maximal aerobic exercise, but a secondary consideration is that significant reductions in mood alone, even if mood remains slightly positive, may be enough to make the experience less desirable.

It has become increasingly clear that in-task mood responses are relatively potent determinants of future exercise behavior. That is, while the creation of a positive mood after exercise is desirable and good, how we feel during exercise has been shown to be more strongly related to future exercise behavior than how we feel after exercise.[50] This research estimates that a one-unit shift in pleasure during exercise impacts weekly physical activity 12 months later by more than 40 minutes. These findings give voice to the power and importance of feeling good during the exercise we participate in.

In conclusion, it seems that the more thoughtful post-exercise positive feelings we get from all different types and intensities of exercise are less important than how we feel during exercise. This reality perhaps links back to the difference between the more automatic and faster type 1 processes and the more deliberate and slower type 2 processes. Though behavior is in part impacted by elaborated and highly cognitive factors, it is also heavily impacted by more visceral and subconscious factors related to momentary perceptions of pleasure and displeasure. Discussion on how to modify and monitor the exercise prescription is provided in Section 10.3.

10.3   PRACTICAL APPLICATION

For practical application, we will focus on "using strengths." Personal strengths are key, individual traits or qualities that are presumed to lead to higher levels of self-actualization, and can be harnessed for successful self-regulation when medical triggers and lifestyle prescriptions are connected to one's personally meaningful needs, values, self-worth, and self-determination.

Progressing through the hierarchies of self and needs gratification is also seen as progressing in value, autonomy (self-determination), purpose, health, and well-being – termed *gratification health*. From this perspective, the role of the practitioner is to remove hindrances to patient growth toward self-actualization and self-determination, providing hope, buffering weaknesses, and helping the patient gain the knowledge and skills that enable successful self-regulation of the prescribed lifestyle prescription. This approach conforms to basic tenets of *Positive Psychology*, a discipline focusing on building positive qualities that allow individuals to grow and flourish (well-being, contentment, and satisfaction *in the past*; hope and optimism *for the future;* flow and happiness *in the present*), rather than a preoccupation only with repairing what is wrong or focusing on worst qualities.[51]

10.3.1   Using Strengths

The *Values in Action* (VIA) classification of strengths includes six broad virtue classes, made up of 24 valued character strengths (Table 10.1). When assessed, the patient is sharing his or her current, perceived endorsement of each strength. In general, character strengths have a positive impact on life satisfaction and health (For a full review of up-to-date research, visit the VIA Institute viacharacter.org). However, to guide application, the question is whether or not character strengths correlate with healthy lifestyles? While more research is still needed, Proyer and colleagues (2013)

TABLE 10.1

Values in Action Classification of Character Strengths

1. **Wisdom and knowledge**: cognitive strengths that entail the acquisition and use of knowledge
   creativity: thinking of novel and productive ways to do things
   - *curiosity*: taking an interest in all of ongoing experience
   - *open-mindedness*: thinking things through and examining them from all sides
   - *love of learning*: mastering new skills, topics, and bodies of knowledge
   - *perspective*: being able to provide wise counsel to others
2. **Courage**: emotional strengths that involve the exercise of will to accomplish goals in the face of opposition, external or internal
   - *authenticity*: speaking the truth and presenting oneself in a genuine way
   - *bravery*: not shrinking from threat, challenge, difficulty, or pain
   - *persistence*: finishing what one starts
   - *zest*: approaching life with excitement and energy
3. **Humanity**: interpersonal strengths that involve "tending and befriending" others
   - *kindness*: doing favors and good deeds for others
   - *love*: valuing close relations with others
   - *social intelligence*: being aware of the motives and feelings of self and others
4. **Justice**: civic strengths that underlie healthy community life
   - *fairness*: treating all people the same according to notions of fairness and justice
   - *leadership*: organizing group activities and seeing that they happen
   - *teamwork*: working well as member of a group or team
5. **Temperance**: strengths that protect against excess
   - *forgiveness*: forgiving those who have done wrong
   - *modesty*: letting one's accomplishments speak for themselves
   - *prudence*: being careful about one's choices; not saying or doing things that might later be regretted
   - *self-regulation*: regulating what one feels and does
6. **Transcendence**: strengths that forge connections to the larger universe and provide meaning
   - *appreciation of beauty and excellence*: noticing and appreciating beauty, excellence, or skilled performance in all domains of life
   - *gratitude*: being aware of and thankful for the good things that happen
   - *hope*: expecting the best and working to achieve it
   - *humor*: liking to laugh and tease; bringing smiles to other people
   - *spirituality*: having coherent beliefs about the higher purpose and meaning of life

Source: From Peterson (2006).[66]

---

found numerous positive correlations of strengths with a self-reported active life-style with the highest being *zest* ($r=0.56$), *hope* ($r=0.42$), *humor* ($r=0.41$), *curiosity* ($r=0.40$), and *bravery* ($r=0.39$).[52] Interestingly, there was only one significant cor-relation among strengths and self-reported healthy eating, *self-regulation* ($r=0.40$). These specific strengths will be the focus of application.

10.3.1.1 Prescribing with Strengths

The VIA classification can be administered to the patient beforehand, so that the prac-titioner has all strengths, including "signature strengths" available – the 3–7 strengths (out of 24) that characterize the patient best. From here, lifestyle prescriptions can be modified toward one's current strengths. For example, with physical activity:

- If the patient is high in *team work*, you might first prescribe a group exercise experience.
- If the patient in high in *love*, prescribe an active volunteer option in service to someone.
- If the patient is high in *curiosity*, prescribe the patient choose 3 new activi-ties that they have always wanted to try.

10.3.1.2 Prescribing for Strengths

The practitioner can also prescribe *for* strengths, in order to directly put strengths into practice in daily life (i.e., *strength exercises*; Table 10.2). Gander and col-leagues (2021) summarized important "functions" of character strengths, which asks what each strength is used for.[53] The daily enacting of each function was assessed using daily diaries, with the goal to experience more functions throughout the day (Table 10.3), and correlated with greater levels of specific strengths. Thus, these functions can be a simple, helpful checklist for a lifestyle prescription to build strengths, which then can be harnessed to guide and improve self-regulation of life-style prescriptions.

10.3.2 Teachable Moments

Teachable moment (TMs) can be an advantageous approach or tool for the practi-tioner to help connect health concerns, medical triggers, and lifestyle prescriptions to *personally meaningful* values, needs, and past experiences of the patient in an effort to then increase willingness and commitment to change behaviors. In general, a TM is a particular event or circumstance that leads an individual to alter his or her behavior positively, and the practitioner–patient interaction has been highlighted as central to creating TMs for health behavior change.[54–56] While TMs have reported to only occur during 10%–15% of practitioner–patient interactions on lifestyle-related factors (i.e., smoking, exercise, fruit/vegetable consumption, height, weight), signifi-cant differences have been found in patient recall of health information and percent movement in one's stage of change versus missed attempts.[54,57]

TMs in primary care have been described and evaluated by meeting the following three key elements during the patient–practitioner interaction.[57]

TABLE 10.2
Prescribing for Strengths

Strength	Exercises	Functions
Zest	Do something (e.g., physical activity) because you want to, not because you are told; go for a brisk, 10-minute morning walk; do a physical activity that you enjoy or have always wanted to try	Mastery, health, engagement, pleasure, optimism
Hope	Write down what doors opened after important doors were closed; record decision you made each day that will positively impact your life; forgive yourself; notice your negative thoughts, and counter them with positive thoughts; reaffirm yourself; Mentally rehearse your next anticipated challenge	Optimism, pleasure, mastery
Humor	Make someone smile; cheer up a gloomy friend; learn a new joke; watch a funny movie; go for a walk with a friend who has a good sense of humor; be active for fun	Pleasure, humanity, optimism
Curiosity	Learn something new that you have always wanted to learn; Try a new physical activity; Learn a new healthy recipe	Wisdom, engagement, optimism
Bravery	Be respectful of other opinions without backing down from yours; Introduce yourself to someone; Add an extra day of exercise this week; Fast from junk or fast food for 3 consecutive days; Try a more difficult recipe or exercise	Courage, positive thinking, accomplishment, self-efficacy
Self-regulation	Pay attention on purpose to your behavior and emotions; set a new, small goal and keep it; track your diet and physical activity for 3 days; find the positive in a negative situation	Courage, accomplishment, wisdom

Functions from Gander et al. (2021).[53] Example exercises modified from Haidt (2002)[67] and https://www.utsc.utoronto.ca/projects/flourish/building-your-strengths/.

Note: The first function listed was the highest correlate to each strength (range: $r \approx 0.20$–0.40).

1. *Linked Salient Patient Concern*: A symptom, worry, or life issue discussed during the visit that is meaningful to the patient and can be linked to the unhealthy risk factor (e.g., smoking, lack of exercise) as something that is exacerbated by or made worse by the health risk factor.
2. *Motivation to Change Talk*: Discussion about a health behavior in which the clinician attempts to persuade, motivate, or support a decision to change the health behavior.
3. *Commitment to Change*: The patient displaying a willingness and engagement to undertake a behavior change.

Cohen and colleagues (2011) provide a helpful, question checklist for efficiency in practice[54]:

TABLE 10.3

Description of Character Strength Functions

Function	Description
Wisdom	Today I applied existing knowledge or acquired new knowledge
Courage	Today I overcame inner and/or outer resistance through willpower in order to reach a goal
Humanity	Today I had loving interactions with other people
Justice	Today I contributed to the welfare of the community
Temperance	Today I counteracted excessive behavior
Transcendence	Today I felt connected to something greater and experienced meaningfulness
Meaning	Today I used my potential for a higher cause
Engagement	Today I was absorbed in an activity and lost myself in it completely
Pleasure	Today I could enjoy, was happy, or had joy
Health	Today I felt fit and healthy
Optimism	Today I was optimistic and positive about what was to come
Accomplishment	Today I made progress with something personally important to me
Mastery	Today it was easy for me to cope with everyday challenges
Positive thinking	Today I influenced my perceptions or thoughts in order to take a positive view of myself, others, or the world
Independence	Today I felt free and independent
Understanding	Today I could understand myself, other people, and the world, and thus experience competence and control
Self-efficacy	Today, I experienced that I could make a difference with my actions

Source: From Gander et al. (2021).[53] Character Strengths Functions Rating (CSFR) scale.
Each item was rated on a 7-point Likert scale, from 1 = "not at all" to 7 = "all the time."

1. Is there the presence of a concern that is salient to the patient that is either obviously relevant to an unhealthy behavior or through conversation comes to be seen as relevant?
2. Is there a link that is made between the patient's salient concern and a health behavior that attempts to motivate the patient toward change?
3. Is there a patient response indicating a willingness to discuss and commit to behavior change?

We recommend reviewing real-life scripts of a TM, an attempted TM, and a missed opportunity from primary care from Cohen and colleagues (2011).[54]

10.3.3 CONNECT-CONFLICT-CHOICE

From a self-determination approach to motivation to regulate behavior, *internalization* is the process of identifying with, accepting, and incorporating a behavior into one's values, identify, and self-concept/-worth. While there is question as to how we might facilitate internalization in practice, three contextual events are proposed (modified from Deci et al.[58]).

10.3.3.1 Connect

Connecting to a rationale that is personally meaningful to the patient can aid in understanding why adoption of the lifestyle prescription would have personal utility and benefit. If, for example, a patient does not want to reduce sugar intake, a rationale for doing it might be "so you can reduce your medications." Ideally, with ongoing patient interactions, slight additions can be made to ensure that the rationale is personally meaningful to each patient.

> ... so you can reduce your medications, and reduce the financial burden and stress they are causing you.
> ... so you can reduce you medications, *and get rid of the [side effect] that has been bothering you so much, lately.*
> ... so you can reduce your medications, *and put that money back into your children.*

10.3.3.2 Conflict

Here, the practitioner acknowledges the conflict, tension, and associated feelings that arise when a rationale for a requested behavior highlights that one's current behavior is contrary to their current values and beliefs.

10.3.3.3 Choice

Free choice is required to promote autonomy in changing behavior, thus the practitioner can use this time to provide options for the patient on how they would like to modify and engage the lifestyle prescription to support personal choice, autonomy, feelings, and values.

10.3.4 THE RESPONSE

There are a few simple recommendations to help ensure modification of exercise prescriptions to maximize potential of positive experiences both during and after exercise for each patient.

10.3.4.1 Prescribing Intensity

Exercise that is more modest or moderate is likely a good option for anyone, especially for relatively unfit and inactive patients commonly seen in healthcare settings. These intensities are "safer" when aiming to provide exercise that will be deemed tolerable and more likely to be repeated. Moderate can be defined in numerous ways but essential in any prescription of this intensity of exercise is to encourage work rates that do not cause exhaustion or the inability to carry on a conversation.

More intense exercise can be appropriate for individuals with a healthy mindset, and extremely intense exercise should be considered carefully and is perhaps most appropriate for individuals with a history of tolerating high intensity exercise, namely fitness enthusiasts and athletes.

10.3.4.2 Regulating Intensity

Next, teaching the patient to regulate intensity during exercise may facilitate improved adherence to the exercise prescription. Frameworks for exercise prescriptions have focused rather exclusively on regulating exercise intensity based on physiological parameters, such as heart rate and metabolic rate. For example, the patient could identify specific heart rate values that correspond to particular exercise intensities and metabolic rates, but such methods can seem burdensome to many individuals.

More contemporary guidelines now specifically recognize the value of more exercise regulation by way of perceptual factors.

1. *Perceived Exertion:* A self-report that aims to combine physiological and perceptual signals into a holistic view of exercise intensity. Several different scales exist to rate perceived exertion and exercise recommendations now routinely promote moderate exercise, which produces significant health-related benefits without inducing a physiological response that may be perceptually uncomfortable. One scale that may be particularly helpful in a clinical setting is the OMNI 0–10 scale which contains both verbal and pictorial descriptors, with 5–7 representing moderate intensity exercise.[59]

2. *Mood Monitoring:* Monitoring mood response to guide exercise intensity operates in a manner similar to perceived exertion. This approach recommends that exercise intensity be manipulated upwards and downwards, so as to elicit a positive mood state. The implication is that optimum exercise is associated with the greatest intensity that feels good and intensity should be adjusted to maintain mood from the beginning of exercise until the end. The single-item Feeling Scale is commonly used to measure mood and ranges from –5 for displeasure to +5 for pleasure (see Section 10.4).[60] This tool could prove helpful for practitioners and patients given the research indicating that exercise intensity can be regulated and maintained simply by adjustments aimed at maintaining a positive mood.[61]

Such novel and innovative approaches are worthy pursuits as part of a goal to leverage our increased understanding that human behavior is impacted by psychological processes that are both cognitively elaborate and rudimentary.

10.4   MEASUREMENT STRATEGIES

The key strategy is to use pre-existing measures that will help you gauge key concepts discussed in this chapter, which can be done as a part of pre-assessments before the practitioner–patient interaction (e.g., a part of initial paperwork in the waiting room, online survey before visit).

- *Character Strengths:* The VIA inventory of character strengths (VIA-IS), a 240-item (24 strengths, 10 items each) self-report questionnaire, is the current standard of measurement in adults (and a version for children). See Table 10.1 for a summary. For more information, visit: https://www.authentichappiness.sas.upenn.edu
- *Functions of Character Strengths:* The functions provided in Table 10.3 are from the larger Character Strengths Functions Rating (CSFR) scale, which

assesses enactment of each function on a 7-point Likert scale, from 1 = "not at all" to 7 = "all the time."

- *Values of Living:* The Valued Living Questionnaire[62] presents specific domains to then rate their importance (1 = *not important at all* to 10 = *extremely important*): family, marriage/relationship, parenting, friends/social life, professional life, academic life, recreation or leisure, spirituality/religion, community life, physical self-care. Results can then be displayed to give the practitioner a quick reference to the leading values of the patient, to not only respect such values but to allow for autonomy support in a personal connection (rather than trying to manipulate the patient).
- *Exercise Mood Monitoring:* The Feeling Scale[60] for monitoring mood at any given point during exercise and physical activity to guide intensity ranges from –5 for displeasure to +5 for pleasure. Verbal anchors are provided at all odd integers (+5 = very good, +3 = good, +1 = fairly good, 0 = neutral, –1 = fairly bad, –3 = bad, and –5 = very bad).

10.5 SUMMARY

When working to empower people to change, identifying their strengths will help to add energy to the behavior change journey. Self-regulation is an important place to start, triggered by a perceived discrepancy between where individuals believe they are and where they want to go (or who they want to be). Such discrepancies are not benign, and they are often discovered in terms of a health setback or falling short with clinical guidelines for a healthy behavior. Acknowledging how the patient feels about their current position or situation will give the individual the time and space to go deeper into their journey of change. To go deeper and further, the individual will need strengths. Finding their strengths is the key and modifying lifestyle prescriptions that not only meet individuals where they are but are also prescribed in a positive way to build and use strengths.

10.6 KEY TAKEAWAYS

Utilizing this approach, the practitioner can:

- Self-regulation, i.e., a process of monitoring and changing behavior to stay in line with a goal, such as a lifestyle prescription, and is commonly initiated when normalcy is interrupted by awareness of a health concern or discrepancy from a personally held or clinical standard.
- Recognize patients' feelings and responses to health concerns, discrepancies, diagnoses, and (un)healthy behavior, and use this understanding to help guide feedback and modify lifestyle prescriptions.
- Focus on patient strengths rather than their weaknesses or deficits.
- Be positive. Your demeanor and words matter. Use more promotion or gain-framed messages (benefits of changing, engaging, or adopting behavior) versus loss-framed messages (costs or consequences of not changing, not engaging, or not adopting behavior).[63,64] For example:

- *Gain frame*: "Getting more physical activity can help you lose weight/ reduce disease risk."
- *Loss frame*: "Not getting enough physical activity can make you gain weight/increase disease risk."
- Be flexible in your lifestyle prescription to meet each individual patient where they are, instead of sticking to a generic or rigid protocol (e.g., only prescribing a standard "best case scenario" lifestyle recommendation, without modification).
- Consider your lifestyle prescription as an innovation to be adopted by the patient (diffusion of innovation theory), and specifically "compatibility" with (1) patient values, (2) past experiences, and (3) current needs.
- Support patient autonomy, by providing options on how to modify and engage a lifestyle prescription for free-will choice.
- Encourage "signature strengths" in your prescription.
- Prescribe "using strengths," as a part of your lifestyle prescription, giving the patient options of strength exercises to choose from.[65]
- To maximize positive response, prescribe exercise that is perceived by the unfit, inactive patient as modest or moderate, and teach the patient to regulate intensity during exercise through perceived exertion and mood monitoring.

10.7   RESOURCES

- https://www.authentichappiness.sas.upenn.edu
- https://www.utsc.utoronto.ca/projects/flourish/building-your-strengths

REFERENCES

1. Moilanen, Kristin L. "The adolescent self-regulatory inventory: The development and validation of a questionnaire of short-term and long-term self-regulation." *Journal of Youth and Adolescence* 36, no. 6 (2007): 835–848.
2. Hennessy, Emily A., Blair T. Johnson, Rebecca L. Acabchuk, Kiran McCloskey, and Jania Stewart-James. "Self-regulation mechanisms in health behavior change: A systematic meta-review of meta-analyses, 2006–2017." *Health Psychology Review* 14, no. 1 (2020): 6–42.
3. Spring, Bonnie, Katrina E. Champion, Rebecca Acabchuk, and Emily A. Hennessy. "Self-regulatory behaviour change techniques in interventions to promote healthy eating, physical activity, or weight loss: A meta-review." *Health Psychology Review* 15, no. 4 (2021): 508–539.
4. Carver, Charles S., and Michael F. Scheier. *On the Self-regulation of Behavior.* Cambridge: Cambridge University Press, 2001.
5. Wing, Rena R., and Suzanne Phelan. "Long-term weight loss maintenance." *The American Journal of Clinical Nutrition* 82, no. 1 (2005): 222–225.
6. Wray, Linda A., A. Regula Herzog, Robert J. Willis, and Robert B. Wallace. "The impact of education and heart attack on smoking cessation among middle-aged adults." *Journal of Health and Social Behavior* (1998): 271–294.

7. Faries, Mark D., and John B. Bartholomew. "Coping with weight-related discrepancies: Initial development of the WEIGHTCOPE." *Women's Health Issues* 25, no. 3 (2015): 267–275.

8. Gorin, Amy A., Suzanne Phelan, James O. Hill, and Rena R. Wing. "Medical triggers are associated with better short-and long-term weight loss outcomes." *Preventive Medicine* 39, no. 3 (2004): 612–616.

9. LaRose, Jessica Gokee, Tricia M. Leahey, James O. Hill, and Rena R. Wing. "Differences in motivations and weight loss behaviors in young adults and older adults in the National Weight Control Registry." *Obesity* 21, no. 3 (2013): 449–453.

10. Maslow, Abraham Harold. "A theory of human motivation." *Psychological Review* 50, no. 4 (1943): 370–396.

11. Zalenski, Robert J., and Richard Raspa. "Maslow's hierarchy of needs: A framework for achieving human potential in hospice." *Journal of Palliative Medicine* 9, no. 5 (2006): 1120–1127.

12. Shih, Chiung-Yu, Chiu-Ya Huang, Mei-Lun Huang, Chyong-Mei Chen, Chih-Ching Lin, and Fu-In Tang. "The association of sociodemographic factors and needs of haemodialysis patients according to Maslow's hierarchy of needs." *Journal of Clinical Nursing* 28, no. 1–2 (2019): 270–278.

13. Beran, David. "Developing a hierarchy of needs for type 1 diabetes." *Diabetic Medicine* 31, no. 1 (2014): 61–67.

14. Poirier, Therese I., and Radhika Devraj. "Pharmacy in an improved health care delivery model using Maslow's hierarchy of needs." *American Journal of Pharmaceutical Education* 83, no. 8 (2019): 1664–1667.

15. Ştefan, Simona Cătălina, Ştefan Cătălin Popa, and Cătălina Florentina Albu. "Implications of Maslow's hierarchy of needs theory on healthcare employees' performance." *Transylvanian Review of Administrative Sciences* 16, no. 59 (2020): 124–143.

16. Hale, Andrew J., Daniel N. Ricotta, Jason Freed, C. Christopher Smith, and Grace C. Huang. "Adapting Maslow's hierarchy of needs as a framework for resident wellness." *Teaching and Learning in Medicine* 31, no. 1 (2019): 109–118.

17. Xu, Ji-Xue, Lin-Xue Wu, Wei Jiang, and Gui-Hong Fan. "Effect of nursing intervention based on Maslow's hierarchy of needs in patients with coronary heart disease interventional surgery." *World Journal of Clinical Cases* 9, no. 33 (2021): 10189–10197.

18. Idler, Ellen L., ed. *Religion as a Social Determinant of Public Health.* New York: Oxford University Press, 2014.

19. Idler, Ellen, John Blevins, Mimi Kiser, and Carol Hogue. "Religion, a social determinant of mortality? A 10-year follow-up of the Health and Retirement Study." *PLoS One* 12, no. 12 (2017): e0189134.

20. VanderWeele, Tyler J. "Religious communities and human flourishing." *Current Directions in Psychological Science* 26, no. 5 (2017): 476–481.

21. Lucchetti, Giancarlo, Alessandra LG Lucchetti, and Harold G. Koenig. "Impact of spirituality/religiosity on mortality: Comparison with other health interventions." *Explore* 7, no. 4 (2011): 234–238.

22. Fortes, Marina, Grégory Ninot, and Didier Delignières. "The hierarchical structure of the physical self: An idiographic and cross-correlational analysis." *International Journal of Sport and Exercise Psychology* 2, no. 2 (2004): 119–132.

23. Moore, Justin B., Nathanael G. Mitchell, Marcus W. Kilpatrick, and John B. Bartholomew. "The physical self-attribute questionnaire: Development and initial validation." *Psychological Reports* 100, no. 2 (2007): 627–642.

24. Crocker, Jennifer, Amara T. Brook, Yu Niiya, and Mark Villacorta. "The pursuit of self-esteem: Contingencies of self-worth and self-regulation." *Journal of Personality* 74, no. 6 (2006): 1749–1772.

25. Gruenewald, Tara L., Margaret E. Kemeny, Najib Aziz, and John L. Fahey. "Acute threat to the social self: Shame, social self-esteem, and cortisol activity." *Psychosomatic Medicine* 66, no. 6 (2004): 915–924.

26. Lamarche, Larkin, Gretchen Kerr, Guy Faulkner, Kimberley L. Gammage, and Panagiota Klentrou. "A qualitative examination of body image threats using social self-preservation theory." *Body Image* 9, no. 1 (2012): 145–154.

27. Frazier, Leslie D., Bennett L. Schwartz, and Janet Metcalfe. "The MAPS model of self-regulation: Integrating metacognition, agency, and possible selves." *Metacognition and Learning* 16, no. 2 (2021): 297–318.

28. Faries, Mark D., Elizabeth Espie, Erik Gnagy, and Kyle P. McMorries. "Experiences with weight loss triggers in women prescribed to lose weight by their physician." *Women's Health Bulletin* 3, no. 1 (2015): e30166.

29. Dionigi, Rylee A., and Jack Cannon. "Older adults' perceived changes in physical self-worth associated with resistance training." *Research Quarterly for Exercise and Sport* 80, no. 2 (2009): 269–280.

30. Fernández-Bustos, Juan Gregorio, Álvaro Infantes-Paniagua, Ricardo Cuevas, and Onofre Ricardo Contreras. "Effect of physical activity on self-concept: Theoretical model on the mediation of body image and physical self-concept in adolescents." *Frontiers in Psychology* 10 (2019): 1–11.

31. Haugen, Tommy, Reidar Säfvenbom, and Yngvar Ommundsen. "Physical activity and global self-worth: The role of physical self-esteem indices and gender." *Mental Health and Physical Activity* 4, no. 2 (2011): 49–56.

32. Govindaraju, Thara, Alice J. Owen, and Tracy A. McCaffrey. "Past, present and future influences of diet among older adults–A scoping review." *Ageing Research Reviews* 77 (2022): 1–11.

33. Stevens, Courtney J., Austin S. Baldwin, Angela D. Bryan, Mark Conner, Ryan E. Rhodes, and David M. Williams. "Affective determinants of physical activity: A conceptual framework and narrative review." *Frontiers in Psychology* 11 (2020): 1–19.

34. Egger, Garry. "Defining a structure and methodology for the practice of lifestyle medicine." *American Journal of Lifestyle Medicine* 12, no. 5 (2018): 396–403.

35. Egger, Garry J., Andrew F. Binns, Bob Morgan, and John Stevens. "Adverse childhood experiences as "upstream" determinants of lifestyle-related chronic disease: A scoping perspective." *American Journal of Lifestyle Medicine* 16, no. 6 (2021): 15598276211001292.

36. Egger, Garry J., Andrew F. Binns, and Stephan R. Rossner. "The emergence of "lifestyle medicine" as a structured approach for management of chronic disease." *Medical Journal of Australia* 190, no. 3 (2009): 143–145.

37. Egger, Garry, John Stevens, Andrew Binns, and Bob Morgan. "Psychosocial determinants of chronic disease: Implications for lifestyle medicine." *American Journal of Lifestyle Medicine* 13, no. 6 (2019): 526–532.

38. Godoy, Lucas C., Claudia Frankfurter, Matthew Cooper, Christine Lay, Robert Maunder, and Michael E. Farkouh. "Association of adverse childhood experiences with cardiovascular disease later in life: A review." *JAMA Cardiology* 6, no. 2 (2021): 228–235.

39. Spencer, Rhonda, Fatimah Alramadhan, Alaa Alabadi, and Nichola Seaton Ribadu. "The call for lifestyle medicine interventions to address the impact of adverse childhood experiences." *The Journal of Family Practice* 71, no. 1 Suppl Lifestyle (2022): eS73-eS77.

40. Korotana, Laurel M., Keith S. Dobson, Dennis Pusch, and Trevor Josephson. "A review of primary care interventions to improve health outcomes in adult survivors of adverse childhood experiences." *Clinical Psychology Review* 46 (2016): 59–90.

41. Czajkowska, Zofia, Hui Wang, Nathan C. Hall, Maida Sewitch, and Annett Körner. "Validation of the English and French versions of the brief health care climate questionnaire." *Health Psychology Open* 4, no. 2 (2017): 2055102917730675.
42. Boylan, Sinead, Jimmy Chun Yu Louie, and Timothy P. Gill. "Consumer response to healthy eating, physical activity and weight-related recommendations: A systematic review." *Obesity Reviews* 13, no. 7 (2012): 606–617.
43. Faries, Mark D., Wesley C. Kephart, and Devin Graham. "The intention–behavior gap." In *Lifestyle Medicine*, edited by James M. Rippe, 241–252. Boca Raton: CRC Press (in press; first print in 2019).
44. Kahneman, Daniel. *Thinking, Fast and Slow.* London: Penguin Books, 2011.
45. Mossman, L.H., G. R. Slemp, K. J. Lewis, R. H. Colla, and P. O'Halloran. "Autonomy support in sport and exercise settings: A systematic review and meta-analysis." *International Review of Sport and Exercise Psychology* (2022): 1–24. doi:10.1080/1750 984X.2022.2031252.
46. Moustaka, Frederiki C., Symeon P. Vlachopoulos, Chris Kabitsis, and Yannis Theodorakis. "Effects of an autonomy-supportive exercise instructing style on exercise motivation, psychological well-being, and exercise attendance in middle-age women." *Journal of Physical Activity and Health* 9, no. 1 (2012): 138–150.
47. Yeung, Robert R. "The acute effects of exercise on mood state." *Journal of Psychosomatic Research* 40, no. 2 (1996): 123–141.
48. Ekkekakis, Panteleimon, Eric E. Hall, and Steven J. Petruzzello. "Variation and homogeneity in affective responses to physical activity of varying intensities: An alternative perspective on dose–response based on evolutionary considerations." *Journal of Sports Sciences* 23, no. 5 (2005): 477–500.
49. Kilpatrick, Marcus, Robert Kraemer, John Bartholomew, Edmund Acevedo, and Denise Jarreau. "Affective responses to exercise are dependent on intensity rather than total work." *Medicine and Science in Sports and Exercise* 39, no. 8 (2007): 1417–1422.
50. Williams, David M., Shira Dunsiger, Joseph T. Ciccolo, Beth A. Lewis, Anna E. Albrecht, and Bess H. Marcus. "Acute affective response to a moderate-intensity exercise stimulus predicts physical activity participation 6 and 12 months later." *Psychology of Sport and Exercise* 9, no. 3 (2008): 231–245.
51. Seligman, Martin EP, and Mihaly Csikszentmihalyi. "Positive psychology: An introduction." In *Flow and the Foundations of Positive Psychology*, edited by Mihaly Csikszentmihalyi, pp. 279–298. Dordrecht: Springer, 2014.
52. Proyer, René T., Fabian Gander, Sara Wellenzohn, and Willibald Ruch. "What good are character strengths beyond subjective well-being? The contribution of the good character on self-reported health-oriented behavior, physical fitness, and the subjective health status." *The Journal of Positive Psychology* 8, no. 3 (2013): 222–232.
53. Gander, Fabian, Lisa Wagner, Lukas Amann, and Willibald Ruch. "What are character strengths good for? A daily diary study on character strengths enactment." *The Journal of Positive Psychology* 17, no. 5 (2021): 1–11.
54. Cohen, Deborah J., Elizabeth C. Clark, Peter J. Lawson, Brad A. Casucci, and Susan A. Flocke. "Identifying teachable moments for health behavior counseling in primary care." *Patient Education and Counseling* 85, no. 2 (2011): e8–e15.
55. Lawson, Peter J., and Susan A. Flocke. "Teachable moments for health behavior change: A concept analysis." *Patient Education and Counseling* 76, no. 1 (2009): 25–30.
56. Pierce, John P., and Alice L. Mills. "Using teachable moments to improve nutrition and physical activity in patients." *American Family Physician* 77, no. 11 (2008): 1510–1511.
57. Flocke, Susan A., Elizabeth Clark, Elizabeth Antognoli, Mary Jane Mason, Peter J. Lawson, Samantha Smith, and Deborah J. Cohen. "Teachable moments for health behavior change and intermediate patient outcomes." *Patient Education and Counseling* 96, no. 1 (2014): 43–49.

58. Deci, Edward L., Haleh Eghrari, Brian C. Patrick, and Dean R. Leone. "Facilitating internalization: The self-determination theory perspective." *Journal of Personality* 62, no. 1 (1994): 119–142.

59. Robertson, Robert J. *Perceived Exertion for Practitioners: Rating Effort with the OMNI Picture System.* Champaign: Human Kinetics, 2004.

60. Hardy, Charles J., and W. Jack Rejeski. "Not what, but how one feels: The measurement of affect during exercise." *Journal of Sport and Exercise Psychology* 11, no. 3 (1989): 304–317.

61. Rose, Elaine A., and Gaynor Parfitt. "Can the feeling scale be used to regulate exercise intensity." *Medicine and Science in Sports and Exercise* 40, no. 10 (2008): 1852–1860.

62. Wilson, Kelly G., Emily K. Sandoz, Jennifer Kitchens, and Miguel Roberts. "The valued living questionnaire: Defining and measuring valued action within a behavioral framework." *The Psychological Record* 60, no. 2 (2010): 249–272.

63. Gallagher, Kristel M., and John A. Updegraff. "Health message framing effects on attitudes, intentions, and behavior: A meta-analytic review." *Annals of Behavioral Medicine* 43, no. 1 (2012): 101–116.

64. Updegraff, John A., and Alexander J. Rothman. "Health message framing: Moderators, mediators, and mysteries." *Social and Personality Psychology Compass* 7, no. 9 (2013): 668–679.

65. Schueller, Stephen M. "Preferences for positive psychology exercises." *The Journal of Positive Psychology* 5, no. 3 (2010): 192–203.

66. Peterson, Christopher. *A Primer in Positive Psychology.* New York: Oxford University Press, 2006.

67. Haidt, Jonathan. "It's more fun to work on strengths than weaknesses (but it may not be better for you)." Accessed March 6 (2002). http://people.stern.nyu.edu/jhaidt/strengths_analysis.doc

11 Accountability

Simon Matthews, MHlthSc

11.1 INTRODUCTION

The only person you are destined to become is the person you decide to be.

Ralph Waldo Emerson

When people hear the word accountability, they often think of "accountability part-ner", which features in many addiction and sobriety programs and related self-help publications, such as this recent work by Surdyka.[1] Such ideas of accountability or "sponsorship" may allude to an unequal power relationship, where the person being accountable is considered to be at a particular point on the journey of recov-ery, whereas the "sponsor" is typically considerably further along this journey. Accountability might also invoke the idea of "cheerleader" – the popular notion of "having someone on your team"; however, this notion is essentially external motiva-tion and perhaps even punitive – when a person is "succeeding" at the task at hand, they may receive cheerleading from the accountability partner (also external moti-vation). When they "fail" in their efforts, the individual may apprehend feelings of shame or judgment from the accountability partner. After all, despite its seeming positivity, "cheerleading" in behavior change is a form of judgment. And if "positive judgment" can be expressed, so can "negative judgment".

This chapter examines the notion of how best to support a person to remain committed to what they say they want, and to do so in a way that honors the well-established principles of human behavior change, such as autonomy as articu-lated into Self-Determination Theory.[2]

11.2 WHAT IS ACCOUNTABILITY?

Accountability refers to the notion that an individual may be called upon to justify his or her actions or inactions.[3–5] In the area of health behavior change, this leads to an immediate disconnect with other elements of the change process – that the behavior change goal is ideally set by the client, not the provider[6]; that the primary human need for autonomy is a main driver of change[7] and that motivating forces which are external to the person are less likely to result in sustainable behavior change.[8] Accountability that arises from an expectation that another might be "checking" or "verifying" that the action has occurred is perhaps better thought of as compliance. It is an example of the research phenomenon of the "Hawthorne Effect",[9,10] first observed in industry in the early 20th century.[11] Applied to a health behavior change setting, the Hawthorne Effect may result in compliance with a health care provider in controlled clinic or treatment conditions, but a reversion to other behavior in the "real world."

DOI: 10.1201/9781003161226-11

In fact, Oussedik et al.[10] argue that the notion of accountability is broadly missing from notable theories of health behavior change and motivation, including Andersen's Behavioral Model,[12] the Health Belief Model,[13] the Integrated Behavior Model,[14] the Theory of Planned Behavior[15] and the Theory of Reasoned Action.[15] How then to best understand accountability?

Accountability may be conceptualized along a continuum from "controlled accountability" to "autonomous accountability".[10] Controlled accountability is entirely extrinsic and may be to a healthcare provider, or a sponsor, or even a relative, friend or acquaintance. Although not implicit in the idea, controlled accountability may be punitive, like a harsh supervisor whose main focus is regular checks on progress and who acts to humiliate, shame or punish if established goals are not met. Autonomous accountability rests entirely within the person engaging in the change in behavior. At first glance, this would seem ideal – since the goal behavior is also autonomously driven, patients and clients may share their outcomes willingly with another person. The client's efforts represent a personal choice to act in a particular way and are likely informed by a broader vision, sense of purpose or expression of personal values; however, patients and clients can be their "own worst enemies" and engage in harsh judgment and self-criticism for perceived failure to achieve goals. Furthermore, there is some evidence that external accountability results in greater persistence in treatment.[16]

Regardless of the type of accountability, the factor that stands out as necessary for any accountability to exist, is *relationship*.

The model of Supportive Accountability[17] provides a means of understanding and operationalizing the accountability process in a way that enhances patient autonomy through the vehicle of the therapeutic alliance. It has long been established that one of the primary drivers of "drop-outs" in treatment, or treatment nonadherence, is a poor therapeutic alliance.[18]

In this model, accountability is not a demand from one person that another gives an account of his or her conduct – rather it is a process in which one person can support another to maintain visions, goals, processes, structures, and supports to enable them to achieve what they have set out to. In the Supportive Accountability model, the patient's health behavior is immediately supported by visions, clear goals, progress and performance monitoring, and the knowledge of the presence of another person to be accountable to. These factors in turn are supported by the idea of "legitimacy" – a concept akin to *therapeutic alliance*,[17] as well as "*bond*" – the emotional attachment of the patient to the person they are being accountable to. These primary human factors are supported by the patient's own motivators and the idea of "bandwidth" – the number of communication cues available in a particular medium (and therefore the putative strength of that medium to support behavioral change). Together, these factors ultimately support the "adherence" of the person to their stated intentions (Figure 11.1).

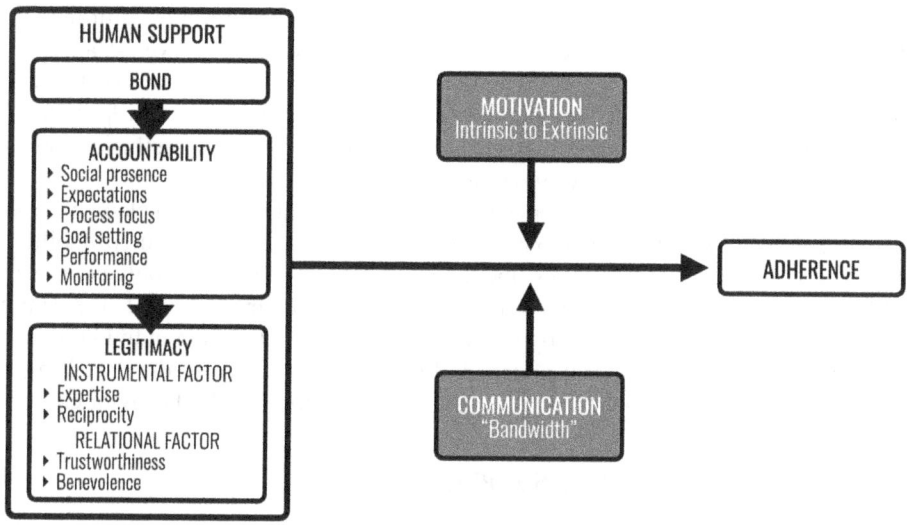

FIGURE 11.1 Supportive accountability. (Modified from Mohr et al., 2011.[17] doi: 10.2196/ jmir.1602. ©David Mohr, Pim Cuijpers, Kenneth Lehman. Originally published in the Journal of Medical Internet Research (http://www.jmir.org), 10.03.2011. This is an open-access article distributed under the terms of the Creative Commons Attribution License (http://creativecommons.org/licenses/by/2.0/), which permits unrestricted use, distribution, and reproduction in any medium, provided the original work, first published in the Journal of Medical Internet Research, is properly cited. The complete bibliographic information, a link to the original publication on http://www.jmir.org/, as well as this copyright and license information must be included.)

11.3 HOW IS ACCOUNTABILITY BEST CONCEPTUALIZED?

The common idea of accountability as *the implicit or explicit expectation that individuals may be called upon to justify their actions or inactions* immediately presents a difficulty when considering notions of autonomy, collaborative decision making and shared power – all key to an effective therapeutic alliance.[19] Such a notion is likely to invoke fear of judgment or shame of perceived failure at the prospect of an unmet goal. It further invites the view that the person to whom an individual is accountable may at any time call on the person for an account – leaving the person in a reactive position, rather than an initiating position.

11.4 ATTRIBUTION, CULPABILITY AND MODIFIABILITY

Any discussion of accountability must begin with an understanding of causal attribution, and in particular fundamental attribution error.[20] This is the tendency for a person to over-emphasize personal culpability for an outcome and under-emphasize environmental, contextual and societal factors which may be at play. In the current context, this attribution error is likely to lead a health practitioner to unconsciously form views that a person with obesity, or diabetes or a number of other medical conditions is solely responsible for its onset, management and ultimate elimination. This tendency has been demonstrated empirically, for example by Evers-Casey and colleagues[21] who showed a strong association among views of clinicians on tobacco smoking and the word "guilt," rather than "innocence." Vishwanath[22] similarly found that a large percentage of individuals misattribute causality (by seeing the individual as responsible) in relation to juvenile diabetes.

It is unhelpful to frame behavior change to an individual in terms of elements over which they have little to no personal control. Rather, the notion of "modifiability" must be incorporated into thinking about accountability – this is the only context in which it makes sense for a person to be accountable for their behavior. If the health behavior in question is significantly influenced by factors outside the individual, then this must be reflected in causal understandings of the presence of disease. It must also be reflected in approaches to cultivating and evaluating health behavior change.

11.5   ACCOUNTABILITY AS A PROCESS

For the purpose of health behavior change (and perhaps for other contexts) accountability may be better conceptualized as *the explicit desire of an individual to describe their goal progress to a significant person in their life*. In this way, the person assumes not only the responsibility for reporting progress but also decides when and how this may be done and values the role that accountability plays in their goal progress and attainment.

Rather than being considered a strategy or simple action, accountability is best thought of as a series of structures and practices woven into the person's environment and goal design, which supports them to maintain a continuous awareness of their goal progress and development.

Furthermore, rather than being an action that a person may take, accountability is best considered the system of processes, structures, and supports which enables the individual to maintain a continuous awareness of their goal progress. In this way, accountability may encompass the therapeutic alliance, goal design, social support, environmental support, and appreciative explorations of goal-directed actions (see Chapter 6).

11.6   ACCOUNTABILITY AND DETERMINANTS OF HEALTH

While some authors such as Glannon[23] have argued that personal responsibility for disease is reasonable (in this case liver disease arising from alcohol consumption), others such as Friesen[24] view the inclusion of personal responsibility in healthcare policy "unethical and ineffective." Friesen argues in particular that such a basis for health resource allocation is likely to not impact patient-level health behavior change in any positive way and will also increase inequity and worsen outcomes over time, as a result of significant determinants of health not being addressed through the lens of personal responsibility. Friesen also contends that discussions around personal responsibility are not underpinned by principles of causal or moral responsibility but by personal biases toward stigmatized behaviors. These polarized positions demonstrate the importance of developing a framework for accountability which supports a patient to assume responsibility and develop accountability for their behavior, rather than compelling them to do so, through an actual or apprehended negative outcome for not doing so.

11.7   EVIDENCE SUMMARY

Two commonly cited studies into goal setting and accountability have dominated the goal setting literature for many years – the 1953 Yale Study and the 1979 Harvard Study.[25] Extraordinarily, the Harvard study reportedly found that of the MBA graduate cohort at the time of the study, only 3% had committed their goals to paper and they ended up earning a staggering 10 times as much as the other 97% put together, just 10 years after graduation!

After extensive research, Kraus[26] and Matthews[27] established that no such research had ever taken place and that the cited papers were mythical. As a result, Matthews[27] elected to conduct her own research into the influence of writing goals, commitment and accountability on goal achievement.

Of the 267 participants recruited for the study from businesses, organizations, and business networking groups, 149 completed the study. The age of respondents ranged from 23 to 72 years, with 37 males and 112 females. Participants from the USA, Belgium, England, India, Australia, and Japan were included. Participants were randomly assigned to various experimental goal conditions, including having an unwritten goal; a written goal; a written goal & action commitment; a written goal and action commitment to a friend; and a written goal, action commitment, and progress reports to a friend.

While the simple act of writing goals led to higher rates of goal achievement (6.08 goals achieved compared with 4.28 for the unwritten goals group), the act of writing goals and making a commitment to a friend led to even greater goal achievement (6.41 goals achieved compared with 4.28 for the unwritten goals group); however, those who made weekly progress reports to a friend achieved significantly more than those with unwritten goals, written goals, commitment to action and announcement to a friend (7.6 goals achieved compared with 4.28, 6.08, 5.08 and 6.41 goals achieved). Thus, the positive effect of accountability on goal attainment was supported.

A recent review[28] of digital approaches to health behavior change broadly supported the principle of digital and online platforms in assisting patients to undertake and reach their behavioral change goals. While noting that any "virtual" component of a digital behavior change intervention must create accountability, it is possible to develop this accountability within a digital approach. The fact that accountability *can* be created and incorporated does not imply that it always is. With a vast number of digital and online approaches available, and more being developed all the time, practitioners should consider the evidence for a particular digital solution and not see the entire field of "digital health" as a solution. Milne-Ives et al.[29] in their systematic review of 52 randomized controlled trials of interventions health behavior change in physical activity, diet, drug and alcohol use, and mental health, found that although patient perceptions were positive, there was no strong evidence

TABLE 11.1
Research Summary

Study	Area of Focus	Outcomes
Matthews[27]	Impact of accountability on goal achievement	Average 7.6 goals achieved compared with 4.28 for no written goals and no accountability
Santarossa et al.[28]	Goal progress studied but not accountability specifically	Unable to describe particular contribution of accountability
Cimmarusti and Gamero[35]	Compassionate accountability in residential settings	Improved relationships and improved mastery over trauma symptoms
Milne-Ives et al.[29]	Goal progress studied but not accountability specifically	Unable to describe particular contribution of accountability
Meyerhoff et al.[39]	Supportive accountability	Development of a validated supportive accountability inventory

of difference in intervention groups and control groups using the various mobile apps studied. Clearly, further research into digital behavior change platforms is required and the role of accountability is a significant factor in this (Table 11.1).

11.8 ACCOUNTABILITY AND PSYCHOLOGICAL SAFETY

Like many concepts and ideas in the field of health behavior change (such as appreciative inquiry), the idea of psychological safety first emerged in the area of organizational functioning more than 50 years ago.[30] It's been a particular focus of research again since the 1990s.[31] Psychological safety describes the beliefs and perceptions that organizational employees might have about the risk to their work relationships of particular behaviors such as speaking up, suggesting new ideas or critiquing the work of another. It involves the extent to which a person feels able to be honest, without artifice, and also without fear of shame, humiliation, loss of respect or loss of status.

The concept of psychological safety has since been drawn into the world of health care, particularly to investigate the operation of healthcare systems and how they can better ensure patient safety and positive patient outcomes.[32,33]

Organizational constructs are often better thought of as "systemic constructs" – since this is what they typically describe: the interdependent operation of elements of a system to produce particular outcomes. The physician/patient relationship, of course, can also be thought of as a relational system. Indeed, when elements of social support, societal expectations and customs, and environmental and contextual structures are added, the system of physician/patient healthcare becomes very complex.

In interpersonal relationships, the term "emotional safety"[34] is sometimes used. An extensive and systematic review by Kim and White[34] identified three themes critical to interpersonal communications which enhance healthcare outcomes. Trust and a sense of *emotional safety* was one of these and promoted open and engaging communication – a necessary prerequisite for accountability.

There are often times in health care when the patient may have difficulty identifying a suitable person to act in the role of "friend" to whom one can report goal progress. Elderly and/or socially isolated patients, sole parents, those newly relocated and without the establishment of a reliable and trustworthy network are all examples. In these situations, the physician or health care provider may also form an important element of the process of patient accountability.

Therefore, all healthcare providers and practitioners must be mindful of the role that psychological or emotional safety plays in behavioral change – from a patient feeling confident enough to engage in a new or uncertain behavior, to reporting efforts to do so which may not have unfolded as planned or desired.

For the physician, the capacity to create a relationship of genuine trust, positive regard, curiosity about the outcomes the patient is uncovering, and an underlying view that the patient is doing his or her best to manage changes within their own capacities and consistent with their own values is vital. The initiation and maintenance of this relationship style by the physician can be achieved by practicing the skills of full presence and attention, practicing open, curious inquiry, reflecting understanding, reflecting with empathy when a patient has not met their stated goal and engaging in discussions about what has been learnt from the experience (rather than viewing the attempt as a "failure").

11.9   A MATURING ACCOUNTABILITY

As noted already, structures of accountability involving another person may be limited in a number of circumstances. Even if a patient is having regular twice-a-month contact with a physician or other health practitioner, this still likely represents only one brief exchange every 336 hours! Additionally, as a patient moves further along the route of long-term, sustainable behavior change, the less likely they may be to want to provide an account to another, and the more likely they may be to want to build internal systems of accountability – to experience mastery in not only the doing of health behavior, but also in tracking its progress, modifying it as required and maintaining it.

The word accountability comes to us by way of Latin and Old French, literally meaning to "provide a report to" [*another*]. The autonomous accountability referred to above might be better described as "***auto-countability***" – a reporting to self. While this may represent a departure from common notions of accountability (and common practices of accountability in health care), it nevertheless represents an important dimension of the range of possible supports and structures to facilitate a person's goal pursuit. In the context of a patient who has struggled to make and maintain new health behaviors over a long period of time, the idea of auto-countability might seem like the proverbial appointment of the fox to guard the henhouse. Early in the behavior change process, this may be the case – a little like asking a very newly qualified driver to navigate their way across the country in arduous and challenging driving conditions; however, the undertaking of, and indeed completion of, such a voyage can be one of the richly rewarding experiences of efficacy and achievement – the feeling of having had minimal reliance on external supports in order to achieve a significant personal challenge.

Therefore, auto-countability may be too demanding early in a behavior change process, but the concept may be introduced and gradually moved toward, so that the person exits the behavior change process with a stronger sense of their own internal capacity to monitor, adjust and strategize around their behavior over time. Using monitoring techniques helps to encourage this auto-countability.

11.10 COMPASSIONATE ACCOUNTABILITY

The idea of compassionate accountability has been explored to some extent in both residential care and behavior management programs for young people[35] and organizational management.[36] It involves the principle of maintaining a focus on accountability, while seeking to understand the psychological and emotional experience of the person *being* accountable – in other words, using an approach of developing empathy for and expressing understanding of the person's situation, while simultaneously working toward the completion of the task or goal that is the focus of accountability. In practice, the beginning difference between a more common or usual approach and a compassionate approach might look like this:

Physician: How did you do with your goals this past week?
Patient: To be honest, I didn't do them at all...
Physician: Oh...why not? What went wrong?
Patient: Well...I needed to care for my Mom...
Physician: And who cares for you if you don't?   **(Common approach)**

Physician: Tell me about your progress toward your goals this past week
Patient: Actually...there wasn't any
Physician: Uh-huh...help me understand a little more about your week and how it
    unfolded...
Patient: My Mom was nearly admitted to hospital on Monday – we kept her out by
    me dropping everything and helping her monitor her meds more closely.
Physician: I can see how important this relationship is to you and how much you
    value it.   **(Compassionate approach)**

While the differences may, at first glance, seem subtle and nuanced, the common approach will often evoke a somewhat defensive response from the patient, since it is really a call to "justify oneself." It may also evoke *sustain talk* – explored in more detail in Chapter 4. Asked to explain why a goal has not been reached, or perhaps even attempted, a patient will often advance reasons why the change is hard, or unmanageable or in some other way unrealistic. It may even evoke a *"righting reflex"* from the physician (see also Chapter 4). In the second example, the response of the physician is an immediate desire to understand the full experience of the patient – not just reasons for not completing a goal. In doing this, the patient may share other aspects of their situation which can further inform the physician in his or her efforts to support the patient. Furthermore, the patient likely feels understood, unjudged, and valued.

Finally, compassion has been shown, through the important work of Neff[37,38] to be a strong predictor of health and well-being and psychological well-being in particular.

11.11   MEASUREMENT STRATEGIES

A valuable means of understanding one's own level of compassion is to take a validated inventory, such as this one developed by Dr Kristin Neff: https://self-compassion.org/test-how-self-compassionate-you-are/

Additionally, Meyerhof et al.[39] are developing and validating the Supportive Accountability Inventory (SAI) as a means of supporting digital coaching interventions. While in the early stages of development, among other psychometric properties, the SAI has an internal consistency described by the authors as "acceptable" of $\alpha = 0.68$.

While subjective, even simple rating scales of various dimensions of the behavior change process can support all parties to identify strengths and areas for growth in accountability. The following simple self-report scales could all encompass a "0–10" range, with the higher end representing the strongest belief or commitment to the idea. Rating scales are valuable ways of supporting people to identify progress and change over time.

- *I have a vision in place for my health and well-being*
- *I am solely responsible for this goal behavior*
- *I understand the connection between this behavior and my vision*
- *I regularly check my goal progress*
- *I look for opportunities to develop my skills*
- *I seek the support of others when I need it*
- *I incorporate useful feedback from others*

The self-check item "*I look for opportunities to develop my skills*" is worthy of particular explanation since it invokes the idea of "growth mindset".[40,41] Further, mindset research has demonstrated that the development of growth mindset in students builds resilience to adversity and challenge[42] and that growth mindset can modify the impact of a social determinant such as poverty, on academic achievement.[43] This invites further questions such as the extent to which growth mindset may mediate and modify the influence of social determinants that may ordinarily impede and limit behavioral change. A 2009 study, for example, demonstrated that growth mindset is as potent as nicotine replacement therapy in cultivating motivation in a smoker to cease tobacco.[44]

11.12   PRACTICAL TIPS AND APPLICATION

The idea of accountability should be introduced early in any behavior change discussion – and in a way that avoids the expression of doubt that the person will be able to maintain their commitment to change. Expressing doubt is demotivating. Rather, a patient could be informed that accountability has been shown to support goal attainment, with an ensuing discussion about what such an accountability structure may look like to the patient. This could involve having a clear vision for change, clearly stated behavior goals, milestone markers for full or partial goal attainment, people to share progress with, means of recording progress such as apps, pen and paper notes and visual or pictorial charts.

The notion of "*auto-countability*" can also be introduced early in a process of change – this also introduces concepts such as efficacy and independence of behavioral choice – the ultimate goal of any health behavior intervention. The best outcome a physician or health practitioner could hope for in relation to any patient, is that they, as a provider, become redundant!

11.13 CASE STUDY

Mr G is a 43-year-old man with a family history of cardiovascular disease, diabetes, hypertension, and stroke. His current weight is 245 pounds and his recent lab results suggest that he is pre-diabetic and has hyperlipidemia and hypercholesterolemia. He is strongly opposed to using any prescribed medication to manage these conditions, and he indicates that he watched the health of both of his parents slowly decline until their premature deaths.

He mentions to you that in the preceding year, his workplace made three health coaching consultations available to all staff. He said that he found these very helpful and was disappointed when they ended. He wonders whether he might be able to engage in a similar coaching relationship to manage his health conditions.

Since you are a certified health coach, you agree to work with him provided that he also has the support and approval of his family physician and you agree that six initial sessions would be helpful.

Across the first two sessions, you work with Mr G to create a vision for his own health and well-being as well as supporting him to identify strengths, supports, past successes and best experiences of his health and well-being to this point.

In Session 3, you begin working with Mr G on setting SMART goals. Mr G explains that two goals which immediately come to mind for him which would support his longer-term health vision are to increase his cardiovascular endurance and to reduce the amount of highly- and ultra-processed food that he eats. Specifically, he creates the following goals:

1. Every weekday, when I arrive home from work at 5:30 pm, I will walk in my neighborhood for 45 minutes, before returning home to eat dinner.
2. Five days out of seven, I will prepare my own lunch and dinner, including at least 1½ cups of vegetables at each meal.

While the goals themselves are SMART and also consistent with the vision that Mr G has for his own health, you engage him in discussion around goal success. In particular, you ask him what the best way for him would be to monitor his progress toward these goals so that he can make timely adjustments to his behavior if necessary.

He volunteers that committing his goals to paper would be helpful – he said he knows from experience at work, that he is much more likely to achieve tasks that he has written, rather than those which he simply carries in his mind. He also mentions the "reminder" function on his smartphone, although he then adds that he is unsure if this would be helpful, because he knows he is able to ignore this at work, from past experience.

You ask him if you can share some information that may be useful. When he agrees, you tell Mr G that there is evidence that reporting progress regularly to a friend has been shown to improve goal attainment. He considers this, then nominates his wife, before expressing concern that if he has been struggling to meet his goals, his wife may remonstrate with him that he does not value his health and well-being sufficiently. You concur and reinforce to him that accountability is likely unhelpful if it is punitive in nature. On reflection, he nominates a friend with whom he goes fishing regularly as someone he would be happy to report his progress to. Mr G adds that his friend also went through his own significant weight loss journey 2–3 years before. You affirm this choice and add that the opportunity to learn from people who are personally significant in some way is a valuable means of building skill and confidence to make behavioral changes.

During the fourth session 3 weeks later, you review with Mr G his progress toward the goals that he has been working on. He reports to you that he made weekly reports of his goal progress to his friend, which was met with encouragement and an invitation to reach out to the friend for further support if necessary. Mr G said he found this very uplifting and noted that it helped him commit strongly and purposefully to his goals.

11.14   SUMMARY

Accountability is one of the keys to behavior change. Empowering people to change is accomplished with compassion, not force, facts, or fear. Holding people accountable for goals without holding a space for compassion will not empower, but will likely be experienced as judgmental. The ultimate goal is auto-countability where the patient learns how to hold themselves accountable for goals within the spirit of self-compassion. Setting goals, creating a methodology for accountability, and sharing the process with another is a powerful setup for behavior change, as research has demonstrated.

11.15   TAKEAWAYS

1. There is a continuum of accountability from entirely extrinsic to deeply internalized accountability.
2. The practitioner can play a central role with regard to accountability, as the relationship and therapeutic alliance created with the patient impacts the success of accountability efforts.
3. Providing an environment of trust and emotional safety allows the individual to embark on their accountability journey.
4. Compassion is critical when working on accountability with individuals.
5. Some individuals continue to connect with friends and others to keep themselves accountable and others reach auto-countability where the patient has internalized means of self-referential accountability.

REFERENCES

1. Surdyka, Michael J. 2021. *Fully Alive: Using Your Individuality to Conquer Addiction.* Michael J. Surdyka.
2. Deci, Edward L, and Richard M Ryan. 1985. *Intrinsic Motivation and Self-Determination in Human Behavior.* Berlin: Springer Science & Business Media.
3. Scott, Marvin B, and Stanford M Lyman. 1968. "Accounts." *American Sociological Review* 33(1): 46–62.
4. Tetlock, Philip E. 1992. "The impact of accountability on judgment and choice: Toward a social contingency model." *Advances in Experimental Social Psychology* 25:331–376.
5. Lerner, Jennifer S, and Philip E Tetlock. 1999. "Accounting for the effects of accountability." *Psychological Bulletin* 125 (2):255.
6. Moore, Margaret, Bob Tschannen-Moran, and Erika Jackson. 2016. *Coaching Psychology Manual.* 2nd ed. Wolters Kluwer Health/Lippincott, Williams & Wilkins, Philadelphia, PA.
7. Deci, Edward L, and Richard M Ryan. 2010. "Self-determination." In E. W. Craighead and C. Nemeroff (Eds.). *The Corsini Encyclopedia of Psychology,* Wiley, New Jersey, pp. 1–2.
8. Deci, Edward L, Richard Koestner, and Richard M Ryan. 1999. "A meta-analytic review of experiments examining the effects of extrinsic rewards on intrinsic motivation." *Psychological Bulletin* 125 (6):627.
9. McCarney, Rob, James Warner, Steve Iliffe, Robbert Van Haselen, Mark Griffin, and Peter Fisher. 2007. "The Hawthorne Effect: A randomised, controlled trial." *BMC Medical Research Methodology* 7 (1):1–8.
10. Oussedik, Elias, Capri G Foy, EJ Masicampo, Lara K Kammrath, Robert E Anderson, and Steven R Feldman. 2017. "Accountability: A missing construct in models of adherence behavior and in clinical practice." *Patient Preference and Adherence* 11: 1285.
11. Roethlisberger Fritz J, and William J Dickson. 1939. *Management and the Worker, Management and the Worker.* Harvard University Press, Oxford, England.
12. Andersen, Ronald M. 1995. "Revisiting the behavioral model and access to medical care: does it matter?" *Journal of Health and Social Behavior* 36(1):1–10.
13. Rosenstock, Irwin M. 1974. "Historical origins of the health belief model." *Health Education Monographs* 2 (4):328–335.
14. Fishbein, Martin, and Marco C Yzer. 2003. "Using theory to design effective health behavior interventions." *Communication Theory* 13 (2):164–183.
15. Ajzen, Icek. 1985. "From intentions to actions: A theory of planned behavior". In J. Kuhl and B. Jurgen (Eds.). *Action Control: From Cognition to Behavior.* Springer-Verlag, Berlin, pp. 11–39.
16. van Onzenoort, Hein AW, Frederique E Menger, Cees Neef, Willem J Verberk, Abraham A Kroon, Peter W de Leeuw, and Paul-Hugo M van der Kuy. 2011. "Participation in a clinical trial enhances adherence and persistence to treatment: A retrospective cohort study." *Hypertension* 58 (4):573–578.
17. Mohr, David, Pim Cuijpers, and Kenneth Lehman. 2011. "Supportive accountability: A model for providing human support to enhance adherence to eHealth interventions." *Journal of Medical Internet Research* 13 (1):e30.
18. Mohl, Paul C, Diane Martinez, Christopher Ticknor, Milton Huang, and Linda Cordell. 1991. "Early dropouts from psychotherapy." *Journal of Nervous and Mental Disease* 179(8):478–481.
19. Hubble, Mark. A., Barry L Duncan and Scott D Miller. 2007. "Common factors and the uncommon heroism of youth." *Psychotherapy in Australia* 13 (2):34.

20. Ross, Lee. 1977. "The intuitive psychologist and his shortcomings: Distortions in the attribution process." In L. Berkowitz (Ed.). *Advances in Experimental Social Psychology*. Orlando, FL: Elsevier, pp. 173–220.
21. Evers-Casey, Sarah, Robert Schnoll, Brian P Jenssen, and Frank T Leone. 2019. "Implicit attribution of culpability and impact on experience of treating tobacco dependence." *Health Psychology* 38 (12):1069.
22. Vishwanath, Arun. 2014. "Negative public perceptions of juvenile diabetics: Applying attribution theory to understand the public's stigmatizing views." *Health Communication* 29 (5):516–526.
23. Glannon, Walter. 1998. "Responsibility, alcoholism, and liver transplantation." *The Journal of Medicine and Philosophy* 23 (1):31–49.
24. Friesen, Phoebe. 2018. "Personal responsibility within health policy: Unethical and ineffective." *Journal of Medical Ethics* 44 (1):53–58.
25. Acton, Annabel. 2017. "How To Set Goals (And Why You Should Write Them Down)." Accessed May 17, 2021. https://www.forbes.com/sites/annabelacton/2017/11/03/how-to-set-goals-and-why-you-should-do-it/?sh=7f16f589162d.
26. Kraus, Stephen. 2002. *Psychological Foundations of Success: A Harvard Trained Scientist Separates the Science of Success from Self-help Snake Oil*. San Francisco, CA: Next Level Sciences, Inc.
27. Matthews, Gail. 2015. "The effectiveness of four coaching techniques: writing goals, formulating action steps, making a commitment, and accountability." *Paper Presented at the 9th Annual International Psychology Conference*, Athens, Greece.
28. Santarossa, Sara, Deborah Kane, Charlene Y Senn, and Sarah J Woodruff. 2018. "Exploring the role of in-person components for online health behavior change interventions: Can a digital person-to-person component suffice?" *Journal of Medical Internet Research* 20 (4):e144.
29. Milne-Ives, Madison, Ching Lam, Caroline De Cock, Michelle Helena Van Velthoven, and Edward Meinert. 2020. "Mobile apps for health behavior change in physical activity, diet, drug and alcohol use, and mental health: Systematic review." *JMIR mHealth and uHealth* 8 (3):e17046.
30. Rogers, Carl R. 1954. "Toward a theory of creativity." *ETC: A Review of General Semantics* 11(4):249–260.
31. Kahn, William A. 1990. "Psychological conditions of personal engagement and disengagement at work." *Academy of Management Journal* 33 (4):692–724.
32. O'Donovan, Róisín, and Eilish McAuliffe. 2020. "Exploring psychological safety in healthcare teams to inform the development of interventions: Combining observational, survey and interview data." *BMC Health Services Research* 20 (1):1–16.
33. Torralba, Karina D, Donna Jose, and John Byrne. 2020. "Psychological safety, the hidden curriculum, and ambiguity in medicine." *Clinical Rheumatology* 39 (3):667–671.
34. Kim, Bora, and Kate White. 2018. "How can health professionals enhance interpersonal communication with adolescents and young adults to improve health care outcomes?: Systematic literature review." *International Journal of Adolescence and Youth* 23 (2):198–218.
35. Cimmarusti, Rocco A, and Soe L Gamero. 2009. "Compassionate accountability in residential care: A trauma informed model." *Residential Treatment for Children & Youth* 26 (3):181–193.
36. Regier, Nate. 2017. *Conflict without Casualties: A Field Guide for Leading with Compassionate Accountability*. Oakland, CA: Berrett-Koehler Publishers.
37. Neff, Kristin D. 2004. "Self-compassion and psychological well-being." *Constructivism in the Human Sciences* 9 (2):27.
38. Neff, Kristin D. 2011. "Self-compassion, self-esteem, and well-being." *Social and Personality Psychology Compass* 5 (1):1–12.

39. Meyerhoff, Jonah, Shefali Haldar, and David C Mohr. 2021. "The supportive accountability inventory: Psychometric properties of a measure of supportive accountability in coached digital interventions." *Internet Interventions* 25:100399.
40. Dweck, Carol. 2016. "What having a 'growth mindset' actually means." *Harvard Business Review* 13:213–226.
41. Dweck, Carol. 2017. *Mindset-Updated Edition: Changing the Way You Think to Fulfil Your Potential*. Boston, MA: Hachette.
42. Yeager, David Scott, and Carol S Dweck. 2012. "Mindsets that promote resilience: When students believe that personal characteristics can be developed." *Educational Psychologist* 47 (4):302–314.
43. Claro, Susana, David Paunesku, and Carol S Dweck. 2016. "Growth mindset tempers the effects of poverty on academic achievement." *Proceedings of the National Academy of Sciences* 113 (31):8664–8668.
44. Johnson, Vicki D. 2009. *Growth Mindset as a Predictor of Smoking Cessation*. Doctoral Dissertation, Cleveland State University.

12 Five-Step Cycle for Collaboration

Beth Frates, MD FACLM DipABLM
and Tracie McCargo, PhD

12.1 FIVE-STEP CYCLE

The chapters in this book provide the background, the theories, and the evidence about behavior change basics. Chronic conditions like heart disease, diabetes, and obesity are multifactorial, but all of them have a component of lifestyle at their root cause. This is why lifestyle medicine and its six pillars are important for each clinician to be aware of and work with. By assessing and addressing the six pillars of lifestyle medicine including adding movement, nutritious food, sound sleep, stress reduction techniques, supportive social connections, and the avoidance of risky substances to the care of people living with and often struggling with chronic conditions, their suffering can be minimized and their disease process can be halted or even reversed in some cases. Guidelines for each pillar are shared in Chapter 14. People know they need to exercise and eat vegetables, but this knowledge does not usually translate into action. For this reason, practitioners need to focus on the act of empowering people to make healthy changes, one step at a time. Small steps lead to big rewards.

There are a number of people on this planet who will have the opportunity to empower individuals to adopt and sustain healthy habits: The list includes but is not limited to physicians, nurses, dentists, physical therapists, occupational therapists, nutritionists, fitness professionals, health and wellness coaches, social workers, teachers, mentors, sports coaches, parents, and grandparents. Clinicians need training to be successful in counseling or coaching. Knowledge is important and it is power. Knowing the behavior change principles, theories, practices, techniques, strategies, and skills is essential. But, practice is paramount because knowledge is not powerful enough to instill lasting change in most people. The clinicians or change agents need to practice these skills. This chapter presents a five-step cycle that can be used as a roadmap to guide practitioners while they practice behavior change counseling or coaching.

There is great power in collaboration. Practitioners' collaboration with patients can be a key factor in helping them change their lifestyle patterns and adopt healthy changes.[1] Building on the information from the 11 chapters that come before this one, this chapter introduces the -five-step cycle of collaboration for behavior change. Clinicians who are used to the EXPERT Approach™ as opposed to the COACH

Approach™ will be able to focus on these five steps to move them into a collaboration, negotiation, and co-creation way of working with patients. The five-step cycle of collaboration utilizes tools of empathy, aligning motivation, building confidence, setting smart goals, and setting accountability (Figure 12.1).

12.1.1 STEP 1: BE EMPATHETIC

Empathy is defined as "the action of understanding, being aware of, being sensitive to, and vicariously experiencing the feelings, thoughts, and experience of another of either the past or present without having the feelings, thoughts, and experience fully communicated in an objectively explicit manner".[2] Sympathy is defined as "the act or capacity of entering into or sharing the feelings or interests of another".[3] Each term carries with it certain connotations. The difference between the terms is often explained in this way "sympathy is when you share the feelings of another; empathy is when you understand the feelings of another but do not necessarily share them".[4] People long to be understood. Thus, expressing an understanding of a person's situation is the key point of communication. Note in the definition of empathy it starts with "the action of understanding." Communicating this action comes in different forms. Eye contact, head nods, facial expressions, body language like leaning in, quiet listening, and stating reflections that reveal an understanding are all actions that will communicate empathy.

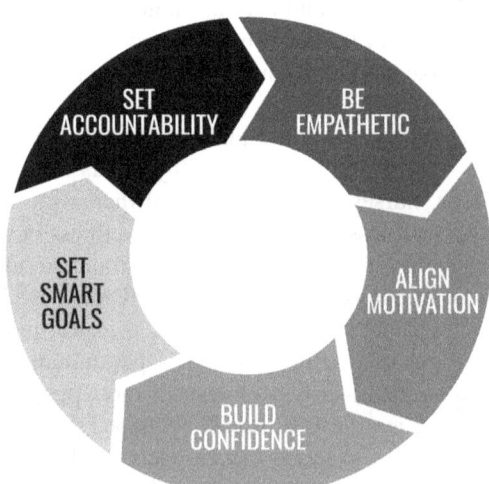

FIGURE 12.1 Five-step cycle (i.e., "Be empathetic," "align motivation," "Build confidence," "set smart goals," "set accountability" depicted in a joined circle). (Modified with permission from Frates, B., Bonnet, J., Joseph, R., Peterson, J. 2020. *Lifestyle Medicine Handbook: An Introduction to the Power of Healthy Habits*. Healthy Learning, p. 101.)

Research on empathy has revealed that patient satisfaction scores improve when their physician has high levels of empathy.[5] Empathy can be rated by the physician on a self-report scale called the Jefferson Scale of Empathy. Patients can report their impression of their physician's level of empathy with the Jefferson Scale of Patient's Perceptions of Physician empathy. Research from Hojat and colleagues reported in 2011 revealed that empathy from physicians may have a positive influence on the health outcomes of patients.[6] Diabetic patients treated by family physicians who self-reported high empathy scores on the Jefferson Scale of Empathy had LDL and Hemoglobin A1C levels that were under better control than the patients whose physicians had lower self-reported scores on the Jefferson Scale of Empathy.[6] Years later, the study design was replicated by Chaitoff and colleagues. This study did not show a correlation between physician self-reported empathy levels and LDL or Hemoglobin A1C levels.[7] Empathy may not have a direct impact on clinical outcomes, but it seems to have an impact on patient satisfaction. Most people want to be understood and appreciated. By expressing empathy, the provider lets the patient know that they are important and valued. Giving someone time and undivided attention is a gift in itself.

Empathy helps build caring relationships. When someone shares their painful stories as well as their physical and mental symptoms with a healthcare professional, they are trusting that person. They hope to be met with non-judgmental understanding. When the healthcare professional listens intently and responds compassionately, trust builds between the patient and the healthcare professional. Compassion is a close cousin to empathy and was discussed in Chapter 1 with the COACH Approach™. With compassion there is the desire to take action. In this five-step cycle, these are action steps so compassion is inherent as by engaging with this road map, the clinician is expressing empathy and then taking action. Before taking action, one must feel safe and trust needs to be built between two people. Trust is key to any therapeutic alliance, and empathy is essential for trust. That is why it is the first step in the five step cycle.

According to Dan Goleman and his book *The Brain and Emotional Intelligence*, there are three types of empathy.[8] Practitioners use all three types which include cognitive, emotional, and empathic need. Cognitive empathy demonstrates to the patient that the provider can see and understand their perspective. Emotional empathy demonstrates to the patient that the practitioner shares their feelings, and this type of empathy is used to build rapport. The use of empathic need relays that the practitioner senses what the patient needs and is spontaneously willing to help.

Being empathetic requires mindful listening. To listen to another, one must focus on the other. The phone, the to-do list, personal worries and concerns must all be left behind. At the forefront is the patient. Listening to understand is different than listening to respond. Listening to understand is a requirement for one to express empathy.

According to the authors of *Co-Active Coaching: New Skills for Coaching People toward Success in Work and Life*, Laura Whitworth, Karen Kimsey-House, Henry Kimsey-House, and Phillip Sandah, listening occurs on three levels: internal listening which focuses on oneself, listening focused on others, and global listening which uses all of the senses to deepen understanding.[9] These three levels parallel the three levels of empathy. The use of reflections deepens understanding of the patient's needs.

When the clinician uses reflections, they are demonstrating that they are listening carefully. A clinician's genuine curiosity reveals a level of authentic concern and helps to build trust. Patients can be distrustful of healthcare professionals because in their past, they may have been dismissed, judged, or threatened with death or disease if they did not change their unhealthy habits like smoking. For a conversation and clinic visit that fosters lifestyle changes, there needs to be mutual respect and trust. When a patient feels non-judgmental support, they are more likely to open up and share their honest feelings and accurate reports of their actions with the clinician.

Someone may feel empathy, but they may not be expressing it. This can happen when someone is distracted and not fully focused on the person in front of them. At times, people involved in a conversation may start thinking about how the words of another relate to their own circumstances. In this way, they can get lost in their own thoughts and their own troubles which may mimic those of the person in front of them. This is natural. It can distract the clinician from the patient. Staying focused on listening to the patient and their exact situation, thinking about how they are expressing their emotions and what they are feeling helps the clinician to stay focused. Remembering that it is important to reflect back what they hear helps to keep clinicians focused.

Feeling empathy and not expressing it to the patient is like wrapping a gift and not giving it. This is similar to the quote by William Arthur Ward, "Feeling gratitude and not expressing it is like wrapping a present and not giving it".[10] Practitioners can express empathy by reflecting what they hear, listening intently, looking the patient in the eye, leaning in toward the patient, nodding, and using appropriate facial expressions that demonstrate surprise, sadness, happiness, confusion, or other emotions that mirror the words the patient is sharing.

If the patient is in the pre-contemplation stage of change discussed in Chapter 2, then expressing empathy is one of the most important actions for a provider (Tables 12.1–12.3).

12.1.2 TRAINING IN EMPATHY

Obesity management training is a helpful tool that assists medical residents to support patient needs. The obesity management framework consists of the 5As: ask, assess, advise, agree, and assist.[30,31] This framework is effective in improving resident attitudes toward people living with obesity, competency, confidence, ability to assess causes of obesity, assist in addressing barriers, and counsel patients on weight gain.[31]

Patients often quit therapy or counseling prematurely, especially during the initial sessions. It is important for clinicians to pay attention during these sessions to ensure that patients are engaged early on. This includes building collaborative relationships where clinicians and patients work together to establish and accomplish goals.[32] Building trust and mutual respect is extremely important during initial sessions and throughout the relationship. Engaging patients to participate in their treatment plans and health goals is not an easy task. This includes acknowledging that the patient has expert knowledge of what strategies may work best and using a non-judgmental approach to elicit this information.

TABLE 12.1
Empathy Studies Chart

Study	Number of Participants	Primary Outcomes
Bernardo et al.[11]	945 patients and 51 physicians from radiology, clinical and surgical specialties	Jefferson scale of patient's perceptions of physician empathy and consultation and relational empathy scale had a positive correlation between physicians' self-assessed empathy and patience measures of physicians' empathy (0, 56; $p > 0,000$).
Hojat et al.[6]	891 diabetic patients	Patients with empathetic physicians had significantly better control of A1c (56%) than those with physicians with low empathy scores (40%).
Chaitoff et al.[7]	4,176 primary care patients	Mean physician Jefferson Scale of Empathy score was 118.4 (standard deviation (SD) = 12). Median patient HgbA1c was 6.7% (Interquartile range (IQR) = 6.2–7.5) and median LDL concentration was 83 (IQR = 66–104).
Menendez et al.[12]	112 consecutive new patients	Physician empathy accounted for 65% of the variation in patient satisfaction in the hand surgery office setting.
Mercer et al.[13]	3,044 patients	Patients' perceptions of physician empathy are of key importance in patient enablement. Perceived GP empathy had a positive effect on enablement in both affluent and underserved patients.
Sanders et al.[14]	89 oncology patients	Oncology patients' perspectives on physician empathy (listening and understanding) may help to refine patient experience.
Simões et al.[15]	456 primary health care patients	There were significantly higher enablement scores for younger, more educated, and professionally active patients ($P < 0.001$). Patient's taking chronic medication had a slight but significantly higher median score on empathy than patients not taking them (6.70 vs. 6.60, $P = 0.049$).
Steinhausen et al.[16]	120 trauma surgery patients	Patients with ratings of 41 points or higher have a twentyfold higher probability to have better medical treatment outcomes. A well-functioning relationship between position is important.

A meta-analysis reviews empathy and psychotherapy outcomes in 3,599 patients.[33] Empathy is found to be a strong predictor of therapy outcomes. However, empathy perceptions of the patients and observers are more accurate than those of therapists in predicting patient outcomes. The therapist may rate themselves with high empathy, whereas the patient may rank that same provider as low. When the patient views the therapist as high on empathy, there is a more positive connection to empathy scores and outcomes. This information helps to highlight the different ways that empathy is experienced within the patient–clinician relationship.

TABLE 12.2
Patient Satisfaction Chart

Study	Number of Participants	Primary Outcomes
Kim et al.[17]	550 outpatients at a university hospital	Patient perception of physician empathy had significant influence on patient compliance and satisfaction.
Naoum et al.[18]	126 patients who visited an outpatient facility	Physician empathy scores were very high (21.2 out of 25) and positively affected overall patient satisfaction. Correlations between physician empathy and patient satisfaction with medical, nursing, and secretarial staff were statistically significant ($p < 0.001$).
Walsh et al.[19]	140 patients with chronic pain between the ages of 30 and 70	Patient perception of physician empathy is positively correlated with patient satisfaction in a pain clinic. Physician education to enhance empathic communication is recommended.
Byrd et al.[20]	28 emergency physicians and 423 patients	Patient satisfaction is correlated with patient assessed physician empathy ($p = 0.60$), has a weak correlation with physician assessed empathy ($p = 0.11$), and no correlation with physician assessed burnout ($p < 0.1$).
Wang et al.[5]	41 emergency medicine (EM) residents and physicians, 1,308 patients	Senior physicians had higher empathy scores (69% – very satisfied) on self-reported measures. EM residents scored lowest (very satisfied 65%). Modest correlation was found between physical self-reports and patient satisfaction.

TABLE 12.3
Patient-Rated Empathy vs. Physician-Rated Empathy Chart

Study	Number of Participants	Primary Outcomes
Abdulkader et al.[21]	30 physicians and 390 patients from family medicine, internal medicine and surgery	Average scores of patient-rated physician empathy are 26.6, and that of physician self-rated empathy 111. No correlation was found between physician and patient empathy ratings.
Chittem et al.[22]	50 patients with type 2 diabetes and their family practice medicine physicians, and 25 physicians	Barriers to self-monitoring and medication adherence include confusion, forgetting and reduced motivation, family recommendations of alternative therapies, stigma and cost of taking insulin. Medical training should address physician empathy and communication.
Elliott et al.[23]	Meta-analysis of 82 independent samples and 6,138 clients	Review of the relationship between therapist empathy and client outcomes found that patient, observer, and therapist perceptions predicted patient outcomes better than empathic accuracy instruments.

(Continued)

TABLE 12.3 (*Continued*)
Patient-Rated Empathy vs. Physician-Rated Empathy Chart

Study	Number of Participants	Primary Outcomes
Surchat et al.[24]	61 primary care physicians using 244 patient experience questionnaires	Female physicians had higher self-ratings for empathy than male physicians. Male physicians were more vocally synchronized with their patients. Vocal synchronization alone significantly predicted patient outcomes.
Sperandeo et al.[25]	23 patients who received in-person and online psychotherapy with different levels of severity of pathology	Patient perceptions of therapist empathy during remote sessions viewed therapists as significantly more empathic and supportive. This differed from perceptions of the psychotherapists.
Farber et al.[26]	Meta-analysis review with 64 studies	A multilevel meta-analysis indicates a strong relationship between therapists' positive regard and patients' clinical outcomes ($g = 0.36$).
Hansen et al.[27]	26 general practitioners and 60 patient ratings for empathy	Median CARE Measure scores were 40, median Patient Enablement Instrument scores were 5.5, and 44.9% of patients achieved healthier lifestyles. No significant association was found between CARE scores, patient enablement, and healthy lifestyle changes.
Geyer[28]	Review article	Clinician communication goes beyond delivering scientific information to include an understanding of the patient and their values. Patients who are treated with respect are more likely to follow through with recommendations, leading to improved health.
Derksen et al.[29]	Six focus groups with 35 general practitioner (GP) trainees	GP trainees face obstacles with personal affective reactions and balance between empathic involvement and task responsibilities. Trainees suggest the need for empathic training in medical curriculum.
Mert et al.[30]	70 physicians and 420 patients who received care from the physicians	Internal medicine physicians and new physicians had higher levels of empathy. Patient perception is directly related to empathy developed by physicians.

12.1.3 Step 2: Align Motivation

In the expert approach, the clinician often is focused on their agenda. The clinician has motivators as to why the patient should change behaviors. Like for quitting smoking, the clinician might be thinking about avoiding heart disease and cancer. This would be the clinician's motivation for change. The key in behavior change counseling and coaching is to figure out what the patient's own motivations are. For example, for smoking, a patient might want to quit smoking because their grandchildren refuse to ride in their car because it smells like smoke, their spouse will not hug them until they shower and put on fresh clothes after smoking, or because cigarettes are expensive. These are the motivators for the patient. It is not possible to predict the motivators of any particular patient. The clinician learns by asking open-ended questions. This is where motivational interviewing enters the five-step cycle. Chapter 4 discussed motivational interviewing in detail.

The key to motivational interviewing is to explore the patient's own reasons for wanting to reach a goal.[1,9] Evoking change talk is one of the main goals. Through change talk, the patient provides their own reasons for change. They share their own motivators. This is how a clinician can align motivation. To align motivation, a clinician asks questions like "What would life be like if you quit smoking?" or "How would life be different if you exercised five days a week?" Inviting the patient to explore these questions with non-judgmental interest and mindful listening, the clinician can guide the patient to appreciate their own motivators for making a lifestyle change. Asking "what is your motivation for quitting smoking?" will allow some patients to identify a powerful motivator. Other patients will need more open-ended questions and more time to align motivation.

Self-Determination Theory by Ryan and Deci explains that people need three main ingredients for sustained motivation: relatedness or connection, competence, and autonomy.[34] It is important that patients feel they have autonomy. Chapter 5 described autonomy in detail. Patients need to be given choices and feel that they have choices. Helping patients identify many different ways forward enters the equation in the fourth step of the five-step cycle with setting SMART goals. This feeds the need for autonomy. Patients also will experience a sense of competence if they select SMART goals that are within reach, meaning they are realistic. Having a real connection with someone like the clinician or coach performing the motivational interviewing and behavior change counseling helps fulfill these three requirements for sustained motivation in the self-determination theory. A non-judgmental approach to the patient enables the process of aligning motivation to flow.

Approaching this step in the five-step cycle with curiosity is key. The patient's reasons are personal and varied. Exploring the patient's own motivation and working to fully understand what the patient prioritizes and cherishes in their life right now is of paramount importance. Even asking, "What do you cherish most in this world right now?" or "What is your main priority?" can help the patient focus on motivation to make a change. The clinician learns a great deal about the patient through aligning motivation (Tables 12.4 and 12.5). While aligning motivation, the clinician uses the COACH Approach described in Chapter 1 with curiosity, openness, appreciation, compassion, and honesty.

12.1.4   STEP 3: BUILD CONFIDENCE

Confidence is defined as "a feeling or consciousness of one's powers or of reliance on one's circumstance".[50] Self-efficacy is the belief that one can be successful at a specific task like ballroom dancing, setting SMART goals, quitting smoking, or jumping rope. Self-esteem is the feeling that you are worthy and feel good about yourself. Self-efficacy and self-esteem play into confidence. Confidence is basically

TABLE 12.4
Motivational Interviewing Chart

Study	Number of Participants	Primary Outcomes
Barrett et al.[35]	10 randomized controlled trials involving 1,949 participants	Motivational interviewing with cognitive behavior therapy significantly increased physical activity (SMD: 0.18, 95% CI: 0.06–0.31, $p < 0.05$).
Dorstyn et al.[36]	10 randomized controlled trials with 987 adults	Motivational interviewing provides significant improvements in physical and psychological and social benefits when used with other counseling or rehabilitation techniques in adults with progressive multiple sclerosis and mild to moderate impairment (range: $g = .34$–2.68).
Ekong and Kavookjian[37]	159 studies identified, 14 retained studies	Motivational Interviewing positively influenced dietary behaviors
Frost et al.[38]	104 review journals, including 39 meta analyses	Motivational interviewing was found effective in stopping unhealthy behaviors, such as alcohol abuse, smoking, and substance abuse, and in promoting physical activity in those with chronic health conditions.
Hedegaard et al.[39]	532 Patients recruited from 3 hospital outpatient clinics	The combined clinical endpoint of stroke, cardiovascular death, or acute myocardial infarction was reached by 1.3% in the intervention group and 3.1% in the control group. Medication nonadherence was 20.3% in the intervention group and 30.2% in the control group receiving usual care ($P = .02$).
Lindson-Hawley et al.[40]	28 studies with 16,000 participants	Motivational interviewing significantly increased smoking quitting (risk ratio 1.26). MI delivered by primary physicians had the greatest effect when compared to delivery by hospital clinicians, nurses, or counselors (RR 3.49).
Lundahl et al.[41]	48 studies of 9,618 participants in medical settings	Motivational interviewing significantly improves patient behavior change to improve health outcomes in areas such as sedentary behavior, alcohol and tobacco use, body weight, alcohol and tobacco use, body weight, self-monitoring, confidence in change, HIV viral load, death rate, and approach to treatment, odd ratio = 1.55 (CI: 1.40–1.71), $z = 8.67$, $p < .001$.
Masterson Creber et al.[42]	67 participants hospitalized with heart failure	Motivational interviewing provides significant and clinically meaningful improvements in heart failure patients' self-care maintenance 90 days post hospital discharge.
Palacio et al.[43]	17 Randomized clinical trials	Improvements in medication adherence was associated with exposure times and counselors' educational level. The pooled risk ratio for medication adherence was higher for MI compared with control (1.17; 95% CI 1.05–1.31; $p < 0.01$).

(Continued)

TABLE 12.4 (*Continued*)
Motivational Interviewing Chart

Study	Number of Participants	Primary Outcomes
Pudkasam et al.[44]	Breast cancer survivors	Motivational interviewing, considering the transtheoretical model, theory of planned behavior, social cognitive theory, and self-determination theory, is shown to improve physical activity in breast cancer survivors.
Soderlund[45]	Nine studies on motivational interviewing in those with diabetes mellitus type 2	Motivational interviewing significantly increases physical activity in those with diabetes mellitus type 2 by targeting a minimal number of self-management behaviors when delivered by proficient counselors, emphasizing frequent MI sessions lasting a minimum of 30–45 minutes each.

TABLE 12.5
Motivational Interviewing and Behavior Change Chart

Study	Number of Participants	Primary Outcomes
Michaelsen and Esch[46]	Review of motivation and seven-stage behavior change process	Day-to-day health behavior is often determined by self-directed motives rather than by reflective thinking and self-control. Understanding the role of internal resources, such as the importance placed on possible outcomes, provides opportunities for understanding behavior change and in developing effective interventions.
Flannery[47]	Review of self-determination theory	Motivation is an essential component of behavioral change. Intrinsic motivation is supported when basic psychological needs of autonomy, competence, and relatedness are met. Intrinsic motivation reinforces enhanced well-being and lasting behavioral change.
Fisher et al.[48]	Review of self-determination theory	Self-determination theory can be used to address the motivational needs of those with diabetes. Using a three-step framework recognizing a person's need for autonomy, competence, and relatedness throughout the clinical encounter can improve providers' relationship building skills and the use of behavioral tools.
Teixeira et al.[49]	Systematic review includes 66 empirical studies	Self-determination theory is used to explore the connection between motivation and physical activity. Short-term adoption of the desired activity and intrinsic motivation positively support the prediction of physical activity across a range of samples and settings.

believing in yourself and your abilities. To be confident, a person needs to recognize their personal power. A person's power is wrapped up in their unique strengths which may be talents they were born with, skills they have honed, or personality traits that help them reach their goals. Chapter 3 reviewed building confidence and Chapter 10 covered building strengths.

This third step in the five-step cycle centers on building confidence. How can a clinician help a patient build confidence? Asking a person about their strengths is a straightforward way to help increase their confidence. A simple question like "What are your strengths?" may work to bring this information to the forefront. However, many people are uncomfortable talking about their strengths. Some people claim they do not have any strengths. Other ways to help people explore this area include saying "Tell me about a time when you reached a goal." When the person is done with this story, then the clinician can ask, "What strengths do you think you used to reach that goal?" Another tactic is to make the request, "Please tell me about a time when you were at your best, a time when you were really shining." If these prompts do not work, the clinician can invite the patient to take the Virtues In Action (VIA) online questionnaire, which is free and easily available. It takes about 10 minutes. (https://www.viacharacter.org). The patient receives a report about their signature strengths. This can open up a conversation about the results.

When people feel confident, they feel a sense of pride. Pride is a positive emotion that helps people feel creative. The next step of the five-step cycle is to set SMART goals, and this often takes creativity in addition to confidence. In this way, step three opens the door for step four (Table 12.6).

12.1.5 Step 4: Set SMART Goals

After the clinician has set the stage with empathy and the patient feels understood and appreciated, they align motivation, identify strengths, build confidence, and are ready for setting goals. Goal setting helps people make progress. Goals were covered in Chapter 4. Feeling motivated is fuel for change. Action is needed to make change. Goals are those action steps that lead to new patterns, practices, and healthy lifestyles. When people achieve goals, they experience the release of dopamine into the reward center of the brain, the ventral tegmental area and nucleus accumbens. People who create video games know this well which is why most games have different levels to reach. Each level reached is like achieving another goal and dopamine is released. With the behavior change process, it is helpful if the process is enjoyable. Reaching goals and releasing dopamine helps to reinforce this behavior change.

Setting SMART goals helps patients achieve success.[1] The acronym SMART represents goals that are: S – Specific; M – Measurable; A – Action Oriented; R – Realistic; and T – Time sensitive. Some people use S – Specific; M – Measurable; A – Achievable; R – Relevant; and T – Time sensitive. That can work too. It is used in business a lot. In the workplace, goals are often set by a manager or boss. In this case, it is important to make sure the goal is relevant to the employee. However, in behavior change counseling, the goal is set by the patient and they make it relevant to their life and lifestyle. Thus, the R changes to realistic. The A is achievable in the

TABLE 12.6
Self-Efficacy and Confidence Chart

Study	Number of Participants	Primary Outcomes
Rabenbauer[51]	224 Patients with back pain	High levels of self-efficacy significantly increase the adoption of healthy habits.
Kwarteng et al.[52]	246 Overweight/obese African American breast cancer survivors	Self-efficacy, perceived access to exercise, and social support played a role in behavior change associated with weight loss and improved diet. Self-efficacy and perceived access to exercise showed more consistent effects than social support.
Hu et al.[53]	151 Hemodialysis patients	Self-efficacy significantly impacts changes in sodium intake at 8 and 16 weeks (p-int=0.051 and 0.06, respectively). Low self-efficacy is significantly found in younger patients and those with perceived income inadequacy.
Awick et al.[54]	370 Breast cancer survivors	Those with higher activity at baseline had significantly higher self-efficacy in areas of barriers ($\beta=0.29$) and exercise ($\beta=0.23$). Women with higher self-efficacy reported significantly higher physical self-worth ($\beta=0.26$, 0.16). Higher physical self-worth is significantly related with greater self-esteem ($\beta=0.47$).
Kudoh[55]	198 Patients with type 2 diabetes	Self-efficacy is positively associated with dental consultations among patients with periodontal disease ([OR]=1.26, 95% confidence interval [CI]: 1.10–1.45) and with knowledge among patients without periodontal disease (OR=1.54, 95%, CI: 1.09-2.16).
Jiang et al.[56]	265 Adults with type 2 diabetes	Self-efficacy is found to have the strongest direct effect on diabetes self-management behaviors ($\beta=0.550$, $p=.000$). Self-efficacy plays an important role in subjects' ability to use knowledge to change diabetes self-management (DSM) behaviors and is a predictor of DSM behaviors.
Burger and Samuel[57]	5126 Compulsory-school leavers (55.3% female)	Baseline levels of self-efficacy and stress as well as within-person change in self-efficacy and stress affected life satisfaction in adolescents. Baseline self-efficacy lessened negative effects of stress on life satisfaction.
Sperber et al.[58]	339 Older adults in a lifestyle physical activity program, with arthritis and joint pain.	Physical activity self-efficacy ($\beta=.32$) change is associated with change in physical activity ($\beta=.36$). Changes in pain and depression are associated with changes in physical activity (PA) self-efficacy ($\beta=-.20$ and $-.21$). PA self-efficacy is associated with PA ($\beta=.15$).
Cinar and Schou[59]	186 participants randomly assigned to health coaching ($n=77$) and health education ($n=109$) groups.	Health coaching is shown to be more effective in reducing HbA1c and clinical attachment loss compared with health education. Health coaching improves self-intrinsic motivation, and self-efficacy needed to support behavior for healthy lifestyles.
Strecher et al.[60]	Systematic review	The reviewed studies suggest that self-efficacy is associated with health behavior change and maintenance. Enhancement of self-efficacy is positively associated with health behavior change.

workplace SMART acronym. In behavior change counseling, it is important that the goals are action oriented. The action might be to watch a movie for someone in contemplation or to research yoga studios for someone in preparation.

A goal that is broad and general is difficult to achieve. For example, I will lose 20 pounds is a goal but is not SMART, as it is too general. It is not time sensitive. It is unknown whether it is realistic because there is no time frame associated with it. It is not realistic in one week. It may be realistic for a year's time. It depends on the patient. Most importantly, it is not action oriented. How will this person lose 20 pounds? Will they change their movement, their meals, their sleep pattern or what?

When the patient is ready for action, the goal setting comes into the counseling session. "What do you want to do this week?" is a good question to start the process of goal setting. It is important that the patient determines the goal. It is possible that the patient may spend a great deal of time talking about exercise, and when it comes to goal setting, they may state, "I want to quit smoking. I won't be able to exercise until I can take deep breaths. I want to work on setting a quit date." It will be important that the clinician allows for autonomy in the goal setting by letting the patient identify the focus. The clinician can help hone the goal into a SMART one, but the patient needs to select the lifestyle pattern or behavior they want to address first. And, the patient selects the specifics of the SMART goal that suits their schedule, desires, and needs.

After the SMART goal is co-created, the clinician can check in on how realistic the goal is by asking about confidence. For example, the provider could ask, "How confident are you that you will accomplish this goal this week on a scale of 0–10 with 10 being fully confident?" If the patient says any number that is less than seven, the clinician can ask, "What would it take to move that confidence to an 8 or 9?" Then, the patient can adjust the goal accordingly. This takes practice for the patient and the clinician.

It is important to remember that small successes build confidence needed to achieve larger goals. Keeping the goals simple and small, especially to begin, is essential to keep the patient engaged and rewarded. Remember about the dopamine release that occurs when reaching a goal. The objective is to set goals that are specific, measurable, action-oriented, realistic, and time-sensitive, SMART. Success breeds success. Keep that dopamine flowing naturally by setting and achieving small goals (Tables 12.7 and 12.8).

12.1.6 STEP 5: SET ACCOUNTABILITY

Accountability is defined as "the quality or state of being accountable *especially*: an obligation or willingness to accept responsibility or to account for one's actions".[73] Chapter 11 provides a detailed description of accountability. Accountable is often interchangeable with answerable. One is responsible for answering for one's behavior when one is accountable. Accountability has been researched with regard to patient compliance. There are two types of accountability described in the literature: controlled accountability and autonomous accountability.[74] With controlled accountability, the clinician may make demands on the patient, and there may be an element of

TABLE 12.7

Goal-Setting Chart

Study	Number of Participants	Primary Outcomes
Bailey[61]	Systematic review	Clinicians can help patients in their behavior change efforts through goal setting that includes action and coping plans. Framing of goals and action plans should be challenging, approach and mastery based, and intrinsically motivating. Action plans can help patients understand the steps needed to achieve their goals. This process is not time consuming but requires effort from the clinician and the patient.
Baker et al.[62]	Systematic review	Self-belief is the strongest factor contributing to goal achievement in older adults, enhanced by personal coaching from health staff. Inconsistent goal terminology reduces engagement and results in confusion.
Aaron et al.[63]	212 African American women from a telephone-based asthma self-management program	Goal attainment is associated with fewer depressive symptoms ($p < .01$) and resulted in more goals being achieved during interventions (Estimate [SE] = 1.25 [0.18]; $p < .001$). The use of specific goal attainment methods increases efficacy.
Dörfler and Kulnik[64]	11 stroke rehabilitation clinicians participated in semi-structured interviews	Rehabilitation professionals combine goal-setting strategies with a mindset to involve clients in the process. The goal-setting process is an evolving practice adapted to the changing needs of the client.
Evans[65]	Systematic review	Fostering patient involvement in the goal-setting process does not require significant resources. However, it enhances goal setting that is more meaningful for the patient and improves the patient experience.
Karamanian et al.[66]	98 SNAP-eligible participants enrolled of which 80% were women, 75% were Black/Non-Hispanic, and 39% were 45–54 years of age	Participants significantly improved self-efficacy, knowledge, and health behaviors. Mean daily intake for vegetables ($P < 0.05$) and fruits ($P < 0.05$) increased by one-third of a cup ($P < 0.01$).
Hughes et al.[67]	13 interviews with group facilitators, 20 interviews with group participants	Facilitators support participant goals and perceive them as vital to improving motivation and self-responsibility. Facilitators influence the translation of participants' goals into behavior change activities.
Knittle et al.[68]	Systematic literature search with 89 intervention studies ($k = 200$; $N = 19,212$)	Interventions delivered face-to-face, and in gym settings, that include behavior change techniques, goal setting, self-monitoring, or rehearsal, showed beneficial motivational outcomes (effect sizes ranged from $d = 0.12$ to $d = 0.46$). Increases in intention and stage of change, but not autonomous motivation, were significantly associated with increases in physical activity.

TABLE 12.8
Goal-Setting and Behavior Change Chart

Study	Number of Participants	Primary Outcomes
Barrett et al.[69]	317 overweight/obese participants	Overweight/obese individuals in cardiac rehabilitation benefited from participating in behavioral weight loss classes and setting weight loss goals. This led to more weight loss than a weight loss goal alone. Having a weight loss goal results in greater weight loss than not setting a goal.
Cullen et al.[70]	Review	Goal setting is an effective strategy for behavior change. A four-step process for goal setting identifies: recognizing a need for change; establishing a goal; adopting a goal-directed activity and self-monitoring it; and self-rewarding goal attainment. Incorporating goal-setting strategies to enhance the behavior change process in nutrition education programs is beneficial.
Epton et al.[71]	Review	Goal setting is effective in behavior change and can be considered an essential component of effective interventions. This review adds insight not on how goal setting can be used to augment behavior change.
Ries et al.[72]	485 women aged 18 years and over	Intervention participants were more likely to move from contemplation to action/maintenance for diet improvement goals (58% intervention, 44% comparison, $p = 0.04$) and physical activity (56% intervention, 31% comparison, $p \leq 0.0001$).

shame, fear, or duress. With autonomous accountability, the clinician and the patient share a partnership and the patient is encouraged to perform the behavior to please themselves. There may be an element of pleasing the clinician in this scenario as well. The accountability is often provided at the clinical visits when a clinician is involved. With behavior change counseling and coaching, the accountability used is similar to autonomous accountability. It's possible to set up accountability with a family member, friend, or even online community. Internal accountability, in which the patient logs and tracks for themselves, is another form of accountability.

Face-to-face follow-up with the patient varies. It could be weekly if the patient is working with a health coach or behavior change specialist or it may be after 8–12 weeks if the patient is using follow-up visits for diabetes or heart disease with their physician as their accountability. Research shows that working with a health coach may be one way to increase accountability.[75] Follow-up that keeps patients accountable does not need to be face to face. Telehealth routine visits with health coaches have been reported to keep patients motivated and accountable.[76] Electronic follow-up with emails and texts can help patients with accountability and follow through too. In one specific study with patients managing psoriasis, investigating the use of topical medication for skin plaques, those patients that used an electronic reporting system were more likely to use the medicine.[77]

"What gets measured, gets managed," said Peter Drucker, the founder of modern management. Accountability helps patients to maintain focus on their goals.[1] When patients set goals, they focus. There is a little stress applied to their change process, not too much stress, but some stress that helps push people into action. Just as when there are deadlines for chapter writing, there is a little stress that puts the writer into action. If the goal is a SMART goal, there will be just the right amount of stress to encourage movement toward attaining the end result. If no one ever checks on the goal and the outcome, then the patient is less likely to follow through. If someone is checking in on the goal, then the patient feels supported. This accountability helps people maintain action. If no one checks in on the goal, the patient might even forget about it themselves.

Tracking systems help people stay accountable. Pedometers can be helpful, and these are connected to many phones and wearable devices that may also track heart rate, hours of sleep, and other metrics. Using a pen and paper log on a piece of paper or a calendar may work for some people, while others will want to use their mobile phone or computer to log data. Patients may want to see hours of sleep, number of vegetables consumed, or minutes of moderate physical activity accumulated in the week or other behaviors. Some patients even enjoy making graphs of their progress. Everyone is different. Providing options for tracking is a way to empower patients and provide autonomy.

Part of accountability might include a buddy or friend who is on a similar behavior change journey. Checking in with each other is enjoyable and encouraging. Sharing goals and commitment to change with others helps people stay accountable. These people often check in with the person wanting to make the change out of interest and genuine concern for the person. They may want to help the person reach their goals as much as they want to reach their own goals. This social connection is powerful. Group interventions discussed in Chapter 13 work to harness the power of social connections.

The clinician helps with accountability. After setting a goal, the patient will return to the clinician and report on the progress. Since the clinician and the patient know the goal, as it was co-created at the previous visit, the clinician can initiate a discussion about the behavior change progress. This needs to be accomplished with empathy. The whole five-step cycle starts again with empathy when the patient comes for follow-up. Then, the process starts again with expressing empathy, aligning motivation, building confidence, setting SMART goals, and setting accountability (Table 12.9).

12.2 SUMMARY

Behavior change is an important part of lifestyle medicine. Knowing the guidelines for exercise, the recommendations for a healthy diet, the importance of sound sleep, the methodologies to reduce stress, the ways to cultivate high-quality connections, and the healthy outcomes from smoking cessation and substance use elimination or moderation are critical parts to practicing lifestyle medicine. But, knowing all of that and sharing this knowledge will not create behavior change in patients. Patients need to focus on what those healthy habits mean to them. They need to become aware of their current lifestyle and compare it to the recommendations created by academic

TABLE 12.9
Accountability Chart

Study	Number of Participants	Primary Outcomes
Knittle et al.[68]	Systematic review 89 studies	Beneficial and impactful studies used specific strategies including face-to-face delivery or delivery in gym settings. Behavior change techniques that were effective included: "behavioural goal setting," "self-monitoring (behavior)," "behavioural practice/rehearsal," or a combination of self-monitoring (behavior) with any other behavior change theory derived from control theory.
McDonough et al.[78]	Qualitative review and Meta Study with 39 articles	Supportive behaviors in breast cancer patients that enable physical activity include providing encouragement and accountability.
Ronkko[79]	Field study of 8 youths using a wearable tracking device and 12 staff social workers in an accommodation home in Helsingborg, Sweden	Youths enjoyed the tracking and instant feedback Creating long-term goals was an important factor for positive lifestyle change The information from the trackers allowed for rich conversations and counseling opportunities.
Browne et al.[80]	12-month randomized placebo controlled study with 56 participants	Intervention group with a biometric tracking ring and behavior modification messaging with an app had significant improvements in sleep onset latency, daily step count, % time jogging, VO2max, body fat percentage, and heart rate variability compared to the control group of wellness education. After 3 months, some participants stopped the intervention and they remained at the same level without regression for the next 9 months. The group that continued with the intervention continued to improve.
Oussedik et al.[74]	Descriptive Paper about the importance of accountability in adherence	There is a distinction made between paternalistic type of accountability or controlled accountability in which duress is utilized to encourage people to be compliant and autonomous accountability in which a person's internal desire to please a respected health care provider is the driver of the behavior.
Liddy et al.[75]	Semi-structured interviews of 11 patients enrolled in a pilot health coaching program who were at risk or diagnosed with type 2 diabetes	Subjects reported that the health coaching program helped them better understand how diabetes impacts their health and their bodies, improved their access to care, and also created a structure for accountability for their lifestyle actions that could impact their health.

(Continued)

TABLE 12.9 (*Continued*)
Accountability Chart

Study	Number of Participants	Primary Outcomes
Warner et al.[76]	Semi-structured interview study with 21 patients with chronic kidney disease who participated in a coaching program	Identified themes include: valuing relationships (motivated by accountability), appreciating convenience, empowering actionable knowledge, increasing diet consciousness, and making sense of complexity.
Wang et al.[81]	12-week randomized control trial in 20 patients with prostate cancer to evaluate a web-based lifestyle medicine intervention	Factors driving engagement include: environment, motivation (accountability), preparedness, program design, and program support.
Church and Dawson[82]	Description of a data-driven approach to driving accountability for behavior change at the individual level called the "Development Check-In" system	The Development Check-In system provides leaders and managers with targeted and positive feedback which keeps them accountable and supports development.

organizations like the American College of Lifestyle Medicine which uses evidence-based approaches to patient care. Then, the patient needs to figure out what they want in life, what they desire, what they hold most dear, where they want to be in 10 or 20 years, and how they will get there. Most people are longing to change in some way.

The lifestyle medicine clinician can help empower the patient to adopt and sustain healthy lifestyles by partnering with them, collaborating with them, using the behavior change theories and techniques that work, and following the five-step cycle to work synergistically with the patient. It is the synergy between clinician and patient that is often the secret sauce of lifestyle medicine practices.

This synergy ultimately sets patients free to thrive while continuing on their lifestyle medicine journeys joyfully.

12.3 TAKEAWAYS

The five-step cycle for collaboration can provide a step-by-step approach to working on behavior change with someone.

1. Without empathy, the five-step cycle cannot start.
2. After expressing empathy and listening intently to the patient, guiding the patient to the next step of aligning motivation is possible through asking open-ended questions.

3. A patient needs to feel a sense of confidence before they are ready to consider action steps.
4. Setting SMART goals is a process that takes time and careful attention to the patient's schedule, desires, abilities, and needs.
5. Without accountability, goals may become words without action. Checking in on the patient's goals can come in many different forms.
6. No matter what progress the patient made toward the goals, the practitioner needs to express empathy at follow-up so that the 5 Step Cycle for collaboration can continue to propel forward.

REFERENCES

1. Frates, E. P., Moore, M. A., Lopez, C. N., McMahon, G. T. 2011. Coaching for behavior change in physiatry. *Am J Phys Med Rehabil* 90(12):1074–1082. doi:10.1097/PHM.0b013e31822dea9a.
2. Merriam Webster Dictionary. Empathy. Online accessed January 1, 2022. https://www.merriam-webster.com/dictionary/empathy.
3. Merriam Webster Dictionary. Sympathy. Online accessed January 1, 2022. https://www.merriam-webster.com/dictionary/sympathy.
4. Merriam Webster Dictionary. Sympathy. What's the difference between 'sympathy' and 'empathy'? Online accessed January 1, 2022. https://www.merriam-webster.com/words-at-play/sympathy-empathy-difference.
5. Wang, H., Kline, J. A., Jackson, B. E. et al. 2018. Association between emergency physician self-reported empathy and patient satisfaction. *PLOS ONE* 13(9):e0204113. doi:10.1371/journal.pone.0204113.
6. Hojat, M., Louis, D. Z., Markham, F. W., Wender, R., Rabinowitz, C., Gonnella, J.S. 2011. Physicians' empathy and clinical outcomes for diabetic patients. *Acad Med* 86(3):359–364. doi:10.1097/ACM.0b013e3182086fe1.
7. Chaitoff, A., Rothberg, M. B., Windover, A. K., Calabrese, L., Misra-Hebert, A. D., Martinez, K. A. 2019. Physician empathy is not associated with laboratory outcomes in diabetes: A cross-sectional study. *J Gen Intern Med* 34(1):75–81. doi:10.1007/s11606-018-4731-0.
8. Goleman, D. 2011. *The Brain and Emotional Intelligence;* New Insights. More Than Sound. Florence, MA.
9. Whitworth, L., Kimsey-House, K., Kimsey-House, H., Sandah, P. 2009. *Co-Active Coaching: New Skills for Coaching People toward Success in Work and Life.* Davies-Black Pub, Mountain View, CA
10. Pass it on. Online accessed January 1, 2022. https://www.passiton.com/inspirational-quotes/7841-feeling-gratitude-and-not-expressing-it-is-like.
11. Bernardo, M. O., Cecílio-Fernandes, D., Costa, P., Quince, T. A., Costa, M. J., Carvalho-Filho, M. A. 2018. Physicians' self-assessed empathy levels do not correlate with patients' assessments. *PLOS ONE* 13(5), e0198488. doi:10.1371/journal.pone.0198488.
12. Menendez, M. E., Chen, N. C., Mudgal, C. S., Jupiter, J. B., Ring, D. 2015. Physician empathy as a driver of hand surgery patient satisfaction. *J Hand Surg Am* 40(9):1860–1865.e2. doi:10.1016/j.jhsa.2015.06.105.
13. Mercer, S. W., Jani, B. D., Maxwell, M., Wong, S. Y., Watt, G. C. 2012. Patient enablement requires physician empathy: A cross-sectional study of general practice consultations in areas of high and low socioeconomic deprivation in Scotland. *BMC Fam Pract* 13:6. doi:10.1186/1471-2296-13-6.

14. Sanders, J. J., Dubey, M., Hall, J. A., Catzen, H. Z., Blanch-Hartigan, D., Schwartz, R. 2021. What is empathy? Oncology patient perspectives on empathic clinician behaviors. *Cancer* 127(22):4258–4265. doi:10.1002/cncr.33834.

15. Simões, J. A., Prazeres, F., Maricoto, T. et al. 2021. Physician empathy and patient enablement: Survey in the Portuguese primary health care. *Fam Pract* 38(5):606–611. doi:10.1093/fampra/cmab005.

16. Steinhausen, S., Ommen, O., Thüm, S. et al. 2014. Physician empathy and subjective evaluation of medical treatment outcome in trauma surgery patients. *Patient Educ Couns* 95(1):53–60. doi:10.1016/j.pec.2013.12.007.

17. Kim, S. S., Kaplowitz, S., Johnston, M. V. 2004. The effects of physician empathy on patient satisfaction and compliance. *Eval Health Prof* 27(3):237–251. doi:10.1177/0163278704267037.

18. Naoum, S., Konstantinidis, T. I., Spinthouri, M., Mitseas, P., Sarafis, P. 2021. Patient satisfaction and physician empathy at a hellenic air force health service. *Mil Med* 186(9–10):1029–1036. doi:10.1093/milmed/usab060.

19. Walsh, S., O'Neill, A., Hannigan, A., Harmon, D. 2019. Patient-rated physician empathy and patient satisfaction during pain clinic consultations. *Ir J Med Sci* 188(4):1379–1384. doi:10.1007/s11845-019-01999-5.

20. Byrd, J., Knowles, H., Moore, S. et al. 2021. Synergistic effects of emergency physician empathy and burnout on patient satisfaction: A prospective observational study. *Emerg Med J* 38(4):290–296. doi:10.1136/emermed-2019-209393.

21. Abdulkader, R. S., Venugopal, D., Jeyashree, K., Al Zayer, Z., Senthamarai, K., Jebitha, R. 2022. The intricate relationship between client perceptions of physician empathy and physician self-assessment: Lessons for reforming clinical practice. *J Patient Exp* 9:23743735221077537. doi:10.1177/23743735221077537

22. Chittem, M., Sridharan, S. G., Pongener, M., Maya, S., Epton, T. 2022. Experiences of barriers to self-monitoring and medication-management among Indian patients with type 2 diabetes, their primary family-members and physicians. *Chronic Illn* 18(3):677–690. doi:10.1177/17423953211032251.

23. Elliott, R., Elliott, R., Bohart, A. C., Watson, J. C., Murphy, D. 2018. Therapist empathy and client outcome: An updated meta-analysis. *Psychotherapy (Chic)* 55(4):399–410. doi:10.1037/pst0000175.

24. Surchat, C., Carrard, V., Gaume, J., Berney, A., Clair, C. 2022. Impact of physician empathy on patient outcomes: A gender analysis. *Br J Gen Pract* 72(715):e99–e107. doi:10.3399/BJGP.2021.0193.

25. Sperandeo, R., Cioffi, V., Mosca, L.L. et al. 2021. Exploring the question: "Does empathy work in the same way in online and in-person therapeutic settings?". *Front Psychol* 12:671790. doi:10.3389/fpsyg.2021.671790.

26. Farber, B. A., Suzuki, J. Y., Lynch, D. A. 2018. Positive regard and psychotherapy outcome: A meta-analytic review. *Psychotherapy (Chic)* 55(4):411–423. doi:10.1037/pst0000171.

27. Hansen, C. B., Pavlovic, K. M. H., Sondergaard, J., Thilsing, T. 2020. Does GP empathy influence patient enablement and success in lifestyle change among high risk patients?. *BMC Fam Pract* 21(1):159. doi:10.1186/s12875-020-01232-8.

28. Geyer, C. 2021. Empathy and language in the clinician patient relationship: Improving the translation of evidence to practice. *Am J Health Promot* 35(4):590–592. doi:10.1177/08901171211002328b.

29. Derksen, F. A. W. M., Olde Hartman, T. C., Lagro-Janssen, A. L. M., Kramer, A. W. M. 2021. Clinical empathy in GP-training: Experiences and needs among Dutch GP-trainees. "Empathy as an element of personal growth." *Patient Educ Couns* 104(12):3016–3022. doi:10.1016/j.pec.2021.03.030.

30. Mert, A., Kaptanoğlu, A., Hasan Olmez, E. 2021. Measurement of patient's perception levels with reference to physician's empathy: Private hospitals scenario. *Cureus* 13(10):e18684. doi:10.7759/cureus.18684.

31. Luig, T., Wicklum, S., Heatherington, M., Vu, A., Cameron, E., Klein, D., Sharma, A. M., Campbell-Scherer, D. L. 2020. Improving obesity management training in family medicine: Multi-methods evaluation of the 5AsT-MD pilot course. *BMC Med Educ* 20(1):5. doi:10.1186/s12909-019-1908-0.

32. Spencer, J., Goode, J., Penix, E. A., Trusty, W., Swift, J. K. 2019. Developing a collaborative relationship with clients during the initial sessions of psychotherapy. *Psychotherapy (Chic)* 56(1):7–10. doi:10.1037/pst0000208.

33. Elliott, R., Bohart, A. C., Watson, J. C., Greenberg, L.S. 2011. Empathy. *Psychotherapy (Chic)* 48(1):43–49. doi:10.1037/a0022187.

34. Ryan, R. M., Deci, E. L. 2017. *Self-Determination Theory: Basic Psychological Needs in Motivation, Development, and Wellness.* New York, NY: Guilford Publishing.

35. Barrett, S., Begg, S., O'Halloran, P., Kingsley, M. 2018. Integrated motivational interviewing and cognitive behaviour therapy for lifestyle mediators of overweight and obesity in community-dwelling adults: A systematic review and meta-analyses. *BMC Public Health* 18(1):1160. doi:10.1186/s12889-018-6062-9.

36. Dorstyn, D. S., Mathias, J. L., Bombardier, C. H., Osborn, A. J. 2020. Motivational interviewing to promote health outcomes and behaviour change in multiple sclerosis: A systematic review. *Clin Rehabil* 34(3):299–309. doi:10.1177/0269215519895790.

37. Ekong, G., Kavookjian, J. 2016. Motivational interviewing and outcomes in adults with type 2 diabetes: A systematic review. *Patient Educ Couns* 99(6):944–952. doi:10.1016/j.pec.2015.11.022.

38. Frost, H., Campbell, P., Maxwell, M. et al. 2018. Effectiveness of motivational interviewing on adult behaviour change in health and social care settings: A systematic review of reviews. *PLOS ONE* 13(10):e0204890. doi:10.1371/journal.pone.0204890.

39. Hedegaard, U., Kjeldsen, L. J., Pottegård, A. et al. 2015. Improving medication adherence in patients with hypertension: A randomized trial. *Am J Med* 128(12):1351–1361. doi:10.1016/j.amjmed.2015.08.011.

40. Lindson-Hawley, N., Thompson, T. P., Begh, R. 2015. Motivational interviewing for smoking cessation. *Cochrane Database Syst Rev* 7 (7):CD006936. doi:10.1002/14651858. CD006936.pub3.

41. Lundahl, B., Moleni, T., Burke, B. L. et al. 2013. Motivational interviewing in medical care settings: A systematic review and meta-analysis of randomized controlled trials. *Patient Educ Couns* 93(2):157–168. doi:10.1016/j.pec.2013.07.012.

42. Masterson Creber, R., Patey, M., Lee, C. S., Kuan, A., Jurgens, C., Riegel, B. 2016. Motivational interviewing to improve self-care for patients with chronic heart failure: MITI-HF randomized controlled trial. *Patient Educ Couns* 99(2):256–264. doi:10.1016/j.pec.2015.08.031.

43. Palacio, A., Garay, D., Langer, B., Taylor, J., Wood, B. A., Tamariz, L. 2016. Motivational interviewing improves medication adherence: A systematic review and meta-analysis. *J Gen Intern Med* 31(8):929–940. doi:10.1007/s11606-016-3685-3.

44. Pudkasam, S., Polman, R., Pitcher, M. et al. 2018. Physical activity and breast cancer survivors: Importance of adherence, motivational interviewing and psychological health. *Maturitas* 116:66–72. doi:10.1016/j.maturitas.2018.07.010.

45. Soderlund, P. D. 2018. Effectiveness of motivational interviewing for improving physical activity self-management for adults with type 2 diabetes: A review. *Chronic Illn* 14(1):54–68. doi:10.1177/1742395317699449.

46. Michaelsen, M. M., Esch, T. 2021. Motivation and reward mechanisms in health behavior change processes. *Brain Res* 1757:147309. doi:10.1016/j.brainres.2021.147309.

47. Flannery, M. 2017. Self-determination theory: Intrinsic motivation and behavioral change. *Oncol Nurs Forum* 44(2):155–156. doi:10.1188/17.ONF.155-156.

48. Fisher, L., Polonsky, W. H., Hessler, D., Potter, M. B. 2017. A practical framework for encouraging and supporting positive behaviour change in diabetes. *Diabet Med* 34(12):1658–1666. doi:10.1111/dme.13414.

49. Teixeira, P. J., Carraça, E. V., Markland, D., Silva, M. N., Ryan, R. M. 2012. Exercise, physical activity, and self-determination theory: A systematic review. *Int J Behav Nutr Phys Activity* 9:78. doi:10.1186/1479–5868-9-78.

50. Merriam Webster Dictionary. Confidence. Accessed January 1, 2022. https://www.merriam-webster.com/dictionary/confidence.

51. Rabenbauer, L. M., Mevenkamp, N. 2021. Factors in the effectiveness of e-Health interventions for chronic back pain: How self-efficacy mediates e-Health literacy and healthy habits. *Telemed e-Health* 27(2):184–192. doi:10.1089/tmj.2019.0301.

52. Kwarteng, J. L., Beyer, K., Banerjee, A., Stolley, M. R. 2020. Facilitators of behavior change and weight loss in an intervention for African American Breast Cancer Survivors. *Cancer Causes Control* 31(8):737–747. doi:10.1007/s10552-020-01315-y.

53. Hu, L., St-Jules, D. E., Popp, C. J., Sevick, M. A. 2019. Determinants and the role of self-efficacy in a sodium-reduction trial in hemodialysis patients. *J Renal Nutr* 29(4):328–332. doi:10.1053/j.jrn.2018.10.006.

54. Awick, E. A., Phillips, S. M., Lloyd, G. R., McAuley, E. 2017. Physical activity, self-efficacy and self-esteem in breast cancer survivors: A panel model. *Psycho-oncology* 26(10):1625–1631. doi:10.1002/pon.4180.

55. Kudoh, R., Shibayama, T., Hidaka, K. 2021. The role of knowledge and self-efficacy on dental consultation behavior of patients with type 2 diabetes. *Japan J Nurs Sci* 18(1):e12378. doi:10.1111/jjns.12378.

56. Jiang, X., Jiang, H., Li, M., Lu, Y., Liu, K., Sun, X. 2019. The mediating role of self-efficacy in shaping self-management behaviors among adults with type 2 diabetes. *Worldviews Evid-Based Nurs* 16(2):151–160. doi:10.1111/wvn.12354.

57. Burger, K., Samuel, R. 2017. The role of perceived stress and self-efficacy in young people's life satisfaction: A longitudinal study. *J Youth Adolesc* 46(1):78–90. doi:10.1007/s10964-016-0608-x.

58. Sperber, N., Hall, K. S., Allen, K., DeVellis, B. M., Lewis, M., Callahan, L. F. 2014. The role of symptoms and self-efficacy in predicting physical activity change among older adults with arthritis. *J Phys Activity Health* 11(3):528–535. doi:10.1123/jpah.2012-0030.

59. Cinar, A. B., Schou, L. 2014. The role of self-efficacy in health coaching and health education for patients with type 2 diabetes. *Int Dent J* 64(3):155–163. doi:10.1111/idj.12093.

60. Strecher, V. J., DeVellis, B. M., Becker, M. H., Rosenstock, I. M. 1986. The role of self-efficacy in achieving health behavior change. *Health Educ Q* 13(1), 73–92. doi:10.1177/109019818601300108.

61. Bailey, R. R. 2017. Goal setting and action planning for health behavior change. Am J Lifestyle Med 13(6):615–618. doi:10.1177/1559827617729634.

62. Baker, N., Lawn, S., Gordon, S. J., George, S. 2021. Older adults' experiences of goals in health: A systematic review and metasynthesis. *J Appl Gerontol* 40(8), 818–827. doi:10.1177/0733464820918134.

63. Aaron, M., Nelson, B. W., Kaltsas, E., Brown, R. W., Thomas, L. J., Patel, M. R. 2017. Impact of goal setting and goal attainment methods on asthma outcomes. *Health Educ Behav* 44(1):103–112. doi:10.1177/1090198116637858.

64. Dörfler, E., Kulnik, S. T. 2020. Despite communication and cognitive impairment - person-centred goal-setting after stroke: A qualitative study. *Disabil Rehabil* 42(25):3628–3637. doi:10.1080/09638288.2019.1604821.
65. Evans, J. J. 2012. Goal setting during rehabilitation early and late after acquired brain injury. *Curr Opin Neurol* 25(6):651–655. doi:10.1097/WCO.0b013e3283598f75.
66. Karamanian, V., Zepka, B., Ernst, A., West, C., Grode, G., Miller, C. 2020. Goal-setting program improves nutrition and physical activity among Supplemental Nutrition Assistance Program eligible adults. *Public Health Nutr* 23(11):1924–1930. doi:10.1017/S1368980019004518.
67. Hughes, S., Lewis, S., Willis, K., Rogers, A., Wyke, S., Smith, L. 2020. Goal setting in group programmes for long-term condition self-management support: experiences of patients and healthcare professionals. *Psychol Health* 35(1), 70–86. doi:10.1080/08870446.2019.1623891.
68. Knittle, K., Nurmi, J., Crutzen, R., Hankonen, N., Beattie, M., Dombrowski, S. U. 2018. How can interventions increase motivation for physical activity? A systematic review and meta-analysis. *Health Psychol Rev* 12(3), 211–230. doi:10.1080/17437199.2018.1435299.
69. Barrett, K. V., Savage, P. D., Ades, P. A. 2020. Effects of behavioral weight loss and weight loss goal setting in cardiac rehabilitation. *J Cardiopulmon Rehabil Prev* 40(6):383–387. doi:10.1097/HCR.0000000000000510.
70. Cullen, K. W., Baranowski, T., Smith, S. P. 2001. Using goal setting as a strategy for dietary behavior change. *J Am Diet Assoc* 101(5):562–566. doi:10.1016/S0002-8223(01)00140-7.
71. Epton, T., Currie, S., Armitage, C. J. 2017. Unique effects of setting goals on behavior change: Systematic review and meta-analysis. *J Consult Clin Psychol* 85(12):1182–1198. doi:10.1037/ccp0000260.
72. Ries, A. V., Blackman, L. T., Page, R. A., Gizlice, Z., Benedict, S., Barnes, K., Kelsey, K., Carter-Edwards, L. 2014. Goal setting for health behavior change: Evidence from an obesity intervention for rural low-income women. *Rural Remote Health* 14:2682.
73. Merriam Webster Dictionary. Accountability. Accessed January 1, 2022. https://www.merriam-webster.com/dictionary/accountability.
74. Oussedik, E., Foy, C. G., Masicampo, E. J., Kammrath, L. K., Anderson, R. E., Feldman, S. R. 2017. Accountability: A missing construct in models of adherence behavior and in clinical practice. *Patient Prefer Adher* 11:1285–1294. doi:10.2147/PPA.S135895.
75. Liddy, C., Johnston, S., Irving, H., Nash, K., Ward, N. 2015 Improving awareness, accountability, and access through health coaching: Qualitative study of patients' perspectives. Can Fam Physician 61(3):e158–e164.
76. Warner, M. M., Tong, A., Campbell, K. L., Kelly, J. T. 2019. Patients' experiences and perspectives of telehealth coaching with a dietitian to improve diet quality in chronic kidney disease: A qualitative interview study. *J Acad Nutr Diet* 119(8):1362–1374. doi:10.1016/j.jand.2019.01.023.
77. Alinia, H., Moradi Tuchayi, S., Smith, J. A., Richardson, I. M., Bahrami, N., Jaros, S. C., Sandoval, L. F., Farhangian, M. E., Anderson, K. L., Huang, K. E., Feldman, S. R. 2017. Long-term adherence to topical psoriasis Treatment can be abysmal: A 1-year randomized intervention study using objective electronic adherence monitoring. *Br J Dermatol* 176(3):759–764. doi:10.1111/bjd.15085.
78. McDonough, M. H., Beselt, L. J., Kronlund, L. J., Albinati, N. K., Daun, J. T., Trudeau, M. S., Wong, J. B., Culos-Reed, S. N., Bridel, W. 2021. Social support and physical activity for cancer survivors: A qualitative review and meta-study. J Cancer Surviv 15(5):713–728. doi:10.1007/s11764-020-00963-y.

79. Rönkkö, K. 2018. An activity tracker and its accompanying app as a motivator for increased exercise and better sleeping habits for youths in need of social care: field study. *JMIR mHealth uHealth* 6(12):e193. doi:10.2196/mhealth.9286.
80. Browne, J. D., Boland, D. M., Baum, J. T., Ikemiya, K., Harris, Q., Phillips, M., Neufeld, E. V., Gomez, D., Goldman, P., Dolezal, B. A. 2021. Lifestyle modification using a wearable biometric ring and guided feedback improve sleep and exercise behaviors: A 12-month randomized, placebo-controlled study. *Front Physiol* 12:777874. doi:10.3389/fphys.2021.777874.
81. Wang, E. Y., Graff, R. E., Chan, J. M., Langlais, C. S., Broering, J. M., Ramsdill, J. W., Kessler, E. R., Winters-Stone, K. M., Van Blarigan, E. L., Kenfield, S. A. 2020. Web-based lifestyle interventions for prostate cancer survivors: Qualitative study. *JMIR Cancer* 6(2):e19362. doi:10.2196/19362.
82. Church, A. H., Dawson, L. M. 2018. Agile feedback drives accountability and sustained behavior change. *Strategic HR Rev* 17(6):295–302. doi:10.1108/SHR-07-2018-0063.

13 Group Healthcare Interventions in Lifestyle Medicine

Beth Frates, MD FACLM DipABLM, Hannah Lee, MS, Amy Comander, MD, DipABLM, and Fraser Birrell BA MB BChir MA PhD Dip Clin Ed FRCP FBSLM PFHEA

13.1 INTRODUCTION

Behavior change interventions come in many different shapes and sizes. One method of counseling for behavior change involves utilizing groups. Group interventions typically involve a provider or providers and a set of 8–12 patients. Group interventions have a variety of styles and take advantage of various health experts. Some groups just serve as support sessions and are commonly led by mental health experts and are aptly named "support groups." Others are educational sessions and workshops where patients learn more about their conditions and pathways to change. Group lifestyle medicine interventions often include a mixture of all three: support elements, education elements, and coaching for behavior change. These lifestyle medicine groups are facilitated by a medical provider. Some groups focus on specific chronic conditions like diabetes, breast cancer, stroke, or heart disease. Some groups focus on a theme of healthy living and a desire to enhance wellbeing. Group interventions that focus on the six pillars of lifestyle medicine are the subject of this chapter. This concept and counseling method is not new, as it was documented in practice as early as 1905.[1] The research on these interventions has repeatedly been promising which continues to spark healthcare providers to include group interventions in their offerings. Medical schools and other health professional schools do not currently include training on how to run group sessions. This chapter may serve as an introduction to providers who are planning to incorporate these types of sessions into their practice. For others, this chapter may solidify knowledge, resources, and logistics needed to put the plan into action. And still, for some, this chapter could help add ideas and liven up group interventions that are already underway. This chapter will review the evidence for using group interventions for lifestyle medicine, provide examples of group intervention models, introduce virtual groups, highlight some specific program strategies to empower change, discuss coaching in a group setting, focus on ways to create connections, provide practical tips to get started with programs and how to sustain them.

DOI: 10.1201/9781003161226-13

13.2   DEFINITIONS

Some names for lifestyle medicine group interventions include Shared Medical Appointments, Drop-In Group Medical Appointments (DIGMA), Group Consultations, and Group healthcare interventions. Lifestyle Medicine Group Interventions are distinct from education groups in delivering healthcare, including relevant investigations and treatments as well as behavior change in a group setting (see Figure 13.1).[2]

There are not only a number of names for these visits but also a number of distinct models, including group visits, shared medical appointments, and group antenatal models, such as Centering Pregnancy. While strong opinions are often expressed about the merits and primacy of different models, an accurate understanding of: firstly, the history (as outlined in section b), and secondly, how similar these group models are in their content, structure, and outcomes should inform our acceptance that the overarching terms lifestyle medicine group interventions or group consultations are always correct, unless making distinct granular comparisons. The more we do that, the clearer is the breadth and depth of evidence supporting them meeting healthcare's quadruple aim[3] or recently proposed quintuple aim (see Figure 13.2; adapted from[4]).

The pandemic has brought Virtual Group Consultations (VGCs) to the forefront: these are remote appointments delivering care to a group of people together on a secure platform. "Hybrid group consultations" (HGCs) let people choose to attend the same clinic in-person or virtually. When pregnant women or other patients attend some antenatal or other group care models in-person and some virtually, this is referred to as a "hybrid group care pathway."

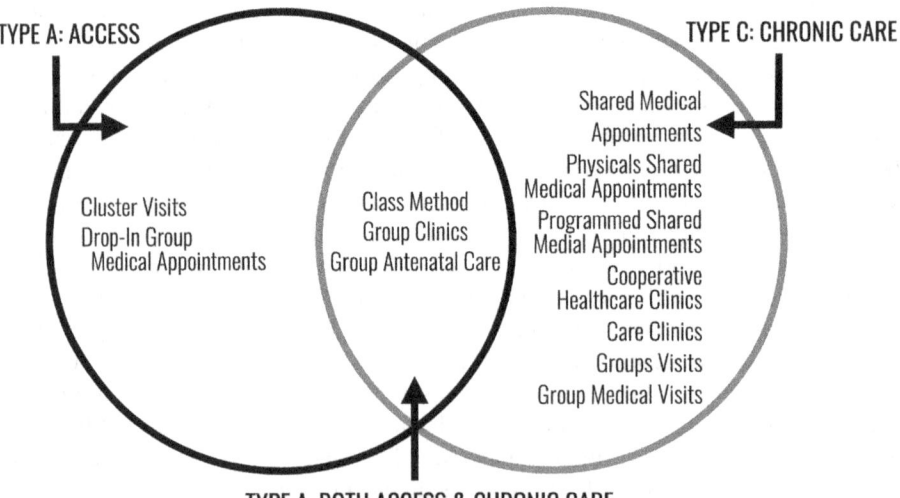

FIGURE 13.1   Group Healthcare Interventions/Group Consultation Models. (Adapted from Jones et al. 2019.[2])

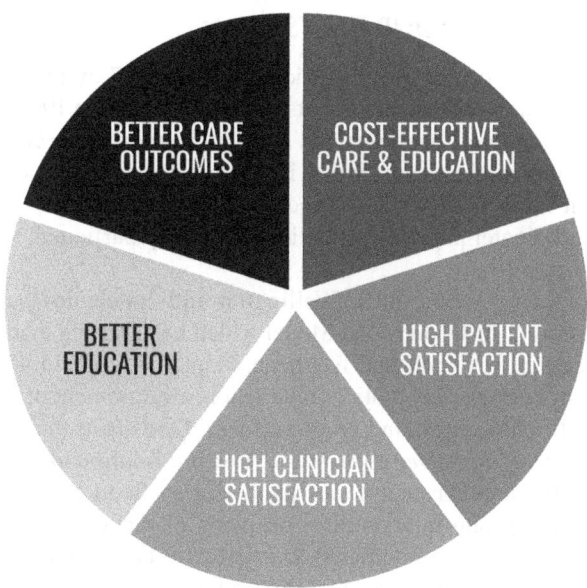

FIGURE 13.2   Healthcare's Quintuple Aim. (Adapted from Birrell et al. 2021.[4])

Shared Medical Appointments are a dominant model in several healthcare systems and regarded by many as the start of group consultation practice, mainly due to the substantial body of work by and sheer force of personality of their founder Dr. Ed Noffsinger.[5,6] This differs from many other models in having serial observed consultations within a group setting and embedding a separate facilitator and often a note-taker within sessions. Noffsinger's philosophy is very much the right people doing the right job and that usually means the expensive clinician only being there for part of the session. However, similar efficiencies can be realized by using group care for undergraduate and postgraduate education and/or doing research where substantial amounts of clinical care can be provided within a randomized controlled trial[7] or observational study.[8]

Other variations of Shared Medical Appointments include Physicals Shared Medical Appointments (with examination in an adjoining space),[9] Drop-In Group Medical Appointments (fairly self-explanatory for self-referral, but these don't always follow a strict observed serial consultation pattern),[10] and Programmed Shared Medical Appointments, which are used in Australia, especially where there is a long-term intervention for an outcome like weight loss.[11]

Group coaching is any coaching that happens in a group, which includes almost all forms of group consultation, where peer-supported and coached behavior change is the norm (an exception would be triage groups, where allocation to coaching interventions is made).

13.3   HISTORY OF GROUP VISITS

The first mention of group visits in medicine was in 1907 by Dr. Joseph Pratt who started this type of intervention for patients with tuberculosis in 1905.[1] An article published about 90 years later that described a research study by Beck and colleagues[12] demonstrated that monthly group visits with a primary care provider indicated fewer emergency room visits, fewer visits to specialists, and fewer hospitalizations. In addition, they showed greater patient satisfaction, and group participants spent about $15 less on care per month.

Almost five years later in 2001, Wellington and colleagues published a study about their Stanford 2-hr Group Visit Model which has a strong evidence base today with over 20 years of research and has been adapted for use in 43 countries. The program had a focus on patient–patient interaction, environment of learning, support for lifelong health challenges, and empowerment. One quote they shared was *"We really can take care of ourselves if we have a little information and support"*.[13] Three years later in 2004, another article was published by Scott and colleagues.[14] They demonstrated that a group intervention consisting of monthly group visits focused on education and caregiving compared to usual care had benefits including higher patient satisfaction, fewer ER visits, and reduced healthcare costs.

Jaber and colleagues published a review of the literature from 1974 to 2004.[15] The patients included in the studies were chronically ill patients, chronically ill low-income patients, diabetic patients, coronary artery disease patients, headache patients, frail elderly, children, mother–infant pairs, and in some studies, all patients in the practice. The review showed that group visits lead to improvements in health behaviors, medication compliance, self-efficacy, and improved quality of life. As for lab tests, the group visits demonstrated improvement in blood pressure and cholesterol, mean blood glucose, and decreased hemoglobin A1c. With regard to the physical exam, there is evidence that these group visits may help reduce obesity. The review highlighted the reduction in healthcare costs noted in earlier trials and cited the reduction in emergency room visits, urgent care visits, and visits to specialists. In terms of the patient–physician relationship, the review reported that there was increased patient satisfaction, improved doctor–patient relations, and improved physician satisfaction. This helps to achieve the quintuple aim mentioned above. Some powerful quotes from this review article include:

> Patients appreciated the physician's unhurriedness, time spent with the physician, and overall quality of care.
>
> Physicians providing group well-child visits covered significantly more American Academy of Pediatrics-recommended content in their education sessions than did control physicians, particularly about safety, nutrition, behavior and development, and sleep.
>
> Physicians who participated in CHCCs (Cooperative Healthcare Clinics—group visits) reported that they greatly enjoyed and were extremely satisfied with their ability to treat group visit patients.
>
> Group visits have been shown to increase physician productivity, which may in turn increase physician satisfaction.

In 2011, Moitra and colleagues published a report on group medical visits in primary care patients with chronic pain and found the group visits often included patients with chronic pain as well as depression and anxiety. The results showed that there were fewer emergency room visits and psychological acceptance of chronic pain as an outcome. Challenges to holding the group visits included reimbursement issues.[16]

Patients with diabetes are often the subjects of group visits and there are many research studies on this population. For example, Housden and colleagues published a review article including studies from 1947 to 2012 which included 26 randomized controlled trials. They concluded that these group visits resulted in significant reductions in hemoglobin A1c.[17] Another review study published by Steinsbekk and colleagues looked at 21 randomized controlled studies in patients with diabetes participating in group visits and found improved clinical, lifestyle, and psychosocial outcomes with groups.[18]

Given the success of the group visits, investigators started to look at specific components of the programs that led to positive outcomes. Thompson and colleagues[19] found that three factors were associated with patient success: a good facilitator, a focus on change as a process, and peer support.

If the group visits are so useful, why weren't all primary care practices implementing them? Careyva and colleagues wondered about and investigated this question.[20] They found that there were barriers to holding group visits including lack of training, staffing issues, and difficulty recruiting patients. Interestingly, they also found that physicians with less than ten years of experience were more likely to hold group visits.

In 2019, the *Journal of Alternative and Complementary Medicines* published a special focus issue on innovations in group-delivered services.[21] They reported that group visits improved access to care and health equity.[22] They noted specifically that there were benefits for cancer survivorship.[23] They mentioned the innovation of adding a teaching kitchen to the group visit model.[24] In addition, they noted that the group visits included patients with depression, working on mindfulness, smoking cessation, chronic diseases, well child care, and low-income groups.

Examples of recent literature in group visits reveal that the target audiences are inclusive of marginalized populations, as demonstrated by Noya in a study assessing the use of shared medical appointments in patients with type-2 diabetes in the Latinx community.[25] The study specifically addressed challenges such as underinsurance and Spanish monolingualism to reach the target population. Recent efforts also include a focus on providing this useful, impactful intervention for free so that it can be accessible to all, like in the case of shared medical appointments for type-2 diabetes at a free student-run clinic in North Carolina.[26]

Investigators are providing the intervention to diverse populations and noting the impact as revealed in a pilot program which brought weight management shared medical appointments to African-Americans with obesity at an urban medical center.[27] Results indicated that the intervention was successful in terms of reducing screen time and thus sedentary behavior in the children. The study revealed that more work needed to be done to engage and retain African-American families with obesity in an urban area. With obesity on the rise, patients with BMI that put them in this category have been subjects in studies evaluating group visits, including one published in 2018 in Cleveland Clinic Journal of Medicine in 2018 titled "Obesity: Are shared medical appointments part of the answer?".[28] The authors concluded that to be successful the group visits with patients with obesity need to address several factors in addition to nutrition including physical activity, appetite suppression, stress management, and sleep.

The idea of group visits has spread to many specialties including dermatology. A 2019 study explored patient satisfaction and physician productivity relative to shared medical appointments for vitiligo. The study found that the intervention was correlated with high patient satisfaction and that more new patients were able to be seen.[29]

For breast cancer survivors, a retrospective study published in 2019 study found that group visits helped participants lose weight, approximately 5 pounds over the course of the 14-week trial, when subjects met for 2 hours every two weeks.[30] This study also demonstrated gains in psychosocial variables including lower rates of depression, lower perceived stress, greater patient activation, and improved quality of life, but these did not reach statistical significance. On average, patients lost 4.9 pounds (-2.6%, $p < 0.01$) and their BMI decreased by 0.8 kg/m^2 (-2.5%, $p < 0.01$). Patients reported a significant decrease in average weekly fat consumption (-31.5%, $p < 0.01$). In terms of nutrition, the subjects reported a reduction in weekly intake of fat. It was noted that "most patients found the program educational, and nearly half of them described it as life changing".[30] With testimonials like that and the evidence quoted, a consensus is emerging that group visits can be so powerful they are truly inspirational. The inspiration allows for life changing transformation. Key drivers are codesign and connections made between participants, with the provider, with the materials, and with themselves and their motivation to change.

In a paper titled "A realist review of shared medical appointments: How, for whom, and under what circumstances do they work?",[31] the authors note that the group visits likely work by combating isolation, vicarious learning, feeling inspired by successful peers, friendships development between patients and providers, provider learning, adequate time allocation, first-hand health knowledge, and increased trust in the physician.

13.4   VIRTUAL GROUP CONSULTATIONS

Before the pandemic, there was limited focus and resource toward virtual group consultations.[32] However, impressive examples include a virtual diabetes study[33] and seamless transition from in-person low carb groups for diabetes/pre-diabetes[34] to virtual group consultation on Zoom with a similar scale (20+ per group) and even more impressive outcomes (achieving >50% remission). Tokuda et al. was not an impressive design, being a small ($n = 100$) non-randomized mixed-methods study of a pharmacist plus nurse practitioner delivered model for managing patients with diabetes (HbA1c $\geq 7\%$). However, the ambition of directly addressing health inequality in poor rural areas of Guam, an extremely remote island which is 4,000–8,000 miles away from the team of health professionals in Hawaii and Rhode Island, must be applauded. The results with significant reduction in HbA1c (-0.8%, $p = 0.03$), emergency department visits (1 vs 16, $p < 0.01$), and blood pressure (9/5 mmHg, $p < 0.05$) in virtual groups were also impressive.[32]

13.5   INEQUITIES

The technological divide is not new, and medicine is not spared from its harsh realities. While virtual visits have remarkably increased access to care for many, they have magnified healthcare inequities for others.[35] Participating in a virtual visit is not always an easy task. Table 13.1 demonstrates barriers to virtual care. There are many resources and skills required that are not required for an in-person visit. An individual needs a compatible technological device, internet connection, the ability to use technology fluently, and a safe place to connect from. Recognizing this allows us

TABLE 13.1
Barriers to Virtual Care

Barrier to Virtual Care	Potential Causes	Questions to Ask Yourself
Lack of compatible device	• Cost is prohibitive • Device is shared/is not always accessible	Are there organizations (community centers, health centers, religious groups) in the community where patients could use computers? Could you partner with such groups to provide financial aid to patients to help purchase devices? Could you offer the meeting over the phone instead?
Lack of reliable internet access	• No internet service at home • Limited or no cellular data plan • Poor connect on (lag, freezing, etc.)	Are there WiFi hotspots in your patient's community you could direct them to? Are you able to distribute pre-paid mobile hotspot gift cards? Could you offer the meeting over the phone instead?
Difficulty using technology/meeting platform	• Older patients may be unfamiliar with device or meeting platform • Platform only available in English • Vision or hearing challenges	Can a member of the team touch base with older patients to personally review using the platform/device? Does using the platform require a high level of technical literacy? Is it feasible to use automatic subtitles or other reasonable accommodations during meetings?
Lack of space to connect from	• Home is not safe • No access to privacy • No access to space with internet service	Are there organizations (community centers, health centers, religious groups) in the community with private, safe spaces that patients could use? Does the patient need assistance in finding a safe place to stay and connect from?

to rethink our approach to begin to lessen the technological divide and create novel approaches to how we include participants for virtual group visits. For example, one could partner with neighborhood health centers, spiritual centers, and community centers to improve community access to shared computers with internet access in a private location. It is crucial to remember that, especially in communities that have been affected by digital redlining.

13.6 PRACTICAL TIPS/APPLICATION

Using the "coach approach" during the group consultations empowers patients to adopt and sustain behavior change. The Introduction chapter and all the chapters in this book will enable readers to facilitate these sessions in a way that invites patients to reflect, review, and renew their intentions around their lifestyle patterns and practices. Making sure that the participants in the group feel safe, especially psychologically safe, is key for the success of these interventions. The first meeting and the information exchanges prior to the first group visit will set the tone for the planned series of sessions whether it is 3 or 12 sessions. The longer the series, the more likely close social bonds will be created and sustained post intervention. The facilitator models the COACH approach by showing curiosity, openness, appreciation, compassion, and honesty from session one and throughout. By modeling this behavior, the participants begin to emulate it with each other and themselves.

There are at least five different connections being created during these group consultations. First, the connection with self. The participants are being asked to consider their health, wellbeing, and lifestyles. This comes with introspection. Without knowing oneself, it is difficult to change. Thus, learning about and experimenting with new patterns of eating, moving, sleeping, managing stress, and connecting socially all allow participants to better understand themselves. This introspection invites connection with oneself, one's core, core values, principles, strengths, and desires. The second connection is the connection between the participant and the facilitator. The facilitator has the opportunity to model a healthy social connection with the participant over the course of the program. By treating each participant with respect, the facilitator helps participants understand what it feels like to be respected and watch similar interactions with other participants. The third connection is the connection between the facilitator and the group as a whole. This makes the facilitators function as the coach of the team. The coach works to find team members' strengths and highlights them. When there is occasion to use the strengths of the participants by asking someone to summarize or encouraging them to help brainstorm solutions around obstacles, that empowers participants and makes them feel appreciated and understood. Everyone wants to feel understood and appreciated. By helping the group feel like a "team" or group of people all on a mission to enhance their health and wellbeing, the facilitator helps foster connections between the members. The fourth connection is connections between group members. Some participants will be naturally outgoing and social. They will seek friendships and make connections. Others are more introverted and will shy away from close contact. With time, all participants tend to open up and share. One way to encourage these social connections between participants is to have them break out into pairs for 1:1 activities.

These could be 8–10 minutes and then there can be a reporting session where groups share lessons learned with the larger group. On Zoom, this can be done in breakout rooms. Some questions for participants could be "What will you do differently this week that will help you adopt a healthy lifestyle? What is one small step you can make to a healthier lifestyle? What are your strengths and how can you use them to adopt and sustain a healthy lifestyle?" The fifth connection is the connection between the participant and the participant's healthy self, who is practicing and sustaining healthy habits. This connection helps patients see themselves as their best selves. Setting a vision of themselves in one year or five years helps to start this connection. Framing this change process as a journey and the journey is one that lasts a lifetime will set them up for long-term success. Long-term success means working on healthy habits and enjoying them each day. These five different connections can be created during a group consultation program.

Five-step cycle is used in groups in-person and virtual. This cycle was described in detail in Chapter 12. Figure 13.3 reviews the cycle and the five steps.

The same Five-Step Collaboration Cycle that is used for one-on-one consultations can be used in group consultations as well.[36] This cycle was first described in the article, "Coaching in Physiatry" in 2011, and it is also incorporated in the Lifestyle Medicine Handbook by Frates et al.[37]. There are five steps to the cycle. The cycle starts with empathy as step one. The facilitators need to prioritize their own self-care so that they can enter the group consultation fully mindful and focused on the process. When facilitators are well rested, nourished with healthy food, energized with routine exercise, fulfilled by high-quality connections, feeling peaceful from using stress reduction techniques like meditation and yoga, and are free from substance use, they are able to tackle the task of facilitating the group consultation. Knowing that the facilitator is there to help the patients reach their own goals is key. Aligning the participants' motivation with their goals will put the program on the path to success. Spending time exploring motivation is time well spent. Then, step three is to build confidence. Treating each participant with respect and honoring

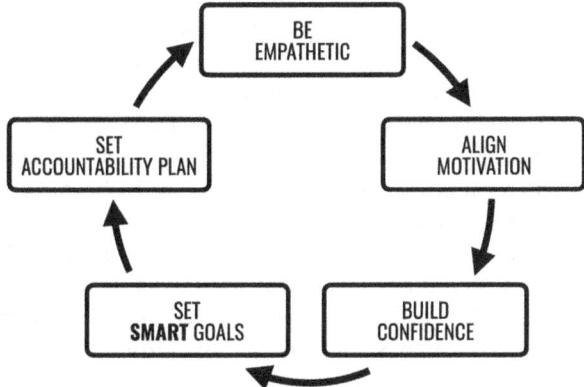

FIGURE 13.3   Five-step cycle for virtual and in-person groups.

their questions, motivations, and goals is an important way to increase self-confidence. Reviewing the strengths of each participant is another powerful way to increase confidence. Setting goals is an integral part of lifestyle medicine interventions one on one and in groups. Making sure to set SMART goals is important with a focus on specific, measurable, action oriented, realistic, and time sensitive. At the end of each session, the participant can write down their weekly goal. They can share it verbally, or if the meeting is by zoom, the participant can share it in the chat box. The chat can be saved for future reference. The last step in the five-step process is to set accountability. With group consultations, accountability is built in as the next group visit is an occasion to share progress on goals. It's important to check in with patients each session to see how they are doing with reaching goals. In addition, in between group meetings, the participants can share their progress in an email group, FaceBook group, or other social media platform that is acceptable to the facilitator and participants. When the group gets back together, it is important to set the tone again and exude empathy. We start and end these sessions with empathy. We work to help patients feel understood and appreciated.

13.7   TRAINING FOR LEADER/CLINICIAN

The training needs for most clinicians are very modest, and many could literally step into a group session and deliver this very competently with expert facilitation. However, the codesign and team buy-in means that clinicians and other key team members will usually attend for some or all of the longer facilitator training. This is usually delivered virtually now for both in-person and virtual group consultations which has advantages for both cost and accessibility. Basic training is available for free (e.g., https://www.groupconsultations.com/), with many providers willing to train whole teams for a fee. This is most effective when used in the context of a peer-supported community of interest to share successes and address challenges together.[2] In some cases, a coaching role may differ slightly from the typical role of a clinician; see Table 13.2 for examples.[38] The expert works on treating and educating the patient. He or she relies on his or her skills and knowledge to find answers to problems and advise the patient. The coach, on the other hand, helps patients to help themselves, builds motivation, confidence, and engagement, relies on patients' self-awareness and insight, strives to help patients find their own answers, focuses on what is working well, and collaborates with patients. Table 13.2 delineates the differences between the two approaches and reveals the importance of using the COACH approach with Group Visit interventions for patients with chronic disease. Table 5.1 from Chapter 5 provides a similar comparison.

Many clinicians are concerned about management of conflict within a group setting. The psychologist Bruce Tuckman developed a model for the formation of groups and published this model in 1965 in a paper entitled "Developmental Sequence in Small Groups".[39] The "Tuckman Model" outlines the different stages of a group formation, and this model is useful in acknowledging the role of conflict within a group setting, and approaches for managing this conflict. According to the "Tuckman Model," the five stages of group development include: forming, storming, norming, performing, and adjourning (see Table 13.3).

TABLE 13.2
EXPERT Approach vs. COACH Approach

EXPERT Approach	COACH Approach
Treats patient	Helps patient to help themselves
Tells patient what to do	Asks patient what they want to do
Patient receives care and plays a passive role	Patient decides next steps and actively engages in decision making and goal setting
Expert's skills, tools, and experience lead the way for treatment	Patient's experience, knowledge, self-reflections, motivations, and interests guide the way forward
Expert educates the patient	COACH may provide just-in-time education on relevant topics
Convince the patient of the treatment plan	Convince the patient that they have the ability to find the best approach and follow through
Goal is for patient to trust provider	Goal is for patient to trust him or herself
Advising is the way	Collaboration is the way

TABLE 13.3
Stages of Group Development Based on Tuckman's Model[39]

Stage	Components	Questions to Consider
Forming	Participants are oriented to new group, identify task/purpose of group, and establish ground rules	What do the group members hope to gain from this group? How can the facilitator(s) help them on the way? How can we make the environment safe and productive?
Storming	Group members do not yet feel united, are resistant to the demands of the task, and may strive to maintain individuality	How can we develop a sense of community within the group? How can we honor the unique experiences and perspectives of each group member? What about the tasks is creating resistance?
Norming	Harmony and unity develop between group members; ideas and perspectives are discussed and exchanged openly	What is the ideal ratio of facilitator guidance to open discussion? Is every group member being heard?
Performing	Group members are able to relate to one another and work together to problem-solve and take constructive action to address task	How can the facilitator(s) best support the group as they work together and form connections? Are tasks being addressed appropriately, or is guidance needed?
Adjourning	Group members self-evaluate their progress and the group concludes and disengages	Will any feedback or assessments be collected from group members? Will the facilitator(s) maintain contact with group members, and if so, how?

TABLE 13.4

Examples of Language Clinicians Can Use during Group Visits

Setting the Tone	Investigating Needs	Encouraging Reflection
We are open and nonjudgmental in this room	What do you need at this moment to embark on your change journey?	What has gone well with your efforts so far?
We will show respect and honor the unique needs, statements, motivations, and goals of each person in this group	What needs to be in place for you to start exercising or quitting smoking or whatever they are working on?	What are you most proud about?
There are no stupid questions or stupid answers	What are some obstacles you are facing and what are some possible solutions around them?	What are your strengths and how can you use those now to help you reach your goals?
We are all learning and growing together on this journey to healthy lifestyles	What can this group do to better support you?	How has this group helped you? What is the best part of this group for you?
The things we discuss in this room will stay in this room	If you could change one thing about this group what would it be?	What was an "AHA" moment you had during this group session?

13.8 EXAMPLES OF TEAM MEMBERS FOR THE GROUP

Group care is by nature a group activity, and it is usual to have at least two people delivering the intervention. There is a core complement for routine delivery, and once embedded and the efficiencies of the scale are seen, it may be possible to move to an ideal complement.

The core delivery team consists of at least one clinician and one facilitator. Occasionally, skilled clinician-facilitators can succeed doing both roles, but this is the exception rather than the rule. This also leaves the session more vulnerable to cancellation since without a facilitator, a single clinician can often deliver a one-off session, but the absence of a single clinician–facilitator requires session cancellation.

The ideal scenario is a clinician with rotating facilitating multidisciplinary input *or* rotating clinical input with consistent facilitator, together with full wraparound support with a note-taker, dedicated secretarial support, and where relevant, research and educational team members. The leaders of the group should determine the tone of the group visits; for ideas, see Table 13.4.

13.9 EXAMPLES OF GROUP INTERVENTION PROGRAMS (LOGISTICS, BILLING, TIMING, PROCEDURES)

13.9.1 LOGISTICS

There are clear pre-session, in-session, and post-session actions (see Figures 13.4–13.6) used with permission from Group Consultations Ltd).

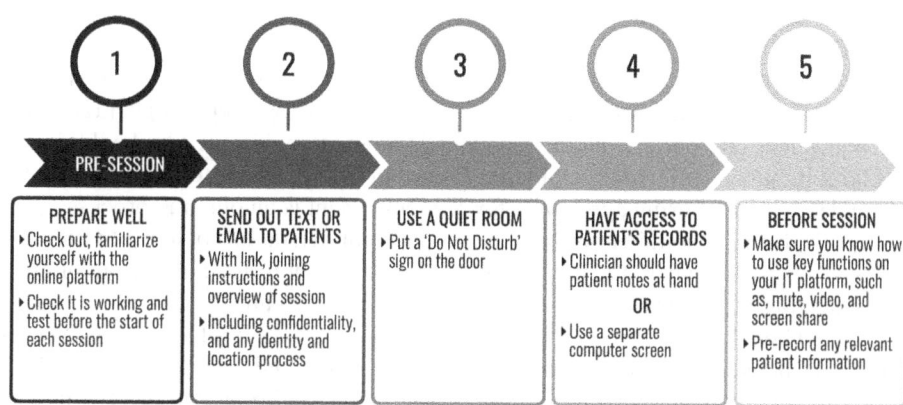

FIGURE 13.4 Pre-session checklist: Preparing for your virtual group consultation.

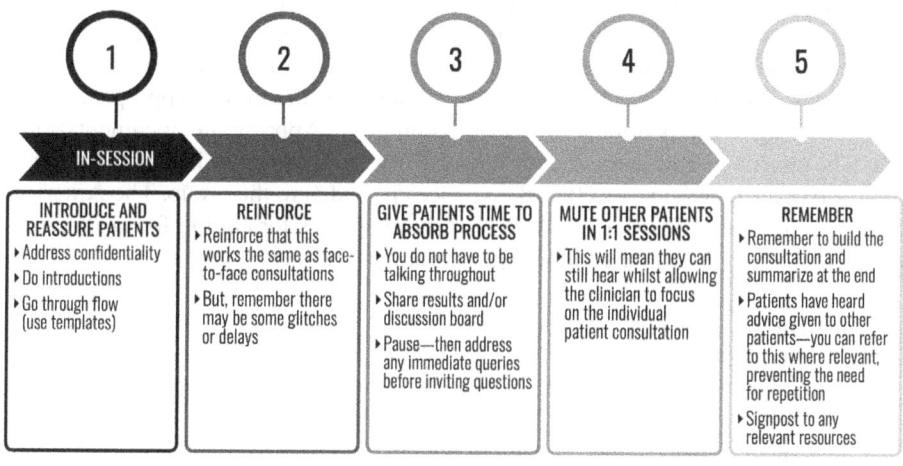

FIGURE 13.5 In-session checklist: Preparing for your virtual group consultation.

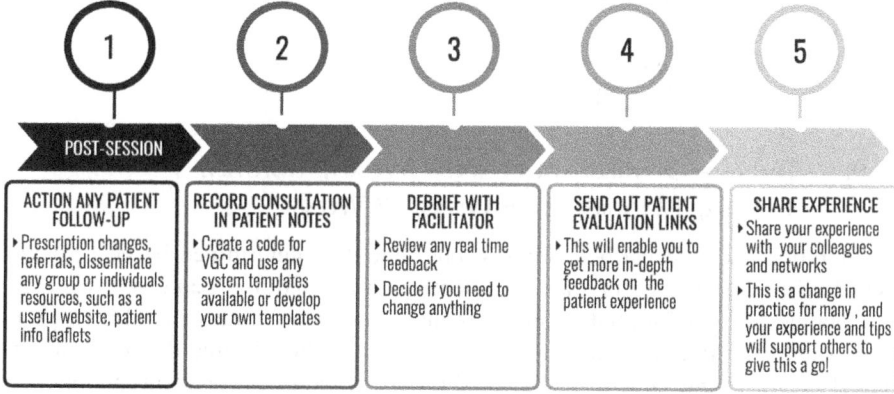

FIGURE 13.6 Post-session checklist: Preparing for your virtual group consultation.

13.9.2 BILLING

It is generally accepted that, due to the quality of care delivered and high satisfaction achieved, group consultations are reimbursed at the same (or rarely a higher rate) than the equivalent one-on-one interaction. This is most often accepted by health insurers for reimbursement. However, there are certain healthcare systems (Australia, for example), where securing agreement for reimbursement is an ongoing process.

Ideally, billing should either be done by the right person or not at all (within the NHS, for example, where the money following the patient is again going out of fashion, encouraging whole system thinking and preventative care).

In the United States, group visits can be billed in a variety of ways. One way is pay out of pocket. Many programs charge $20 a session and even have scholarships for those who cannot pay. Some programs run on philanthropy and there is no fee. This involves the physician and providers finding funding or raising funds with a run for health or selling t-shirts. Creativity goes a long way with this. Another way to offer the programs is to do research and receive funding that way. If the goal is reimbursement, speaking with the hospital or practice manager is critical to make sure that the documentation suits the insurers in the practice or hospital. Commonly used CPT codes include 99212–99215. It is important to pay attention to appropriate time-based leveling which is often allowed for group visits. Appropriate documentation is key. The chart and electronic record must be filled with specific individual services provided to each patient as well as the services provided to the group. The American Academy of Family Physicians (AAFP) shares specifics for coding for group visits. According to the AAFP, the following criteria must be met:

- Patient is established patient of practice
- Disease or condition specific
- Voluntary and patients are entitled to have individual appointments as needed
- Adequate facilities and time are provided
- Appropriate staff members are maintained to facilitate the group discussion and coordinate the meeting
- Individual as well as group interaction must be documented in the patient's medical record
- Patient cannot be new
- Physician must be present

13.9.3 TIMING – OPTIONS/ADVANTAGES – WEEKLY, MONTHLY, 1 HOUR, 2 HOURS, FOR 6 WEEKS, 12 WEEKS

The duration and interval between sessions should be determined by best practice (NICE clinical guidance or the equivalent) for the condition being managed. So, for example, early inflammatory arthritis should be seen monthly in a 2-hour group session until the treatment target is achieved, and stable chronic disease can have annual review in the same or a dedicated group, depending on patient numbers.[8] In contrast, osteoporosis or menopausal patients would be seen once in a 90-minute group session, with optional self-referral or compliance-driven updates if not adherent to treatment or worsening symptoms.[7] More intensive sessions are justified for weight loss[11] or diabetes prevention.[34] A key advantage of the group approach is the flexibility for adding extra patients who have urgent clinical problems (such as flare-ups, decompensation or complications, depending on the condition determining the need for care).

13.9.4 PROCEDURES FOR SUCCESS – TIPS FROM RESEARCH+EXPERIENCE

It is much easier to fail than succeed with group care, so it is especially important to adopt best practice and heed the critical success factors (see Box 13.1), which we have derived from over a decade of training at scale and validated through international collaboration. The other element which might seem self-evident is the importance of codesign with patients[2] and collaboration in both setting and sharing the process and outcomes.[4]

The Coronary Health Improvement Project (CHIP, although CHIP more commonly refers to the Complete Health Improvement Program) incorporates exercise and dietary modification and has a long track record of successful lifestyle medicine change.[40] This has been widely used with consistent positive benefits, but a recent randomized study failed to show regression of coronary atheroma in either arm or significant difference in key cardiovascular risk markers apart from BMI, where CHIP participants lost more weight than Healthy Heart participants.[41]

Dysinger[42] and Mirsky's Center for Organized Research and Education for Health (CORE Health) at Massachusetts General Hospital[43] have shown that other lifestyle medicine group models can also be successful and adaptable even during the pandemic.

Less obvious models which would not generally be recognized as group consultations, but should be, include the UK Diabetes Prevention Programme[44] and ESCAPE Knee pain.[45] Most impressive of all, in terms of whole system change[2] however, is the Fresh Start diabetes program implemented across Northwest London Clinical Commissioning Group, covering all 360 practices and serving 2.5 m population. This has brought virtual group consultation practice into the mainstream, in the same way that the Cleveland Clinic made group care a routine care option. We are hoping to see other areas adopt this model and similar whole system changes in cardiac care and cancer within the next few years.

BOX 13.1   CRITICAL SUCCESS FACTORS

1. Strong leadership, including system and team buy-in
2. Ability to clearly communicate benefits
3. Codesign to meet current challenges
4. Simple/compelling patient recruitment
5. Defined roles and training including facilitation
6. Familiarity with platform and right equipment

13.10 PAVING THE PATH TO WELLNESS WITH STROKE SURVIVORS (STANFORD VA AND SPAULDING)

In 2012, Dr. Beth Frates piloted a PAVING the Path to Wellness for Stroke Survivors group at Spaulding Rehabilitation Hospital.[46] There were three stroke survivors and one caregiver in the group, making a total of four participants. All four attended all 6 hours of the sessions. The topics of discussion were physical activity, attitude, variety, investigations, nutrition, and goal setting. The sessions were broken up into one half lecture and one half discussion with goal setting at the end. Each participant increased their number of fruits and vegetable intake, increased their minutes of physical activity, and reported lowered stress levels and one participant cut down the number of cigarettes he was smoking as well as committed to a quit date. Since this first pilot was successful, the Stoke Institute for Research and Recovery at Spaulding Rehabilitation Hospital funded more programming.

The lifestyle medicine group intervention, PAVING the Path to Wellness, evolved and developed with time at Spaulding Rehabilitation Hospital. One version of the program is a 12-week program addressing all six pillars of lifestyle medicine as well as setting SMART goals, cultivating a sense of purpose, using variety, adopting healthy attitudes, managing energy levels, using timeouts as empowerment moments, and investigating how trying new activities and patterns impacts their health and sense of wellbeing. Figure 13.7 reviews the different steps in the program.

Table 13.5 demonstrates the PAVING questionnaire that was used to evaluate the progress of each participant in 12 steps. The participants take this prior to the start of the program and at the end of the program. It serves to help guide them. The questionnaire was developed by Dr. Beth Frates in collaboration with Harvard Health in 2016.

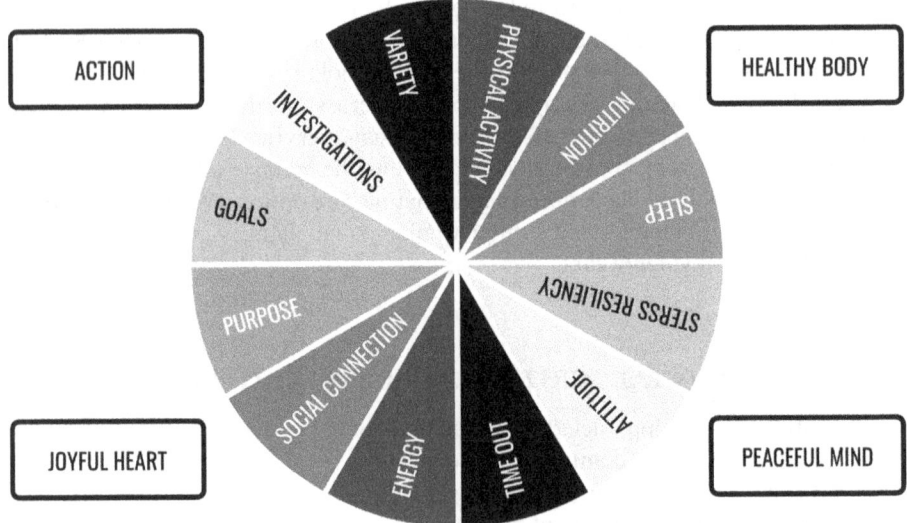

FIGURE 13.7 The PAVING the path to wellness wheel.

TABLE 13.5

PAVING the Path to Wellness Questionnaire

INSTRUCTIONS Rank each item on a scale of 1-5. The Key is below. Calculate the subtotal of each of the 12 sections and plot them on the PAVING Wheel on page 1.

1 Never do this	**2** Only rarely do this	**3** Sometimes do this	**4** Often do this	**5** Do this regularly as part of my routine

MODULE 1 Physical Activity

- I exercise 5 days in the week for about a half an hour.
- I enjoy myself when I exercise.
- I perform strength training exercises twice a week.
- I perform flexibility exercises routinely.
- I perform balance exercises routinely.

Physical Activity Total:

MODULE 1 Stress

- I have learned about stress and its effect on the mind and body.
- I am familiar with stress reduction techniques, and I use at least one when I feel that I am anxious, annoyed, or worried.
- I know about stress resiliency, and I practice enhancing my resiliency on a regular basis.
- I don't get angry easily.
- I meditate, take deep breaths, practice yoga, or do mindfulness based stress reduction (MBSR) regularly.

Stress Total:

MODULE 2 Attitude

- I use mistakes as opportunities to learn and grow.
- I write thank you notes or express my gratitude verbally.
- I celebrate success when it happens.
- I concentrate on the task at hand fully without distraction.
- I am optimistic about the day.

Attitude Total:

MODULE 2 Time outs

- If I sit for over an hour, I stand up and take a break for five minutes each hour.
- If I feel frustrated and annoyed, I take a few deep breaths to calm down.
- I take my vacation every year.
- When I am at home, I make sure to turn off my computer and put my work projects away at least for an hour at dinner time.
- After working on the same project for a few hours, I step away from it to get perspective on it.

Time Outs Total:

MODULE 3 Variety

- I do a variety of different exercises.
- I try to have a rainbow of colors on my plate.
- I enjoy a variety of fruits and vegetables.
- I like to try new activities.
- I spend time and connect with a wide range of friends.

Variety Total:

MODULE 3 Energy

- I have a friend who I know energizes me.
- I have identified at least one activity that brings me joy and energy.
- I am able to avoid situations and people that drain my energy.
- I only drink two cups of coffee a day.
- I don't rely on sugar/sweets or cookies for a quick energy fix.

Energy Total:

MODULE 4 Investigations

- I perform mini experiments on myself regularly.
- I am curious as to what foods are good for my body.
- I am curious as to what effect physical activity has on my body.
- I read about the latest research findings in medicine, nutrition, sleep, stress management, and/or exercise.
- I talk about health with family and friends.

Investigations Total:

MODULE 4 Purpose

- I feel that I have a clear purpose in life.
- I am able to prioritize my activities and projects easily.
- I make sure that my activities and projects are in alignment with my values.
- I have identified the people and activities that are most important to me.
- I am using my strengths to fulfill my purpose.

Purpose Total:

MODULE 5 Nutrition

- I eat 4 fruits a day.
- I eat 5 or more vegetables a day.
- I know proper portions for protein, carbohydrates, and fats, and I eat those portions.
- I think about the food that I eat and ask myself if it is good for my body.
- I view food as fuel, as medicine, and enjoyment too.

Nutrition Total:

MODULE 5 Sleep

- I sleep 7-8 hours a night.
- I don't drink coffee after noon time.
- I have a bedtime routine in which I relax before bed.
- I don't sleep with my phone on in the bedroom.
- I take 20 minute naps when I am over tired.

Sleep Total:

MODULE 6 Goals

- I set long-term goals for myself, share them with someone, and review them.
- I set three-month goals for myself, share them with someone, and work toward them.
- I set monthly goals and share them with someone.
- I set weekly goals and share them with someone.
- I set daily goals for myself and keep myself accountable for them.

Goals Total:

MODULE 6 Social

- I can name at least one person who brings me strength.
- I am involved with a group (activity, exercise class, art class, religious affiliation or the like)
- I visit with friends on the phone or in person at least 5 times a week.
- I have a healthy relationship with my spouse, partner, or best friend.
- I have a pet or plant that I can nurture and spend time with every day.

Social Total:

The different formats for PAVING the Path to Wellness include a 12-month program, a 12-week program, and a 6-week program. There are usually between 8 and 12 participants in the groups and the groups meet between 1 and 2 hours depending on the format. There is an administrator who helps with marketing, referrals from physicians, email announcements, obtaining consent, describing the program as a coaching program not a medical visit, helping with logistics of parking, and answering questions. For the programs at Spaulding, the fee is 20 dollars per session, as is the case with all their group offerings. The Stroke Institute for Research and Recovery has funds to cover any participant who cannot afford this fee.

With a 12-month program, the group meets twice a month, the first and second Thursday of each month. Each month there is a different focus. The focus follows the PAVING STEPSS mnemonic.

P – Physical Activity
A – Attitude
V – Variety
I – Investigations
N – Nutrition
G – Goal Setting
S – Stress Resilience
T – Timeouts
E – Energy Management
P – Purpose
S – Sleep
S – Social Connections

The first meeting is one in which the facilitator describes the research, guidelines, and importance of the step. Then, there is discussion about how the participants are using that particular step and how they are feeling about their accomplishments and proficiency with it. The second meeting in the month focuses on the same topic, but it is an active meeting where the participants engage in the action of the step. For example, if the step is physical activity, the group takes a walk together. If it is nutrition, the chef in the hospital does a cooking demonstration; if it is stress reduction, the group practices some deep breathing or meditation. With a 12-month program, the group has a great deal of time to create high-quality connections and gel together.

Another format is to meet 12 weeks in a row. In this format, the meetings run 2 hours weekly. The first hour is informational and the second is discussion as well as action, depending on the topic. For exercise, the group may stand and do stretches or gentle chair yoga. For diet, the group may review recipes and share a healthy snack. For stress, they may try different deep breathing techniques. At the end, they craft goals for the week.

In the six-week format, the meetings last 2 hours and occur weekly. In this format, 2 of the 12 steps are covered together. This can also be completed in 1 hour. About half of the time is educational and half is discussion. Massachusetts General Hospital Cancer Center adopted this format for their patients. Their groups are run by a Nurse Practitioner and a Registered Dietician. The payment model for this group is shifting to CPT coding much like shared medical appointment models.

Stanford University Medical Center physician, Jeff Krauss MD, adopted the PAVING the Path to Wellness Program and used it for Stroke Survivors at the Palo Alto VA. Dr. Krauss called his program a comprehensive lifestyle medicine program for post-stroke patients, and it was based on the twelve steps of the PAVING the Path to Wellness model.[47] In his program, he received IRB approval to study the outcomes of the participants. In his 12-week program involving 17 participants, he included exercise, healthy cooking, meditation, and education sessions with discussion at each meeting. He tested cardiovascular fitness, body composition, vital signs, and quality of life pre and post the intervention. The results revealed that 14 patients improved their fitness levels. Other improvements included increased exercise duration, longer distance traveled in the 6-minute walk test, improved 30-second sit to stand, grip strength, and balance. For the patients who had high blood pressure, there was a mean decrease in systolic blood pressure of 11 mmHg. It was noted that participant satisfaction was high. And, Dr. Krauss reported enjoying the process of facilitating the groups.

With COVID, there was a shift in formatting. The groups went virtual for the Stroke Institute of Research and Recovery. This was found to be feasible and acceptable by the participants. They also reported improvements in minutes of physical activity, increased vegetable consumption, improved mood, and a strong connection to the other participants in the group. Some even stated that because of this virtual PAVING the Path to Wellness Program, they planned to get more involved with virtual groups so they could sustain social connections during the pandemic. The format for the virtual groups involved 2-hour sessions for six weeks.

13.10.1 A Case Study: The PAVING the Path to Wellness™ Program for Breast Cancer Survivors

Group interventions are a powerful tool for providing care for specific populations, and recently, we have demonstrated the role of a group intervention for breast cancer survivors. In the United States alone, there are currently over 3.8 million breast cancer survivors, and there is a need to address the unique medical and psychosocial needs of this population. Groups such as the American Society of Clinical Oncology (ASCO) and American Cancer Society (ACS) have provided evidence-based guidelines for breast cancer survivorship care.[48] In terms of the role of health promotion in breast cancer survivorship, there is growing evidence that poor diet, obesity, and inactivity are associated with an increased risk for recurrence and mortality from breast cancer.[49] Given this evidence, an important component of breast cancer survivorship care includes proactive assessment of diet, exercise, and other lifestyle factors, as well as empowering survivors with the education and tools to adopt these lifestyle behaviors.

A recent ASCO survey demonstrated that, during routine oncology follow-up visits, the majority of oncologists do not address the importance of diet, physical activity, and other lifestyle factors in a comprehensive fashion.[50] There is a need for lifestyle medicine education in cancer survivorship.

TABLE 13.6

PAVING the Path to Wellness Steps

Physical Activity: Aerobic exercise, strength training, and stretching are covered, as well as strategies to incorporate more movement into daily living.

Attitude: Participants are introduced to "growth mindset" concept and encouraged to have an attitude of openness throughout the sessions.

Variety: Whether trying new vegetables, a different form of physical activity, or a new stress resiliency practice, "Variety" is emphasized throughout the lifestyle pillars.

Investigations: Participants enjoy investigating which lifestyle behaviors feel best for their body and are empowered to lead healthier lives.

Nutrition: content encourages increasing nutrient density, preferring whole foods over processed foods, and helps participants gain skills through cooking classes.

Goal Setting: Through learning to set SMART goals, successful behavior change becomes more likely.

Stress Resiliency: Participants are introduced to a variety of stress resiliency tools including deep breathing, the relaxation response, and mindfulness-based stress reduction.

Time Outs: Participants learn the benefits of taking breaks from unhealthy influences, prolonged sitting, difficult conversations, and negative self-talk. A "time out" allows for increased clarity and overall wellbeing.

Energy: Increasing the use of natural sources of energy such as healthful foods, exercise, and connecting with friends, allows participants to increase vitality through healthy behaviors.

Purpose: Identifying priorities, examining life's meaning, and seeing the bigger picture in life, allows participants to align their behaviors with their purpose.

Sleep: Through evaluation of the quantity and quality of their sleep and what enhances/detracts from sleep, participants are prepared to make their nights more restful.

Social Connections: Throughout the course, high-quality connections with family, friends, and community are emphasized and meaningful connections with others in the cohort are experienced.

Developed by Dr. Beth Frates, the PAVING the Path to Wellness is an innovative, evidence-based program based on the tenets of lifestyle medicine. The program focuses on 12 key topics (Table 13.6), and the program empowers participants to pursue lifestyle behaviors that enhance their overall health and wellbeing. The PAVING the Path to Wellness program has been adapted for breast cancer survivors, with the goal to provide a proactive assessment of diet, exercise, and other lifestyle factors.[51]

Each of the topics covered in the 12 weekly sessions of the PAVING program includes a didactic component, group discussion, exercises, and goal setting. Each participant in the program is provided with a workbook. During the first session, the participants assess their lifestyle behaviors and wellbeing by using the PAVING Wheel (see Figure 13.8). Over the course of the 12-week program, participants learn in the group setting, support one another, and develop meaningful social connections.

Prior to the COVID-19 pandemic, the PAVING the Path to Wellness program was delivered to participants in-person only. During the pandemic, the program was transitioned to a virtual format using Zoom. At the beginning of each weekly session, the participants reflect on the lessons learned from the previous week and share successes and struggles in a supportive group environment. Following this discussion,

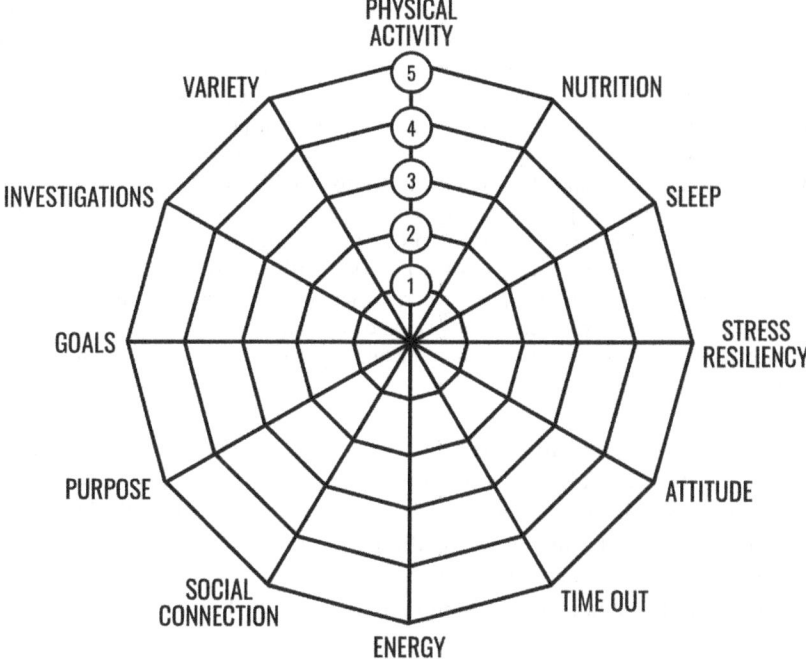

FIGURE 13.8   PAVING the path to wellness self-assessment wheel.

the physician leader or guest expert presents content on the PAVING step for that week. This presentation is followed by a group exercise, discussion, and often the use of "breakout" rooms. During the final session, each participant completes a second PAVING Wheel and reflects on progress made during the program. The final week of the program focuses on the importance of "Social Connections," and this component of the program has been quite remarkable. A unique aspect of the program is that these PAVING groups have continued to meet on their own for ongoing support. Transitioning the program to a virtual format presented a number of logistical challenges, and there was concern that participants may not engage as fully with one another and form meaningful social connections. However, participants adjusted well to the online program and appreciated not having to deal with travel time, parking costs, babysitting, eldercare, and other challenges. While there was a loss of being physically present with the group, the feedback from participants was overwhelmingly positive. Use of the "breakout rooms" in Zoom and other techniques enabled the group to engage fully.

The PAVING program has made a meaningful impact on the participants. As one participant stated:

> The PAVING survivorship program has been an essential piece of my breast cancer treatment process for so many reasons. Most importantly, it connected me with others who have been through cancer treatment and understand that the end of active

treatment is the beginning of a new step in the recovery process. My PAVING pals immediately understand what I am talking about when I express a concern or fear at our meetings. In fact, these are the only people whom I can talk to openly about breast cancer and that has been invaluable in helping me move forward with my life. Cancer will always be a part of my life but I want to keep it in perspective and PAVING, and my PAVING pals, have helped me do just that. People who have not experienced cancer think that once your active treatment is finished, it's over for you. In fact, well-meaning friends often implicitly encourage the cancer survivors to move on before they are ready. This makes survivorship programs an even more important aspect of the recovery process. The cancer survivor knows it will be part of his/her life forever so it's really important to have a place where cancer can be interwoven into conversations about your life experiences with ease and without tension. These conversations help me maintain a positive attitude, and the healthy lifestyle habits we learned in the survivorship program.

While the COVID-19 pandemic has presented numerous challenges for cancer survivorship care, there has also been an opportunity to innovate, and telemedicine is playing an increasingly important role. The experience with the PAVING program has demonstrated that the use of telemedicine for group virtual lifestyle medicine interventions for breast cancer survivors has great potential, and it is our hope that this approach can be expanded to other populations as well.

13.11   MEASUREMENT STRATEGIES

Ramdas and Darzi[52] recommended that measured outcomes should include (1) respected patient-centered clinical outcomes, (2) patient satisfaction, (3) provider satisfaction, (4) cost, and (5) productivity. But we would now recommend measurement primarily mapped to the quintuple aim[4]:

1. Better key outcomes
2. Patient satisfaction
3. Clinician satisfaction
4. Low cost
5. Effective education

We recommend centers/practices adopting group models to establish baseline activity data in the exemplar conditions to be included, e.g., diabetes, asthma, musculoskeletal. Prospective collection of key process and outcome data will establish the business case for scaling, as well as enabling sharing of often impressive outcomes.

13.11.1   PROCESS MEASURES INCLUDE:

Total patient number and mean number per group, mean (SD) patient, and clinician time per appointment (group and 1:1)

Attendance and admission metrics for group vs 1:1-only patients in healthcare utilization

Proportion of workload seen in groups vs. 1:1 care to estimate cost and efficiency, wasted slots

Number and proportion of teams/practices: adopting group model for routine care; refusing to adopt; adopting and then failing

13.11.2 OUTCOME MEASURES INCLUDE:

Disease-specific – All routinely available chronic disease indices, e.g., Blood pressure (hypertension), Cholesterol (hypercholesterolemia), HbA1c (diabetes), Serum creatinine (renal failure), exercise tolerance (chronic airflow limitation), hospital admissions + courses of prednisolone, and reliever/preventer inhaler prescriptions (asthma/COPD).

Generic, e.g., Weight or Body Mass Index, Knowledge, Quality of Life (EuroQol – EQ-5D, SF-36), and Patient Activation Measure. The Australasian Society of Lifestyle Medicine has developed a composite set of questionnaires for lifestyle medicine (LM-10, LM-25, LM-67), but unfortunately these are not yet published or widely available, so we hope to include these with permission in future editions.

Satisfaction using optimal patient experience question/tools (e.g., GPAQ or equivalent validated and accepted tools matched to settings). There is no single, optimal, validated tool – versions using Likert (tick boxes) scale, numerical rating scale and visual analog scale have similar validity. Increasingly light touch satisfaction is preferred with a single question, which makes routine collection feasible and efficient. Examples include the friends & family test: "Would you recommend our service to your friends & family." However, increasingly this is being replaced with the patient-centered – "Overall how was your experience of our service?"

For conditions with no agreed outcome/target, patients will be encouraged to choose a personal treatment target – outcome and level – at the first session. This should be recorded in the notes and used as a reference for subsequent comparison, allowing % target achievement and comparison with other conditions and usual care when applied there too.

   a.   PAVING Pre and Post Intervention Self-Assessment Wheel

13.12 SUMMARY

Group healthcare interventions in lifestyle medicine provide a methodology to visit with multiple patients during an hour. There are different names for these visits, shared medical appointments when there is coding and billing for insurance purposes, group visit consultations, lifestyle medicine group interventions, and others. These are not support groups as there is a physician or other healthcare provider there to lead and guide the group. In some cases, the physician will meet with a patient one-on-one in a consultation room or a breakout room in a virtual setting. There are a variety of formats to deliver these group visits. In most group visits, there is a component of education on an aspect of disease or a pillar of lifestyle medicine. The patients are encouraged to share their experiences and questions. The group process is one that empowers patients to change by cultivating connections between the participants and the provider as well as connections between participants. These group visits are a way to help patients have autonomy in setting their goals, competence by crafting specific, measurable, action oriented, realistic, and time sensitive (SMART) goals, and relatedness by connecting to the provider and other participants. Autonomy, competence, and relatedness are the three components of the self-determination theory reviewed in Chapters 1 and 5 of this book. Group sessions are one of the 13 keys to behavior change.

13.13   KEY TAKEAWAYS

1. Group Interventions are feasible and well accepted by patients with a number of different diagnoses.
2. There are a variety of methods to facilitate lifestyle medicine group interventions, but all of them include an aspect of education, social support, coaching, and goal setting.
3. The team approach is helpful. It is helpful to have a team to support the group lifestyle medicine interventions. An administrator to help with paperwork, consent forms, email exchanges, answering logistical questions about the program, finances, and marketing. Nurses, nurse practitioners, health and wellness coaches, other behavioral medicine specialists, nutrition specialist, exercise specialists, social workers, psychologists, and others may be able to play a role in the group sessions.
4. Use a coach approach to help participants adopt and sustain behavior change. The ultimate goal of these lifestyle medicine interventions is that the participants have learned important information about guidelines and developed skills and strategies to adopt and sustain healthy lifestyle practices.

13.14   RESOURCES

a. Websites with a long history and credibility (All)
   https://bslm.org.uk/vgc/
   www.lifestylemedicine.org
   Consider using the LM 101 Curriculum slides as part of your educational section of the group visits. There are 150–200 PowerPoints freely available with a teaching manual and syllabus. The slides follow the Lifestyle Medicine Handbook. There is also a syllabus available on the website.
b. Journal articles that are reviews
   Frates, E. P., Morris, E. C., Dysinger, W. S., et al. 2017. The art and science of group visits in lifestyle medicine. *American Journal of Lifestyle Medicine* 11(5). https://doi.org/10.1177/1559827617698091.
   Booth, A., Cantrell, A., Preston, L., et al. 2015. What is the evidence for the effectiveness, appropriateness, and feasibility of group clinics for

patients with chronic conditions? A systematic review. *Health Services and Delivery Research Journal* 3(46):1–372.

Burke, R. E., Ferrara, S. A., Fuller, A. M., et al. 2011 The effectiveness of group medical visits on diabetes mellitus type 2 (dm2) specific outcomes in adults: A systematic review. *JBI Library of Systematic Reviews* 9(23):833–835.

Edelman, D., Gierisch, J. M., McDuffie, J. R., et al. 2015. Shared medical appointments for patients with diabetes mellitus: A systematic review. *Journal of General Internal Medicine* 30(1):99–106.

Edelman, D., McDuffie, J. R., Oddone, E., et al. 2012. *Shared Medical Appointments for Chronic Medical Conditions: A Systematic Review.* Washington, DC: Department of Veterans Affairs. http://www.hsrd. research.va.gov/publications/esp/shared-med-appt.pdf

Housden, L., Wong, S. T., and Dawes, M. 2013. Effectiveness of group medical visits for improving diabetes care: A systematic review and meta-analysis. *Canadian Medical Association Journal* 185(13):E635–E644.

Riley, S. B. and Marshall, E. S. 2010. Group visits in diabetes care: A systematic review. *The Diabetes Educator* 3(6):936–34.

Steinsbekk, A., Rygg, L. O., Lisulo, M., Rise, M. B., and Fretheim, A. 2012. Group based diabetes self- management education compared to routine treatment for people with type 2 diabetes mellitus. A systematic review with meta-analysis. *BMC Health Services Research* 12:213.

13.14.1 BOOKS

PAVING the Path to Wellness - Frates, E. P., Tollefson, M., Comander, A. 2021. *PAVING the path to wellness workbook.* Monterey: Healthy Learning https://www.amazon.com/PAVING-Path-Wellness-Workbook-Frates/dp/1606795503.

Lifestyle Medicine Handbook - Frates, E. P., Bonnet, J., Joseph, R. et al. 2020. *Lifestyle Medicine Handbook*, 2nd ed. Monterey: Healthy Learning. https://www.amazon.com/Lifestyle-Medicine-Handbook-2nd-ed/dp/1606795147.

Teen Lifestyle Medicine Handbook - Frates, E. P., Plaven, B., Watts, B. et al. 2020. *The Teen Lifestyle Medicine Handbook: The Power of Healthy Living.* Monterey: Healthy Learning. https://www.amazon.com/Teen-Lifestyle-Medicine-Handbook-Healthy/dp/1606795139.

Running Group Visits - Noffsinger, E. B. 2009. *Running Group Visits in Your Practice.* New York: Springer. https://www.amazon.com/Running-Group-Visits-Your-Practice/dp/1441914137.

ABCs of Group Visits - Noffsinger, E. B. 2013. *The ABCs of Group Visits: An Implementation Manual for Your Practice.* New York: Springer. https://www.amazon.com/ABCs-Group-Visits-Implementation-Practice/dp/1461435250/ref=sr_1_1?

MCQs: Monya, I., Ifezulike, A., Adamson, K. et al. 2021. *Lifestyle Medicine: Essential MCQs for Certification in Lifestyle Medicine.* Hoboken: Wiley-Blackwell.

Jaber, R., Braksmajer, A., and Trilling, J. 2006. Group visits for chronic illness care: Models, benefits, and challenges. *Family Practice Management.* https://www.aafp.org/pubs/fpm/issues/2006/0100/p37.html.

Strategy 6M: Group visits. 2017. *Agency for Healthcare Research and Quality.* https://www.ahrq.gov/cahps/quality-improvement/improvement-guide/6-strategies-for-improving/access/strategy6m-group-visits.html.

Houck, S., Kilo, C., and Scott, J. 2003. Group visits 101. *Family Practice Management.* https://www.umassmed.edu/globalassets/diabetes-division-department-of-medicine/resources/groupvisits101.pdf.

Hawes, C., Lorig, K., Scott, J. n.d. Group visit starter kit. *Institute for Healthcare Improvement.* https://www.ihi.org/resources/Pages/Tools/GroupVisitStartKit.aspx.

Thompson-Lastad, A. 2019. Group medical visits as participatory care in community health centers. *Qualitative Health Research* 28(7):1065–76. https://doi.org/10.1177/1049732318759528. https://www.ncbi.nlm.nih.gov/pmc/articles/PMC6500445/.

Geller, J. S., Kulla, J., and Shoemaker, A. 2015. Group medical visits using an empowerment-based model as treatment for women with chronic pain in an underserved community. *Global Advances in Health and Medicine* 4(6):27–31. https://doi.org/10.7453/gahmj.2015.057. https://www.ncbi.nlm.nih.gov/pmc/articles/PMC4653596/.

Maskell, J. 2021. Participatory care: How group visits are essential to its growing popularity. *Fullscript.com.* https://fullscript.com/blog/group-consultations

Shared medical appointments. *Cleveland Clinic.* https://my.clevelandclinic.org/patients/information/shared-medical-appointments

Group visit (shared medical appointment) guidelines. 2021. *BlueCross BlueShield of North Carolina.* https://www.bluecrossnc.com/sites/default/files/document/attachment/services/public/pdfs/medicalpolicy/group_visit_shared_medical_appointment_guidelines.pdf

Medical group visits implementation guide. 2013. *Greater Flint Health Coalition.* http://gfhc.org/wp-content/uploads/2015/07/GR-8D21W1-ImplementationGuide.FINAL_.pdf

Group medical visits. *Accelerating Change Transformation Team.* https://actt.albertadoctors.org/PMH/team-based-care/Pages/Group-Medical-Visits.aspx

Eisenstat, S., Carlson, K., and Ulman, K. 2014. Putting group visits into practice in the patient centered medical home. *Society of General Internal Medicine.* https://www.sgim.org/File%20Library/SGIM/Meetings/Annual%20Meeting/Meetign%20Content/AM%2014%20handouts/WE04-STEPHANIE-EISENSTAT.pdf

REFERENCES

1. Pratt, J.H. 1907. The class method of treating consumption in the homes of the poor. *JAMA* 49:755–759. https://doi.org/10.1001/jama.1907.25320090031001i.
2. Jones, T., Darzi, A., Egger, G., et al. 2019. A systems approach to embedding group consultations in the National Health Service. *Future Healthcare Journal* 6:8–16. https://doi.org/10.7861/futurehosp.6-1-8.
3. Sikka, R., Morath, J. M., and Leape, L. 2015. The quadruple aim: Care, health cost, and meaning in work. *BMJ Quality & Safety* 24:608–610. http://doi.org/10.1136/bmjqs-2015-004160.

4. Birrell, F., Johnson, A., Scott, L., et al. 2021. Educational collaboration can empower patients, support doctors in training and future-proof medical education. *Lifestyle Medicine* 2(4):e49. https://doi.org/10.1002/lim2.49.
5. Noffsinger, E. 2013. *The ABCs of Group Visits*. New York: Springer.
6. Noffsinger, E. B. and Scott, J.C. 2000. Understanding today's group visit models. *Permanente Journal* 4:99–112.
7. Baqir, W., Gray, W. K., Blair, A., et al. 2020. Osteoporosis group consultations are as effective as usual care: Results from a non-inferiority randomized trial. *Lifestyle Medicine* 1:e3. https://doi.org/10.1002/lim2.3.
8. Russell-Westhead, M., O'Brien, N., Goff, I., et al. 2020. Mixed methods study of a new model of care for chronic disease: Co-design and sustainable implementation of group consultations into clinical practice. *Rheumatology Advances in Practice* 4:1–13. https://doi.org/10.1093/rap/rkaa003.
9. Noffsinger, E. B. 2002. Physicals shared medical appointments: A revolutionary access solution. *Group Practice Journal* 51:16–26.
10. Noffsinger, E. 1999. Increasing efficiency, accessibility, and quality of care through drop-in group medical appointments. *Group Practice Journal* 48:12–18.
11. Egger, G., Stevens, J., Ganora, C., et al. 2018. Programmed shared medical appointments. *Australian Journal General Practice* 47:70–75. https://doi.org/10.31128/AJGP-05-19-4940.
12. Beck, A., Scott, J., Williams, P., et al. 1997. A randomized trial of group outpatient visits for chronically ill older HMO members: The Cooperative Health Care Clinic. *Journal of the American Geriatrics Society* 45(5):543–549. https://doi.org/10.1111/j.1532-5415.1997.tb03085.x.
13. Wellington, M. 2001. Stanford Health Partners: Rationale and early experiences in establishing physician group visits and chronic disease self-management workshops. *Journal of Ambulatory Care Management* 24(3):10–16. https://doi.org/10.1097/00004479-200107000-00004.
14. Scott, J. C., Conner, D. A., Venohr, I., et al. 2004. Effectiveness of a group outpatient visit model for chronically ill older health maintenance organization members: A 2-year randomized trial of the cooperative health care clinic. *Journal of the American Geriatrics Society* 52(9):1463–1470. https://doi.org/10.1111/j.1532-5415.2004.52408.x.
15. Jaber, R., Braksmajer, A., and Trilling, J. S. 2006. Group visits: A qualitative review of current research. *Journal of the American Board of Family Medicine* 19(3):276–290. https://doi.org/10.3122/jabfm.19.3.276.
16. Moitra, E., Sperry, J. A., Mongold, D., et al. 2011. A group medical visit program for primary care patients with chronic pain. *Professional Psychology: Research and Practice* 42(2):153–159. https://doi.org/10.1037/a0022240.
17. Housden, L., Wong, S. T., and Dawes, M. 2013. Effectiveness of group medical visits for improving diabetes care: A systematic review and meta-analysis. *Canadian Medical Association Journal* 185:E635–E644. https://doi.org/10.1503/cmaj.130053.
18. Steinsbekk, A., Rygg, L. Ø., Lisulo, M., et al. 2012. Group based diabetes self-management education compared to routine treatment for people with type 2 diabetes mellitus: A systematic review with meta-analysis. *BMC Health Services Research* 12:213. https://doi.org/10.1186/1472-6963-12-213.
19. Thompson, C., Meeuwisse, I., Dahlke, R., et al. 2014. Group medical visits in primary care for patients with diabetes and low socioeconomic status: Users' perspectives and lessons for practitioners. *Canadian Journal of Diabetes* 38(3):198–204. https://doi.org/10.1016/j.jcjd.2014.03.012.

20. Careyva, B. A., Johnson, M. B., Goodrich, S. A., et al. 2016. Clinician-reported barriers to group visit implementation. *Journal of Primary Care & Community Health* 7(3):188–193. https://doi.org/10.1177/2150131916631924.
21. Weeks, J. 2019. Reversing the fields: Do group-delivered services belong closer to the center of a transformed health care system? *Journal of Alternative and Complementary Medicine* 25(7): 666–668. https://doi.org/10.1089/acm.2019.29070.jjw.
22. Abercrombie, P. D. and Hameed, F. A. 2019. Group visits as a path to health equity. *Journal of Alternative and Complementary Medicine* 25(7):669–670. https://doi.org/10.1089/acm.2019.0158.
23. Cohen, J. A., Shumay, D. M., Chesney, M. A., et al. 2019. Survivorship wellness: Insights from an interdisciplinary group-based survivorship pilot program at a comprehensive cancer center. *Journal of Alternative and Complementary Medicine* 25(7):678–680. https://doi.org/10.1089/acm.2019.0080.
24. Kakareka, R., Stone, T. A., Plsek, P., et al. 2019. Fresh and savory: Integrating teaching kitchens with shared medical appointments. *Journal of Alternative and Complementary Medicine* 25(7):709–718. https://doi.org/10.1089/acm.2019.0091.
25. Noya, C. E., Chesla, C., Waters, C., et al. 2020. Shared medical appointments: An innovative model to reduce health disparities among Latinxs with type-2 diabetes. *Western Journal of Nursing Research* 42(4):117–124. https://doi.org/10.1177/0193945919845677.
26. Kahkoska, A. R., Brazeau, N. F., Lynch, K. A., et al. 2018. Implementation and evaluation of shared medical appointments for type 2 diabetes at a free, student-run clinic in Alamance County, North Carolina. *Journal of Medical Education and Training* 2(1):032.
27. Srivastava, G., Palmer, K. D., Ireland, K. A., et al. 2018. Shape-up and eat right families pilot program: Feasibility of a weight management shared medical appointment model in African-Americans with obesity at an urban academic medical center. *Frontiers in Pediatrics* 6:101. https://doi.org/10.3389/fped.2018.00101.
28. Shibuya, K., Pantalone, K. M., and Burguera, B. 2018. Obesity: Are shared medical appointments part of the answer? *Cleveland Clinic Journal of Medicine* 85(9):699–706. https://doi.org/10.3949/ccjm.85a.18006.
29. Tkachenko, E., Refat, M. A., Balzano, T., et al. 2019. Patient satisfaction and physician productivity in shared medical appointments for vitiligo. *Journal of the American Academy of Dermatology* 81(5):1150–1156. https://doi.org/10.1016/j.jaad.2019.03.044.
30. Schneeberger, D., Golubíc, M., Moore, H. C. F., et al. 2019. Lifestyle medicine-focused shared medical appointments to improve risk factors for chronic diseases and quality of life in breast cancer survivors. *Journal of Alternative and Complementary Medicine* 25(1):40–47. https://doi.org/10.1089/acm.2018.0154.
31. Kirsh, S. R., Aron, D. C., Johnson, K. D., et al. 2017. A realist review of shared medical appointments: How, for whom, and under what circumstances do they work? *BMC Health Services Research* 17:113. https://doi.org/10.1186/s12913-017-2064-z.
32. Birrell, F., Lawson, R., Sumego, M., et al. 2020. Virtual group consultations offer continuity of care globally during Covid-19. *Lifestyle Medicine* 1(2):e17. https://doi.org/10.1002/lim2.17.
33. Tokuda, L., Lorenzo, L., Theriault, A., et al. 2016. The utilization of video-conference shared medical appointments in rural diabetes care. *International Journal of Medical Informatics* 93:34–41. https://doi.org/10.1016/j.ijmedinf.2016.05.007.
34. Unwin, D. J., Tobin, S. D., Murray, S. W., et al. 2019. Substantial and sustained improvements in blood pressure, weight and lipid profiles from a carbohydrate restricted diet: An observational study of insulin resistant patients in primary care. *International Journal of Environmental Research and Public Health* 16(15):2680. https://doi.org/10.3390/ijerph16152680.

35. Gergen Barnett, K., Mishuris, R. G., Williams, C. T., et al. 2022. Telehealth's double-edged sword: Bridging or perpetuating health inequities?. *Journal of General Internal Medicine* 37:2845–2848. https://doi.org/10.1007/s11606-022-07481-w.

36. Frates, E. P., Moore, M. A., Lopez, C. N., et al. 2011. Coaching for behavior change in physiatry. *American Journal of Physical Medicine & Rehabilitation* 90(12):1074–1082. https://doi.org/10.1097/PHM.0b013e31822dea9a.

37. Frates, E. P., Bonnet, J., Joseph, R., et al. 2020. *Lifestyle Medicine Handbook*, 2nd ed. Monterey: Healthy Learning.

38. Frates, E. P., Moore, M. A., Lopez, C.N., et al. 2011. Coaching for behavior change in physiatry. *American Journal of Physical Medicine and Rehabilitation* 90:1074–1082. https://doi.org/10.1097/PHM.0b013e31822dea9a.

39. Tuckman, B. W. 1965. Developmental sequence in small groups. *Psychological Bulletin* 63(6): 384–399. https://doi.org/10.1037/h0022100.

40. Diehl, H. A. 1998. Coronary risk reduction through intensive community-based lifestyle intervention: The Coronary Health Improvement Project (CHIP) experience. *American Journal of Cardiology* 82(10B):83T–87T. https://doi.org/10.1016/s0002-9149(98)00746-2.

41. Elkoustaf, R. A., Aldaas, O. M., Batiste, C. D., et al. 2019. Lifestyle interventions and carotid plaque burden: A comparative analysis of two lifestyle intervention programs in patients with coronary artery disease. *Permanente Journal* 23:18. https://doi.org/10.7812/TPP/18.196.

42. Frates, E. P., Morris, E. C., Sannidhi, D., et al. 2017. The art and science of group visits in lifestyle medicine. *American Journal of Lifestyle Medicine* 11(5):408–413. https://doi.org/10.1177.1559827617698091.

43. Mirsky, J. B. and Thorndike, A. N. 2021. Virtual group visits: Hope for improving chronic disease management in primary care during and after the COVID-19 pandemic. *American Journal of Health Promotion* 35(7):904–907. https://doi.org/10.1177/08901171211012543.

44. Marsden, A. M., Bower, P., Howarth, E., et al. 2022. 'Finishing the race' - A cohort study of weight and blood glucose change among the first 36,000 patients in a large-scale diabetes prevention programme. *International Journal of Behavioral Nutrition and Physical Activity* 19(1):7. https://doi.org/10.1186/s12966-022-01249-5.

45. Walker, A., Boaz, A., Gibney, A., et al. 2020. Scaling-up an evidence-based intervention for osteoarthritis in real-world settings: A pragmatic evaluation using the RE-AIM framework. *Implementation Science Communications* 1:40. https://doi.org/10.1186/s43058-020-00032-6.

46. Armstrong, C., Wolever, R. Q., Manning, L., et al. 2013. Group health coaching: Strengths, challenges, and next steps. *Global Advances in Health and Medicine* 2(3):95–102. https://doi.org/10.7453/gahmj.2013.019.

47. Krauss, J., Frates, E. P., Myers, J., et al. 2021. Comprehensive lifestyle medicine program improves fitness, function, and blood pressure in poststroke veteran cohort: A pilot study. *American Journal of Lifestyle Medicine*, 16 (6):765–771. https://doi.org/10.1177/1559827620988659.

48. Runcowicz, C. D., Leach, C. R., Henry, N. L., et al. 2016. American Cancer Society/American Society of Clinical Oncology breast cancer survivorship care guideline. *Journal of Clinical Oncology* 34(6):611–635. https://doi.org/10.1200/JCO.2015.64.3809.

49. Orman, A., Johnson, D. L., Comander, A., et al. 2020. Breast cancer: A lifestyle medicine approach. *American Journal of Lifestyle Medicine* 14(5):483–494. https://doi.org/10.1177/1559827620913263.

50. Ligibel, J. A., Jones, L. W., Brewster, A. M., et al. 2019. Oncologists' attitudes and practice of addressing diet, physical activity, and weight management with patients with cancer: Findings of an ASCO survey of the oncology workforce. *Journal of Oncology Practice* 15(6):e520–e528. https://doi.org/10.1200/JOP.19.00124.

51. Comander, A., Frates, E. P., and Tollefson, M. 2021. PAVING the path to wellness for breast cancer survivors: Lifestyle medicine education and group interventions. *American Journal of Lifestyle Medicine* 15(3):242–248. https://doi.org/10.1177/1559827620986066.

52. Ramdas, K. and Darzi, A. 2017. Adopting innovations in care delivery – The case of shared medical appointments. *New England Journal of Medicine* 376:1105–1107. https://doi.org/10.1056/NEJMp1612803.

14 Lifestyle Medicine
Guidelines and Statistics

*Beth Frates, MD FACLM DipABLM
and Tracie McCargo, PhD*

14.1 LIFESTYLE MEDICINE

As a reminder from Chapter 1 in Introduction to Behavior Change, Lifestyle Medicine is defined as

> "Lifestyle medicine is a medical specialty that uses therapeutic lifestyle interventions as a primary modality to treat chronic conditions including, but not limited to, cardiovascular diseases, type 2 diabetes, and obesity. Lifestyle medicine certified clinicians are trained to apply evidence-based, whole-person, prescriptive lifestyle change to treat and, when used intensively, often reverse such conditions. Applying the six pillars of lifestyle medicine—a whole-food, plant-predominant eating pattern, physical activity, restorative sleep, stress management, avoidance of risky substances and positive social connections—also provides effective prevention for these conditions.[1]"

Sharing the guidelines in the six pillars of lifestyle medicine is an important part of counseling and coaching patients to adopt and sustain healthy lifestyle patterns for their body and brain. Launching into a lecture on these pillars will likely build resistance. Asking permission to share some interesting facts when they are related to the person's conditions and concerns can help to not only educate the patient but also inspire them. Knowing the guidelines and striving to meet them may be a long-term goal, depending on the patient. These behaviors are the root causes of our major killers in the United States and globally. Addressing these behaviors with an empowering approach will help transform healthcare and health in the United States as well as globally.

Table 14.1 is a useful tool to understand the guidelines for the six pillars of lifestyle medicine and their evidence-based background. There are medical societies and specific articles to review which are listed in the key as well as in the references.

14.2 EXERCISE

Guidelines:
The guidelines from the World Health Organization and the United States Department of Health and Human Services recommend that adults accumulate 150–300 minutes of moderate intensity physical activity each week.[2,3]

DOI: 10.1201/9781003161226-14

TABLE 14.1

Lifestyle Medicine Guidelines

Pillar	Guidelines	Source	Questions
Physical activity	Accumulate 150–300 minutes of moderate intensity physical activity each week (you can talk but not sing) and strength train twice a week	WHO and USHHS	How can you meet these?
Nutrition	Consume predominantly a variety of minimally processed vegetables, fruits, whole grains, legumes, nuts and seeds	ACLM and Study 1	How many vegetables do you eat? How can you add more plants to and seeds your plate?
Sleep	7–9 hours of sleep	NSF	How do you feel when you wake up? How would you describe your sleep?
Stress reduction	10–20 minutes of relaxation, meditation, mindfulness-based stress reduction, other mind body practices each day	Study 2	What do you do for stress reduction? What do you do to relax?
Social connection	Connect with six to seven friends each week	Study 3	How do you feel about your relationships?
Substance use	Quit Smoking Alcohol 0–1 drinks for a woman CDC Alcohol 0–2 drinks for a man If you do not drink, do not start	AHA	How much are you drinking?

Key:

WHO World Health Organization.[2]

USHHS United States Health and Human Services Physical Activity Guidelines for Americans.[3]

ACLM American College of Lifestyle Medicine.[1]

Study 1 Hauser ME, McMacken M, Lim A, Shetty P. Nutrition-An evidence-based, practical approach to chronic disease prevention and treatment. J Fam Pract. 2022;71(Suppl 1 Lifestyle):S5–S16.[57]

NSF National Sleep Foundation.[56]

Study 2 Basso JC, McHale A, Ende V, Oberlin DJ, Suzuki WA. Brief, daily meditation enhances attention, memory, mood, and emotional regulation in non-experienced meditators. Behav Brain Res. 2019;356:208–220.[10]

Study 3 Becofsky et al., "Influence of the Source of Social Support and Size of Social Network on All-Cause Mortality."[15]

Center for Disease Control and Prevention: Smoking and Tobacco Use.[22]

AHA American Heart Association guidelines on alcohol.[23]

Statistics:

Physical activity supports normal growth in children, improves wellbeing, physical function, sleep, and reduces the risk of chronic disease.[4] According to the World Health Organization, globally adults over 18 years of age were not getting enough physical activity, as 23% of men and 32% of women did not achieve global recommendations of 150 minutes of moderate intensity or 75 minutes of vigorous activity weekly in 2016.[2] High-income countries average 26% compliance for men and 35% for women compared with 12% and 24%, respectively, in low-income countries.[2] Low rates of physical activity have resulted from increased leisure time and passive modes of transportation.

The Department of Health and Human Services performed a systematic review of their 2018 Physical Activity Guidelines in an Advisory Committee Scientific Report.[4] This review found that 80% of adults and adolescents do not achieve the recommended physical activity.[4] Post-Covid trends of remote work may contribute to further decline in physical activity.

14.3 NUTRITION

Guidelines:
The dietary guidelines for Americans provide nutrition and dietary recommendations to promote health and reduce chronic disease. Updates are conducted every five years to monitor adherence to these guidelines. The 2020–2025 Dietary guidelines for Americans recommends consumption of more fruits and vegetables to achieve a healthy diet. Adult recommendations include consumption of 1.5–2 cups of fruit and 2–3 cups of vegetables daily.

Statistics:
The average healthy eating score increased from 56 to 59 between 2005 and 2016. However, this increase in adherence to the recommended guidelines still falls short of the maximum score of 100.[5]

Since the COVID-19 pandemic, more Americans have become more health conscious. As a result, American consumers have become more aware of the effects of diet on risk factors for chronic illness, susceptibility to coronavirus, and the need to adopt healthy diets.[5] Surveys of 1,800–2,000 consumers representative of the population were conducted on behavior changes to adopt healthy eating habits. Prior to 2020, 27% of people reported regularly including foods that enhance the immune system to their diet. Post pandemic survey results indicate that 47% regularly include immune enhancing foods to their diets.[5] However, only 18% of respondents consider plant based to be an attribute of healthy food. There is still much work to be done.

Healthy diets help combat obesity, support healthy immune function, prevent type 2 diabetes, prevent cancers and COVID-19-related illness and death.[6] The Centers for Disease Control and Prevention (CDC) accessed the 2019 Behavioral Risk Factor Surveillance System (BRFSS) data to estimate consumption of fruits and vegetables by state for 294,566 participants.[6] The Morbidity and Mortality Weekly report from CDC January 7, 2022 by Seung Lee and colleagues reports that overall, 12.3% of participants met the fruit guidelines and 10% fulfilled vegetable guidelines.[6] Latinx adults consumed the most fruit (16.4%), while men consumed the least (10.1%). With respect to age groups, people over 51 years of age consumed the most vegetables

(12.5%). Those with low incomes (6.8%) consumed the least.[6] Women met recommendations for fruit and vegetable consumption at higher rates (14.5% and 12.4%, respectively) than men (10.1% and 7.6%, respectively).[6]

14.4   SLEEP

Guidelines

The National Sleep Foundation recommends sleeping 7–9 hours per night.[7]

Sleep can affect several areas of our health, including glucose regulation, hormone balance, risk of cardiovascular disease, mood, and cognition.

Statistics

Examination of sleep trends includes a US health survey exploring sleep duration in 250,111 US adults from 2004 to 2012 with data from 1985.[8] Reports of averaging less than 6 hours of sleep per night were revealed in 22.35% of respondents in 1985, 28.6% in 2004, and 29.2% in 2012.[8] Research on sleep and cognition in 10,314 adults indicates 48.9% of respondents slept on average less than 6.3 hours per night during the previous month.[9] This amount of sleep is considered chronic partial sleep deprivation and is correlated with impaired cognitive and psychological functioning in laboratory settings. Sleeping less than 4 hours per night is equivalent to aging the brain 8 years.[9]

14.5   STRESS

Guidelines:

It is recommended that people engage in 10–20 minutes of stress resilience activities each day.[10] Stress resilience activities can include relaxation, meditation, mindfulness-based stress reduction, deep breathing, yoga, Tai Chi or other mind-body practices.

Statistics:

The statistics about stress are startling. These were published in a WebMD article titled, "The Effects of Stress on Your Body."[11]

43% of all adults suffer adverse health effects from stress.
75-90% of all doctor's office visits are for stress-related ailments and complaints.
Stress can play a part in problems such as headaches, high blood pressure, heart problems, diabetes, skin conditions, asthma, arthritis, depression, and anxiety.
The Occupational Safety and Health Administration (OSHA) declared stress a hazard of the workplace. Stress costs American industry more than $300 billion annually.
The lifetime prevalence of an emotional disorder is more than 50%, often due to chronic, untreated stress reactions.

The American Psychological Association created a special report titled "Stress in American 2022" which shared data from their "2022 Stress in America™ survey." The survey was conducted online in the United States from August 18 to September

2 in 2022 by The Harris Poll.[12] There were 3,192 people polled who were all over the age of 18 and residing in the US, and interviews were completed in English as well as in Spanish depending on the subjects.

Results revealed that in the month before the interview, 76% of people polled reported experiencing health impacts due to stress including headache (38%), fatigue (35%), feeling nervous or anxious (34%), and feeling depressed or sad (33%). Other results included that 33% of the people reported feeling overwhelmed, 32% experienced a change in sleeping habits, 10% reported using alcohol or cigarettes to relax, and 15% reported using drugs to relax.[12]

As for sources of stress, health care was highlighted. Seventy percent of people identified health care as a significant source of stress in their lives. Adults at the poverty level or below the poverty level were more likely than those above the poverty level to say that health care is a significant source of stress in their lives (75% vs. 68%). Black, Latino/a, and Asian adults were more likely than White adults to agree that health care is a significant source of stress in their lives (74%, 77% and 74% vs. 67%).[12] The poll also revealed that when adults are feeling stressed, it impacts their lifestyle behaviors with 76% of people polled reporting aspects of their lives that were negatively impacted by stress. Thirty-six percent reported their mental health was impacted.

Thirty-three percent reported their eating habits were impacted; 32% reported their physical health was impacted, and 30% reported their interest in hobbies/activities was impacted.

With respect to the question on the poll regarding whether the people polled felt difficulties were piling up so high that they could not overcome them, there was a difference according to race and ethnicity with

27% of Latino/a adults reported very/fairly often
24% of White adults reported very/fairly often
23% of Black adults reported very/fairly often
18% of Asian adults reported very/fairly often.

With respect the question on the poll regarding whether subjects felt so stressed they felt numb there was also a difference according to race and ethnicity with:

35% of Latino/a adults felt this way
31% of Black adults felt this way
28% of White adults felt this way
26% of Asian adults felt this way[12]

With regard to the pandemic and stress statistics, with this poll, the researchers asked about stress levels on a scale of 1–10, with 10 being the highest amount of stress. The average number for the 3,192 subjects polled was 5. Pre-pandemic stress levels on this scale averaged 4.8 for 2016, 4.8 for 2017, 4.9 for 2018, and 4.9 for 2019, and then pandemic and post pandemic years held at 5 for 2020, 2021, and 2022.[12]

Stress experienced during the COVID-19 pandemic has the potential to change decision-making for many. Stress changes the way that people think and make decisions in ways that support impulsive and habitual thinking as opposed to goal orientation.[13] Data from The American Psychological Association's 2021 Stress in America survey indicates that approximately one-third of Americans have difficulty making everyday decisions.[14] Those who have experienced financial difficulties during the pandemic fare worse. Black, Hispanic, and Asian Americans reported experiencing more COVID-19-related stress than their White counterparts. The experience of race-related stress also results in depleted cognitive reserves, increasing stress load, and the difficulty of flexible decision-making[13] for these populations.

Stress management is important for everyone in light of the stress experienced from daily life, the pandemic, fears about the war in Ukraine and its effects on inflation globally. It is important to explore different methods of stress relief to find what works for each individual. This may include trying new physical activities, exploring new walking trails, and trying yoga and meditation. As many of these activities may be more fun when experienced with others, social connection becomes an important component of stress management. This is why this book is so important because the most effective way to help people manage stress is to get to know them and work with them to find what they are willing to try and what will work best for them using coaching and collaboration while counseling the patients.

14.6   SOCIAL CONNECTION

Guidelines for social connection recommend connection with friends and family seven times per week.[15]

Statistics:
Social isolation increased in the U.S. pre pandemic according to the 2003 and 2020 American Time Use Survey.[16] People spent an average of 262 minutes per day with family in 2003, 243 minutes in 2019 and 252 minutes per day in 2020. This represents a decrease of 122 hours between 2003 and 2019, and an increase of 61 hours 2020. Time spent with friends declined from 35 minutes/day in 2003, to 28 in 2019, and 22 minutes in 2020.[16] Black Americans faced social isolation at higher levels (344 minutes/day) than other groups.[16] White Americans experienced an average of 285 minutes/day, and Hispanic Americans experienced 253 minutes/day.[16]

Women were socially isolated an average of 37 hours more per year than men between 2003 and 2019. However, the experience of social isolation in men increased more at 176 hours/year, as compared to 73 hours/year for women.[16]

Social connectedness is the perception of adequate care and support in relationships.[17] Loneliness and social isolation are very different. Social isolation is the deficit of social relationships and contact with others that provide support. Social isolation is considered detrimental to health outcomes in the absence of loneliness.[17] Loneliness is the perception of lack of connection with others.[17] One can have many friends or be in the presence of others and experience loneliness.

Belonging as a basic psychological need is represented on the third tier of Maslow's hierarchy of needs, falling above food and water on the first tier and shelter on the second tier.[18] After Belonging comes esteem needs on the fourth level and self-actualization on the fifth and highest level.

Loneliness and social isolation have been linked with several medical conditions including cardiovascular disease, obesity, high blood pressure, anxiety, depression, dementia, cognitive decline, and cancer.[19] Social isolation and loneliness are associated with unhealthy behaviors which include drinking, tobacco use, poor sleep hygiene, emotional eating, and inactivity.[19]

The effects of COVID-19 pandemic lockdowns on social connection were felt globally. Social distancing guidelines implemented for physical safety had serious psychological consequences for people.[20] Among Medicare recipients, 81.1% of White Americans reported having an internet connection, 65% of Black Americans, and 60% of Hispanic Americans.[20] Social connection is important to the overall health and well-being of a person. Those who are socially isolated experience less support to remain healthy and when experiencing illness. White Americans on average owned 1.71 technological devices, Black Americans 1.21, and Hipsanic Americans 1.08.[20] Those with devices were less likely to feel socially isolated and disconnected from others.[20] Lower income individuals reported feeling more socially isolated.[20] Women and those living in urban areas felt more socially isolated. Black Americans were 30% more likely to experience social isolation when compared to other ethnicities.[20]

Research including a systematic review and meta-analysis of 90 cohort studies on loneliness, social isolation, and mortality with 2,205,199 subjects indicates that social isolation increases the risk of all-cause death by 26% for loneliness and 29% for isolation.[21]

14.7   AVOIDANCE OF RISKY SUBSTANCES: ELIMINATION OR MODERATION OF SUBSTANCE USE

Guidelines for Smoking:

Medical Associations and the Center for Disease Control recommend quitting smoking.

Smoking tobacco results in premature death from preventable disease including cardiovascular disease and cancer.[22] The American Heart Association guidelines on tobacco use recommend smoking cessation for approximately 1.3 billion people globally who use tobacco products.[24] Tobacco use results in over 8 million deaths per year globally from cancer, cardiovascular disease, and respiratory disease.[25] Approximately 1.2 million deaths occur among non-smokers who are exposed to secondhand smoke.[25] Most of these deaths (80%) occur in middle to low income countries where tobacco is marketed intensively. Tobacco use in 2020 included 22.3% of the global population, 7.8% of women and 36.7% of men.[25]

Cigarette smoking was prevalent in 11.5% of adults in the United States over 18 years of age in 2021. This equates to approximately 28.3 million adult smokers in the U.S., of whom 16 million suffer from smoking-related diseases.[26] Within the U.S., men (13.1%) smoke more than women (10.1%) however, U.S. women smoke more when compared to overall global rates of women who smoke.

Cigarette smokers by age:

Adults aged 18–24 years - 5.3%
Adults aged 25–44 years - 12.6%
Adults aged 45–64 years - 14.9%
Adults aged 65+ years - 8.3%

Cigarette smokers by ethnicity:

Other racial groups, Non-Hispanic - 14.9%
Non-Hispanic White adults - 12.9%
Non-Hispanic Black adults -11.7%
Hispanic adults - 7.7%
Non-Hispanic Asian adults - 5.4%

14.7.1 DISEASES

In the U.S., approximately 480,000 people die from smoking.[27] Approximately 35% of these 480,000 deaths are the result of cardiovascular disease including heart disease and stroke.[24,27]

Chronic obstructive pulmonary disease (COPD) causes breathing problems and airflow blockage in the lungs. Cigarette smoking is present in 38% of 16 million COPD diagnoses[28] and is responsible for as many as 8 of 10 COPD-related deaths in the U.S.[29]

14.7.2 HYPERTENSION, CORONARY ARTERY DISEASE AND STROKE

Cigarette smoking increases the risk of hypertension. Each time a person smokes, their blood pressure increases temporarily.[30] Smoking increases the risk of plaque buildup in the arteries (atherosclerosis) which can lead to high blood pressure and cardiovascular disease.[31]

Chemicals in tobacco and cigarette smoke damage blood vessels by causing inflammation, plaque buildup, and blood clots.[32] Plaque buildup contributes to coronary artery disease by blocking arteries to the heart. Resulting blood clots lead to heart attack and death.[32] Cigarette smoking leads to blocked blood flow and clots in arteries leading to the brain, causing stroke, brain damage, and death.[32] Smoking contributes to peripheral artery disease (PAD) as blood flow to the arms and legs is reduced or blocked, resulting in reduced function and limb loss.[31,32]

14.7.3 CANCER

Smoking is the primary cause of cancer, causing 10 million cancer associated deaths in 2020.[33] Approximately 1.31 million cases of lung, bronchus, and tracheal cancer are estimated to have resulted from smoking in 2020.[33] Most lung cancers (9 out of 10) are caused by smoking and exposure to secondhand smoke.[34] Smoking cessation is not only important for cancer prevention; persons who have developed cancer are also advised to stop smoking to improve health outcomes and reduce the incidence of death.[33]

Smoking not only causes cancer but also prevents the body from fighting existing cancer.[35] Chemicals released from cigarette smoke weaken the immune system hindering its ability to fight cancer cells. These chemicals damage cell DNA enabling cancer cells to grow and form tumors.[36]

14.7.4 ERECTILE DYSFUNCTION

Smoking has detrimental effects on men's health as it obstructs blood flow throughout the body including the genitals leading to erectile dysfunction. Upon quitting, blood flow restriction associated with erectile dysfunction starts to improve in 2–12 weeks.[37]

Heated tobacco products and electronic non-nicotine delivery systems may contain nicotine, and are also unsafe and detrimental to one's health.[38] The World Health Organization reports "Brief advice from health professionals can increase quitting success rates by up to 30%, while intensive advice increases the chance of quitting by 84%."[39]

Guidelines for Alcohol: The American Heart Association recommends if you don't drink, don't start. If you do drink, limit yourself to one drink if you are a woman and two drinks if you are a man. One drink is the equivalent of one 12 ounce beer or one 5 ounce glass of wine, for example.[23] The American Cancer Society states "it is best not to drink alcohol" in their Guideline for Diet and Physical Activity for Cancer Prevention.[40]

Alcohol accounts for 6% of all deaths and 4% of cancer-related deaths in the U.S.[40] Health risks of alcohol consumption also include heart disease, stroke, liver disease, high blood pressure and digestive issues.[41] Excessive alcohol consumption weakens the immune system.[42] Alcohol substance use disorder often occurs with mental health issues including anxiety and depression, and it is unclear which comes first in many cases.

Findings from the Global Burden of Disease Study 2020 demonstrate that 59.1% of those aged 15–39 years were drinking alcohol at harmful levels in 2020 globally.[43] During the same period, 76.9% of males consumed alcohol at harmful levels. Injuries accounted for 66.3% disability adjusted life years (DALY's) in men and 47.9% of females globally in 2020. In populations aged 40–64 years, chronic conditions such as cancer and cardiovascular disease were most prevalent among alcohol users. In those over 65 years of age, alcohol use resulted in ischemic heart disease in men and 31.5% of alcohol-related DALY's. Stroke accounted for 10.9% of alcohol related DALY's in women over age 65, and 11.6% in men within the same age group.[43]

If data on exercise, nutrition, sleep, stress management, social connection, and avoidance of risky substances is not motivation enough to focus on behavior change, then statistics on health care costs, COVID, long COVID, diabetes, and heart disease will add inspiration. These health crises can increase the need for health coaching to prevent pandemic related illness and improve overall health outcomes. Reading this book and examining each chapter may be the best activity you can do to help yourself, patients, your community, and the world to lead healthier lives.

14.8   HEALTHCARE COSTS

Healthcare costs in the US increased by 10.3% in 2020 and 2.7% in 2021 to $4.3 trillion.[44] This moderate increase in 2021 is the result of a 3.5% decline in federal spending, following an increase in healthcare costs due to the COVID-19 pandemic. Healthcare costs in the US for 2030 are projected at $157 billion lower than pre-pandemic projections as a result of slower than expected growth.[45] The COVID-19 pandemic strained financial models for hospital and healthcare systems. Rising healthcare costs hinder some from seeking proper medical care jeopardizing health outcomes. National Health Expenditure projections suggest a shift away from institutional settings including hospitals and institutional nursing care.[45]

14.9   COVID-19

COVID-19 has been a wake-up call for health awareness as individuals contemplate new habits to improve health and prevent death from another pandemic. Recent research gives pause to the motives for improved health as it brings an awareness of unknown dangers of contracting COVID-19.

The coronavirus disease 2019 (COVID-19) pandemic is caused by severe acute respiratory syndrome coronavirus 2 (SARS-CoV-2).[46] From a review article by Gao and colleagues in the journal titled Allergy, it is noted that this pandemic has resulted in global impact including unprecedented death, economic and social impact.[46] Risk factors resulting in severe disease include multiple comorbidities, advanced age, diabetes, hypertension, chronic lung disease, heart, kidney and liver diseases, immunodeficiencies, and pregnancy.[46] Complications of COVID-19 include thromboembolism, coagulation disorders, and acute kidney injury.[46]

The virus that causes COVID-19 (SARS-CoV-2) can compromise the cardiovascular system, increasing the risk of cardiovascular events.[47] An article published in Nature Medicine by Xie and colleagues reports on National healthcare databases from the US Department of Veterans Affairs which was used to compile a cohort of 153,760 people with COVID-19 and two control cohorts with 5,637,647 current controls and 5,859,411 historical controls to assess risk of cardiovascular incidents at 1 year.[47] This data indicates an increased risk of cardiovascular incidents including stroke, transient ischemic attacks, ischemic heart disease, and myocardial infarction.[47] When compared to the control group, those who experienced COVID-19 had an overall increased risk of a major adverse cardiovascular event (MACE) including heart attack, stroke, and all-cause mortality.[47] Increased awareness of the need to improve health through diet and exercise increases the need for lifestyle health coaching that educates, motivates, and empowers patients to reach their health goals.

14.10 LONG COVID

Most patients who contract COVID-19 are asymptomatic or have mild to moderate symptoms. Approximately 5%–8% of COVID-19 patients require ventilator support, non-invasive ventilation, and develop decreased lung function.[48] Some patients experience long-term symptoms of shortness of breath, severe fatigue, and decreased quality of life despite negative test results for SARS-CoV-2.[48] Post-Acute COVID-19 (Long Covid) is characterized by persistent symptoms of fatigue, brain fogginess, headache, extended loss of smell or taste, joint pain, muscle pain, dizziness, palpitations, low-grade fevers, and cough beyond four weeks after the initial COVID-19 infection.[48] Long-term effects of hospital treatment include severe weakness, post-traumatic stress disorder, and post-intensive care syndrome.

In terms of lifestyle medicine and long covid, research demonstrates that lifestyle has an impact. There was an analysis of the Nurses' Health Study II titled Adherence to Healthy Lifestyle Prior to Infection and Risk of Post-COVID-19 Condition published in *JAMA Intern Med*.[49] Of the 32, 249 women in the study, 44% developed long covid. Women with healthy lifestyles had a 49% lower risk of long covid. There were six lifestyle factors evaluated including healthy body mass index (BMI) between 18.5 and 24.9, never smoking, achieving at least 150 minutes per week of moderate to vigorous physical activity, moderate alcohol intake (5–15 g/d), a healthy diet demonstrated by a high diet quality (upper 40% of Alternate Healthy Eating Index – 2010 score), and adequate sleep (7–9 h/d). According to this study, the two lifestyle factors that had the biggest impact were sleeping 7–9 hours a night and maintaining a healthy weight.

14.11 CHRONIC CONDITIONS

Obesity increased from 30.5% in 1999–2000 to 41% for the period of 2017–March 2020. Severe obesity increased during the same period from 4.7% to 9.2%.[50] Obesity contributes to heart disease, type 2 diabetes, stroke, and certain cancers. Black (49.9%) and Latinx adults (45.6%) experience obesity at higher rates when compared to those of other races. Prevalence by age is 39.8% for adults aged 20–39 years, 44.3% for those aged 40–59, and 41.5% for adults over 60 years of age.[50]

Dementia is an impaired ability to think, remember, or perform daily activities.[51] Over 55 million people worldwide live with dementia, with 10 million new cases yearly.[52] Dementia is the seventh leading cause of death globally.[52] Alzheimer's disease is the most widely known form of dementia affecting 5.6 million Americans over age 65 and about 200,000 people under age 65.[53]

Alzheimer's disease affects about 60%–70% of people with dementia.[52] Approximately 14 million people are projected to have Alzheimer's by 2060, with minorities estimated to be affected at the highest rates.[53] Cases among Latinx populations are expected to increase seven times and those among African Americans four times by 2060. Disparities in health conditions such as diabetes and heart disease for minorities may contribute to these disparaging increases in Alzheimer's.[53] Conditions such as poverty, lower levels of education, exposure to discrimination and adversity may also contribute to the risk of Alzheimer's.

Diabetes affects approximately 37.3 million (11.3% of the population) diagnosed and undiagnosed Americans.[54] Unfortunately, 8.5 million adults are unaware of their diabetes diagnosis but may still need help managing their weight and diets. Those considered prediabetic make up over 30% of the US population or 96 million people aged 18 or over. Aging populations (65 years or older) are predisposed to diabetes in high numbers (26.4 million).

Around 695,000 people died from heart disease in 2021, which equals around one in five deaths.[55] Heart disease is the leading cause of death for men, women, and all ethnic groups within the US, killing one person every 33 seconds.[55] Coronary artery disease is the most prevalent type of heart disease affecting almost 20.1 million people over age 20 and causing death in 375,476 people in 2021.[55] Someone experiences a heart attack every 40 seconds in the US, affecting approximately 805,000 each year.

These statistics are alarming and motivating to many. Some people are moved by numbers. This data can be useful when counseling these people. Other people are not interested in statistics. However, success stories of people who have changed their behaviors or scary stories about people who follow unhealthy habits move them. It is critical to know the data, the research, and the stories so that practitioners can meet people where they are and provide them what they need to move forward in their journeys of change.

14.12 CONCLUSION

Lifestyle medicine addresses six main pillars including physical activity, nutritious eating patterns, sound sleep, stress resilience, positive social connections, and elimination or moderation of risky substances. These lifestyle behaviors account for the development and progression of a significant number of chronic conditions including obesity, dementia, diabetes, and heart disease to name a few. By assessing and addressing lifestyle behaviors, the suffering from these conditions can be avoided, reduced, or even eliminated. It is clear from the statistics shared in this chapter that people need help. There is a healthcare crisis that needs attention and spending time counseling and coaching people on healthy lifestyles is a critical component of the solution to the crisis. The key is not only knowing the evidence-based guidelines for the six pillars of lifestyle medicine but also using the 13 keys to behavior change, as outlined in this book, to empower patients to adopt and sustain healthy lifestyle patterns and practices through play, joy, and love.

REFERENCES

1. American College of Lifestyle Medicine. https://www.lifestylemedicine.org. Accessed July 2, 2023.
2. World Health Organization. Physical activity. World Health Organization. Published October 5, 2022. https://www.who.int/news-room/fact-sheets/detail/physical-activity. Accessed July 2, 2023.
3. Physical Activity Guidelines for Americans. https://health.gov/our-work/nutrition-physical-activity/physical-activity-guidelines. Accessed July 2, 2023.
4. Piercy KL, Troiano RP, Ballard RM, et al. The physical activity guidelines for Americans. *JAMA*. 2018;320(19):2020. https://doi.org/10.1001/jama.2018.14854
5. Sanders LM, Allen JC, Blankenship J, et al. Implementing the 2020-2025 dietary guidelines for Americans: Recommendations for a path forward. *Journal of Food Science*. Published online December 7, 2021. https://doi.org/10.1111/1750-3841.15969
6. Lee SH. Adults meeting fruit and vegetable intake recommendations - United States, 2019. *MMWR Morbidity and Mortality Weekly Report*. 2022;71(1). https://doi.org/10.15585/mmwr.mm7101a1
7. Suni E. How much sleep do we really need? Sleep Foundation. Published March 9, 2021. https://www.sleepfoundation.org/how-sleep-works/how-much-sleep-do-we-really-need. Accessed July 2, 2023.
8 Ford ES, Cunningham TJ, Croft JB. Trends in self-reported sleep duration among US adults from 1985 to 2012. *Sleep*. 2015;38(5):829–832. https://doi.org/10.5665/sleep.4684
9. Wild CJ, Nichols ES, Battista ME, Stojanoski B, Owen AM. Dissociable effects of self-reported daily sleep duration on high-level cognitive abilities. *Sleep*. 2018;41(12). https://doi.org/10.1093/sleep/zsy182
10 Basso JC, McHale A, Ende V, Oberlin DJ, Suzuki WA. Brief, daily meditation enhances attention, memory, mood, and emotional regulation in non-experienced meditators. *Behavioural Brain Research*. 2019;356(356):208–220. https://doi.org/10.1016/j.bbr.2018.08.023. Accessed July 2, 2023.
11. Web MD. The effects of stress on your body. WebMD. Published February 2007. https://www.webmd.com/balance/stress-management/effects-of-stress-on-your-body. Accessed July 2, 2023.
12. Bethune S. Stress in America 2022. Apa.org. Published 2022. https://www.apa.org/news/press/releases/stress/2022/concerned-future-inflation. Accessed July 2, 2023.
13. Abrams Z. High stress levels during the pandemic are making even everyday choices difficult to navigate. Apa.org. Published 2022. https://www.apa.org/monitor/2022/06/news-pandemic-stress-decision-making. Accessed July 2, 2023.
14. American Psychological Association's 2021 Stress in America. https://www.apa.org/news/press/releases/2021/10/stress-pandemic-decision-making. Accessed July 2, 2023.
15. Becofsky KM, Shook RP, Sui X, Wilcox S, Lavie CJ, Blair SN. Influence of the source of social support and size of social network on all-cause mortality. *Mayo Clinic Proceedings*. 2015;90(7):895–902. https://doi.org/10.1016/j.mayocp.2015.04.007. Accessed July 2, 2023.
16. Kannan VD, Veazie PJ. US trends in social isolation, social engagement, and companionship - nationally and by age, sex, race/ethnicity, family income, and work hours, 2003-2020. *SSM - Population Health*. 2023;21:101331. https://doi.org/10.1016/j.ssmph.2022.101331

17. Centers for Disease Control and Prevention. Social connectedness. Published May 8, 2023. https://www.cdc.gov/emotional-wellbeing/social-connectedness/index.htm. Accessed July 2, 2023.

18. Maslow AH. *Motivation and personality*. Harper and Row. 1954.

19. National Institute of Aging. Loneliness and social isolation - Tips for staying connected. National Institute on Aging. Published January 14, 2021. https://www.nia.nih.gov/health/loneliness-and-social-isolation-tips-staying-connected. Accessed July 2, 2023.

20. Jacobs M, Ellis C. Social connectivity during the COVID-19 pandemic: Disparities among Medicare beneficiaries. *Journal of Primary Care & Community Health*. 2021;12:215013272110301. https://doi.org/10.1177/21501327211030135

21. Wang F, Gao Y, Han Z, et al. A systematic review and meta-analysis of 90 cohort studies of social isolation, loneliness and mortality. *Nature Human Behaviour*. 2023:1–13. https://doi.org/10.1038/s41562-023-01617-6

22. Center for Disease Control and Prevention: Smoking and Tobacco Use. https://www.cdc.gov/tobacco/index.htm. Accessed August 20, 2023.

23. American Heart Ússociation website: Is Drinking Alcohol Part of a Healthy Lifestyle? https://www.heart.org/en/healthy-living/healthy-eating/eat-smart/nutrition-basics/alcohol-and-heart-health. Accessed August 20, 2023.

24. American Heart Association. Tobacco control, prevention, & cessation. Published 2009. https://www.heart.org/en/get-involved/advocate/federal-priorities/tobacco. Accessed July 2, 2023.

25. World Health Organisation. Tobacco. Published 2022. https://www.who.int/news-room/fact-sheets/detail/tobacco. Accessed July 2, 2023.

26. Centers for Disease Control and Prevention. CDC - fact sheet - current cigarette smoking among adults in the United States - smoking & tobacco use. Smoking and Tobacco Use. Published 2020. https://www.cdc.gov/tobacco/data_statistics/fact_sheets/adult_data/cig_smoking/index.htm

27. American Heart Association. The facts about smoking. https://www2.heart.org/khc-assets/g5-aha-facts-about-smoking.pdf. Accessed July 2, 2023.

28. Centers for Disease Control and Prevention. Employment and activity limitations among adults with chronic obstructive pulmonary disease - United States, 2013. www.cdc.gov. https://www.cdc.gov/mmwr/preview/mmwrhtml/mm6411a1.htm. Accessed July 2, 2023.

29. Centers for Disease Control and Prevention. TobaccoFree. 2014 SGR: The health consequences of smoking-50 years of progress. Centers for Disease Control and Prevention. Published June 2, 2021. Accessed July 2, 2023.

30. American Heart Association. Smoking, high blood pressure and your health. Published 2010. https://www.heart.org/en/health-topics/high-blood-pressure/changes-you-can-make-to-manage-high-blood-pressure/smoking-high-blood-pressure-and-your-health. Accessed July 2, 2023.

31. National Institutes of Health. Smoking and your heart - How smoking affects the heart and blood vessels. NHLBI, NIH. Published March 24, 2022. https://www.nhlbi.nih.gov/health/heart/smoking. Accessed July 2, 2023.

32. Centers for Disease Control and Prevention. Smoking and cardiovascular disease. 2014. https://www.cdc.gov/tobacco/sgr/50th-anniversary/pdfs/fs_smoking_CVD_508.pdf. Accessed July 2, 2023.

33. Frazer K, Bhardwaj N, Fox P, et al. Systematic review of smoking cessation inventions for smokers diagnosed with cancer. *International Journal of Environmental Research and Public Health*. 2022;19(24):17010. https://doi.org/10.3390/ijerph192417010

34. Centers for Disease Control and Prevention. CDC - Fact sheet - Health effects of cigarette smoking. Smoking and Tobacco Use. Published October 29, 2021. https://www.cdc.gov/tobacco/data_statistics/fact_sheets/health_effects/effects_cig_smoking/index.htm. Accessed July 2, 2023.

35. Centers for Disease Control and Prevention. Smoking and cancer. Tips from former smokers. Published May 5, 2022. https://www.cdc.gov/tobacco/campaign/tips/diseases/cancer.html. Accessed July 2, 2023.

36. Pezzuto A, Citarella F, Croghan I, Tonini G. The effects of cigarette smoking extracts on cell cycle and tumor spread: novel evidence. *Future Science OA*. 2019;5(5):FSO394. https://doi.org/10.2144/fsoa-2019-0017

37. Web MD. Erectile dysfunction and smoking. https://www.webmd.com/erectile-dysfunction/guide/ed-how-quit-smoking#:~:text=Men%20who%20smoke%20are%20about. Accessed July 2, 2023.

38. World Health Organization. Tobacco. Published May 24, 2022. https://www.who.int/news-room/fact-sheets/detail/tobacco. Accessed July 2, 2023.

39. World Health Organization. Quitting tobacco. https://www.who.int/activities/quitting-tobacco. Accessed July 2, 2023.

40. American Cancer Society Guideline for Diet and Physical Activity. https://www.cancer.org/cancer/risk-prevention/diet-physical-activity/acs-guidelines-nutrition-physical-activity-cancer-prevention/guidelines.html. Accessed July 2, 2023.

41. Centers for Disease Control and Prevention. Alcohol and Public Health. Frequently Asked Questions. https://www.cdc.gov/alcohol/faqs.htm

42. Sarkar D, Jung MK, Wang HJ. Alcohol and the immune system. *Alcohol Research: Current Reviews*. 2015;37(2):153–155. https://www.ncbi.nlm.nih.gov/pmc/articles/PMC4590612/

43. GBD 2020 Alcohol Collaborators. Population-level risks of alcohol consumption by amount, geography, age, sex, and year: a systematic analysis for the Global Burden of Disease Study 2020. *Lancet*. 2022;400(10347):185–235.

44. Centers for Medicare & Medicaid Services. National health spending grew slightly in 2021. CMS. https://www.cms.gov/newsroom/press-releases/national-health-spending-grew-slightly-2021. Accessed July 2, 2023.

45. Miller G, Turner A, Corwin R, Hempstead K. National health expenditures post COVID: Hints of a new normal? Forefront Group. Published online March 28, 2022. https://doi.org/10.1377/forefront.20220324.285437

46. Gao YD, Ding M, Dong X, et al. Risk factors for severe and critically ill COVID-19 patients: A review. *Allergy*. 2021;76(2):428–455. https://doi.org/10.1111/all.14657

47 Xie Y, Xu E, Bowe B, Al-Aly Z. Long-term cardiovascular outcomes of COVID-19. *Nature Medicine*. 2022;28(28):1–8. https://doi.org/10.1038/s41591-022-01689-3

48. Chippa V, Aleem A, Anjum F. Post acute Coronavirus (COVID-19) syndrome. PubMed. Published 2021. https://www.ncbi.nlm.nih.gov/books/NBK570608/

49. Wang S, Li Y, Yue Y, et al. Adherence to healthy lifestyle prior to infection and risk of post-COVID-19 condition. *JAMA Internal Medicine*. Published online February 6, 2023. https://doi.org/10.1001/jamainternmed.2022.6555

50. CDC. Adult obesity facts. Centers for Disease Control and Prevention. Published February 11, 2021. https://www.cdc.gov/obesity/data/adult.html. Accessed July 2, 2023.

51. Centers for Disease Control and Prevention. What is dementia? Centers for Disease Control and Prevention. Published April 5, 2019. https://www.cdc.gov/aging/dementia/index.html. Accessed July 2, 2023.

52. World Health Organization. Dementia. World Health Organization. Published March 15, 2023. https://www.who.int/news-room/fact-sheets/detail/dementia. Accessed July 2, 2023.

53. Centers for Disease Control and Prevention. The truth about aging and dementia. CDC. Published September 26, 2019. https://www.cdc.gov/aging/publications/features/Alz-Greater-Risk.html. Accessed August 20, 2023.

54. Center for Disease Control and Prevention. National diabetes statistics report. CDC. Published 2022. https://www.cdc.gov/diabetes/data/statistics-report/index.html. Accessed July 2, 2023.

55. Centers for Disease Control and Prevention. Heart disease facts. Centers for Disease Control and Prevention. Published October 14, 2022. https://www.cdc.gov/heartdis-ease/facts.htm. August 20, 2023.

56. NSF National Sleep Foundation Website. https://www.thensf.org/how-many-hours-of-sleep-do-you-really-need/. Accessed August 20, 2023.

57. Hauser. Nutrition-An evidence-based, practical approach to chronic disease prevention and treatment. *The Journal of Family Practice.* 2022;71(1 Suppl Lifestyle). https://doi.org/10.12788/jfp.0292.

15 Summary Chapter

15.1 BEHAVIOR CHANGE OPPORTUNITIES INSIDE AND OUTSIDE OF HEALTHCARE

Dean Ornish, MD and other leaders in healthcare have shared a cartoon that depicts a sink faucet flowing over creating a flood in a bathroom. This is a powerful picture. Dr. Ornish then reminds people that there are a few ways to handle the flood. One is to mop up the floor. This option does not address the source of the flood: the sink faucet that is turned on and overflowing with water. The second option to manage the mess is to get to the source: the faucet. Turning off the faucet is the best way to stop the flood in the bathroom and prevent it from continuing. Lifestyle medicine is the specialty that is trying to stop the onslaught of chronic diseases that are killing people like heart disease. The root causes of these diseases are analogous to the faucet in the bathroom flood analogy. The root cause of most chronic conditions is inflammation. There is evidence that this is the case for heart disease, obesity, and diabetes. To address inflammation, clinicians need to address lifestyle. Specifically, exercise, diet, sleep, and stress reduction can help lower inflammation. This means that to help tackle the epidemics of diabetes, obesity, and even dementia, which is also considered to be related to inflammation, clinicians need to empower people to start enjoying regular movement, nourishing foods, sound sleep, and stress resilience techniques like deep breathing, meditating, mindfulness-based stress reduction, yoga, Tai Chi, and other activities that connect breathing and deliberate body movements. The key here is empowering. Empowering people means equipping them not just with knowledge but also with know-how. The know-how includes strategies and tools. Inspiring and motivating people to change is complex and multifactorial as the chapters in this book have clearly demonstrated.

Recent statistics about chronic conditions and lifestyle factors contributing to disease are alarming. They can propel healthcare professionals into action. They may even propel patients into action. However, it is not just the field of medicine that can use the expertise of behavior change, although that is the main target audience for this book. As mentioned in the introduction to the book chapter, teachers, parents, grandparents, clergy, rabbis, friends, partners of loved ones, and even strangers who are having conversations with people looking to change behaviors can utilize the principles and strategies in this book to empower people and accompany them on their journey of change. The COACH Approach™ is a mindset that can be so powerful.[1] Add a COACH Approach™ to behavior change strategies outlined in this book and you have a recipe for a comfortable, collaborative conversation about ways to tackle change.

Many people feel that educating, demanding, threatening, advising, bullying, scaring, or wrestling people are all required in the process of change, but these are far from needed. Education, information, and at times advising may be useful. However, the other strategies in the list do not work. They do not empower people. They do not inspire people. They do not motivate people. In fact, they can build resistance. What does work? A few actions that empower people to change include caring, listening, honoring, respecting, guiding, brainstorming, identifying strengths, using strengths, appreciating, and believing in them. As Dr. Dean Ornish says love is one of the most powerful motivators. Fear may work for a short time, but it is not sustainable. Love is sustainable.

There are many opportunities to use behavior change techniques. They can be used by healthcare professionals in the primary care setting, the rehabilitation setting, the cardiovascular health setting, cancer setting, endocrinology specialty, respiratory medicine setting, nephrology clinics, and even in the ER. It is best used for the care of people with chronic conditions. People with chronic conditions are also present in the ER, and the ER visit might well be the time and place for a behavior change conversation. People are often vulnerable and open to change after a health setback. This is often a good time to connect with a health coach or behavior change specialists. Taking the opportunity to counsel patients on healthy lifestyles prior to any chronic conditions developing is optimal. Working with patients in primary care during wellness visits provides an opportunity to address the pillars of lifestyle medicine including physical activity, nutrition, sleep, stress resilience, positive social connection, and avoidance of risky substances. Pediatricians are uniquely positioned to help young people adopt and sustain healthy lifestyles starting from a young age. Family physicians have the benefit of being able to work with parents, children, and, in some cases, grandparents. Teachers in elementary school, middle school, high school, and college can help too. The Teen Lifestyle Medicine Handbook can be useful for parents and teachers alike.[2] There is a Lifestyle Medicine 101 Curriculum at American College of Lifestyle Medicine and a Teen Curriculum available to download. Both curricula include PowerPoints, syllabi, teachers' manuals, quizzes, handbooks.

Behavior change techniques are used in many ways. Some healthcare professionals need training for proficiency in motivational interviewing. Some clinicians need to focus on using patience and empathy when listening to patients. Some clinicians need to shift their attitudes from expert to coach. When clinicians take the time to reflect on their own behaviors and counseling practices, they can identify areas of strength and areas of weakness. A good strategy is to choose one area of behavior change counseling and build competency in it.

Physicians, nurses, nurse practitioners, physician assistants, social workers, therapists, physical therapists, occupational therapists, psychology therapists, dentists, personal fitness trainers, psychiatrists, behavior change specialists, nurse's aides, teachers, parents, people in relationships, nutrition specialists like registered dietitians, and basically everyone can benefit from having a better understanding of behavior change. Medical students and students in a variety of healthcare professions can benefit from this knowledge. They are the healthcare leaders of the future. Take this opportunity to share your new found knowledge with anyone who you think might benefit.

Clinicians will know that they are using empowering behavior change techniques when people report change, they witness the changes themselves, or the tracking devices the person is using indicate behavior change. Lab results might also reveal the power of these changes. For example, inflammatory markers may be reduced with a whole-food plant-predominant diet. Cholesterol levels can also change with diet changes. Vitamin D levels may rise with time in sunshine (be careful of melanoma so use sunscreen and avoid 12–2 pm sun), dietary changes like adding mushrooms or taking Vitamin D supplements when indicated. Other indicators of change may be lowered blood pressure from exercising regularly or lowering sodium in the diet. Mental health self-report questionnaires may demonstrate significant changes. Perceived stress questionnaires, Hamilton Depression scores, wellbeing questionnaires, and the PAVING the Path to Wellness questionnaire can all be useful. The goal is to increase life satisfaction.

Behavior change is a process for patients and healthcare professionals. It can be a joyful journey. This book can serve as a guide for clinicians working with people to change behavior. It can be read all at once or in sections. There are opportunities to practice the skills and techniques described in these chapters throughout the day at work or even at home. There are online and live courses available for physicians where they can earn CME (Continuing Medical Education) credit for their professional development and learning, and the same or similar courses are available for other healthcare professionals to earn CE (Continuing Education) credits. There are also courses online that do not offer CME credit but may be effective for learning motivational interviewing or reviewing some of the theories presented in this book. For example, ProChange's website (www.prochange.com) is useful and convenient to review the Transtheoretical Model of Change in Chapter 2. Webinars serve to help keep clinicians up to date. Listening to webinars and podcasts on behavior change can help clinicians to learn new theories and skills. There are a number of useful books on this topic too.

Questions to Revisit from the Introduction to this Book Front Matter

1. Before reading this book, you were asked these questions. Take a look at them again now. List behavior change theories you know now.
2. Identify behavior change strategies that you know work for you and those that do not, and
3. List questions you currently have about behavior change.

15.2 THE 13 KEYS TO BEHAVIOR CHANGE

15.2.1 Introduction to Behavior Change: The Patient's Agenda Is the Guide

Effective behavior change counseling relies upon several important factors including coaching. The Frates COACH Approach™ provides a structure of collaboration founded upon respect for the patient's goals and desires. It requires openness, supports growth and learning for both the clinician and the patient. The mnemonic stands for curiosity, openness, appreciation, compassion, and honesty. Landmark and review studies on coaching and health promoting behavior change in areas including cardiac and chronic disease, cardiovascular risk, and diabetes reveal that coached patients exercised more, lost more weight, and achieved lower cholesterol levels than those who did not receive coaching.

15.2.2 WORK WITH THE PATIENT'S STAGE OF CHANGE (PROCHASKA)

Striving to achieve or maintain good health requires adopting healthy habits associated with diet, exercise, smoking cessation, healthy eating, and stress management. Distress experienced by many often derails behavior change goals. The Transtheoretical Model of Behavior Change (TTM) is a tool used to identify stages within the change process. TTM allows healthcare professionals to identify a patient's level of readiness for behavior change through the stages of Precontemplation (not ready to take action), Contemplation (getting ready), Preparation (ready), Action (meeting the healthy behavior change criteria), and Maintenance (keeping up the healthy behavior change). TTM then provides principles and processes of change interventions matched to each stage of change. Self-efficacy is an important component of behavior change throughout the Transtheoretical Model of Behavior Change.

15.2.3 BUILD PATIENT CONFIDENCE

Confidence, or *self-efficacy*, is the belief that one can behave in a way that will successfully produce desired outcomes. It is important that clinicians motivate patients and build confidence in their ability to adopt a healthy behavior change. However, several challenges to building patient confidence are faced throughout the patient-clinician relationship, which can occur during all phases of the behavior change process. To help, clinicians may approach building self-efficacy in patients by providing and/or modifying appropriate lifestyle prescriptions using four key principles for building confidence: (1) mastery experience, (2) vicarious experience, (3) verbal persuasion, and (4) emotional arousal. Clinicians are also challenged to build their own confidence through continued education. Chapter 3 provides practical application suggestions and case studies to help you get started.

15.2.4 TAP INTO THE PATIENT'S MOTIVATION

Building self-efficacy and confidence requires the acknowledgment that there is no one-size-fits-all approach to behavior change. It also requires collaboration between the clinician's expertise in health and patient's expertise in the self, supported by the platform of motivational interviewing (MI). MI allows the clinician to transfer responsibility for goal achievement with the highest regard for the patient's expertise. This allows patients to build confidence by using their own wisdom for problem solving and take ownership in their behavior change successes.

15.2.5   HONOR THE PATIENT'S AUTONOMY

Self-determination theory (SDT) informs us of the three basic psychological needs (autonomy, competence, and relatedness) that affect patients' internal motivation.[3] Consideration of SDT's three basic needs helps healthcare professionals identify and promote the patient motivators. SDT also helps healthcare professionals support patient goals and autonomy and identify strengths to build competence and confidence needed to achieve and sustain healthy behavior change. Interventions with a relatedness component within community settings support intrinsic motivation needed to promote healthy behavior change.[4] SDT provides a framework for motivation where clinicians partner with patients as coaches as opposed to providing advice in the role of expert.

15.2.6   APPRECIATE THE POSITIVE AND WHAT IS WORKING WELL

Healthcare professionals, trained to solve problems of life and death, often carry this approach into non-life threatening situations. One such instance is health behavior change. Behavior change interventions benefit from appreciative inquiry, empowering the patient toward goal setting and self-efficacy. Appreciative inquiry enhances the patient-clinician relationship by acknowledging the power of beliefs, words, vision, capacities, and patient focused action. Appreciative inquiry uses query to promote patient discovery and behavior change. It is used to guide patients to build upon their own self-determined approaches to change through appreciation of what is working well.

15.2.7   CO-CREATE GOALS WITH THE PATIENT

Goal setting is commonly cited in the research on the topic of behavior change.[5] It sets the foundation for both action planning and goal achievement. Goal setting should be conducted collaboratively with the patient to ensure that patient specific factors are evaluated and considered. Co-creating goals with the patient incorporates patients' expertise on self and includes consideration of readiness to change. This ensures contemplation of patients' life span status and overall function. Development of action goals that position the patient for success rests upon the patients' motives for behavior change. Patient-driven goals support increased buy-in and perception of ownership in health outcomes. Patient motivation for healthy behavior change is subjective. Co-creation of goals acknowledges factors that the patient deems as important and uses those values to build and support motivation.

15.2.8   MAINTAIN MOTIVATION

Motivation is a complex, dynamic, and ambivalent driver of behavior and behavior change. Maintaining motivation is a critical focus for the clinician who must embrace its fluctuating, waning, and fluid nature. Exploration of intrinsic and extrinsic motivators increases awareness, collaboration, and creativity for both the clinician and patient. MI helps clinicians prioritize the use of compassion and empathy to meet the patient where they are in their change process and maintain motivation. When patient motivation wanes, clinicians may reflect on whether they have reverted into fixing mode. Clinicians' focus on maintaining motivation strengthens the coaching relationship and improves patient and clinician outcomes.

15.2.9 OVERCOME OBSTACLES

Obstacles or barriers to health-related behavior change are commonly experienced by patients, such as lack of motivation, lack of time, lack of interest, mismatched stage interventions, and so on.[6,7] However, such obstacles are difficult to overcome due to their complexity and uniqueness to each patient. Thus, identification of individual barriers is a patient-centered process that respects the patient's expertise and experiences. This chapter provides practical insights for key steps and tips to help identify and overcome obstacles to healthy living, such as action planning, help sheets, providing feedback, and preparing lifestyle prescriptions that honor patient goals, priority, and preference. Clinician check-ins improve accountability and allow for real-time problem solving.

15.2.10 IDENTIFY AND USE THE PATIENT'S STRENGTHS

The process of self-regulation includes monitoring and redirecting behavior toward goals and lifestyle prescriptions. During this process, patients are guided to embrace flexibility as they plan, monitor, persevere, and inhibit behavior goal directed behavior. The self-regulation process is depicted as a series of gears representing skills and abilities including action and coping planning, emotional regulation, cognitive reframing, and self-talk. Clinicians add oil to the series of gears by aiding the patient throughout the behavior change process. Identification of patient strengths provides input for lifestyle prescriptions. Clinician awareness of patient attitudes toward their health diagnoses and health behaviors provides feedback for lifestyle prescriptions that meet the patient where they are. Allowing the patient to choose components of lifestyle prescriptions supports patient autonomy, which is a key predictor of healthy lifestyle adoption. Clinician flexibility requires an awareness of patient strengths and willingness to use this information to guide prescription activities. Prescription of exercise perceived as moderate by the patient helps build self-regulation skills and allows the patient to adjust intensity during exercise based on mood and energy levels. Focus on strengths, not deficits, includes the use of positive wording intended to motivate the patient.

15.2.11 SET ACCOUNTABILITY

Accountability is the acceptance of responsibility for one's actions. It is often conceptualized as being other-focused, such as to an accountability partner. As a partnership, it opens the door for positive judgment or praise and therefore also has the potential for negative judgment. Accountability is understood with a focus on autonomy as a primary human need and driver of behavior change, where external motivators are less likely to result in lasting behavior change. Viewed on a continuum, controlled accountability or external motivation rests on one end with autonomous accountability vested solely in the individual on the other end. The patient–clinician collaboration must provide an environment of safety in which patients can honestly share their experiences of behavioral change progress. The process of behavior change accountability is further enhanced as the patient describes their goals to a significant person, writes and monitors goals. Patients can be encouraged throughout the behavior change process to develop their own autonomous accountability or "auto-countability."

15.2.12 ENJOY THE PROCESS AND FIVE-STEP CYCLE OF COLLABORATION FOR BEHAVIOR CHANGE

Chronic disease diagnoses share a factor of behavior or lifestyle. The chapters of this book inform on evidence and theory of behavior change in lifestyle medicine. It is not difficult to inform patients of the guidelines for lifestyle changes needed to combat chronic disease. However, behavior change recommendations for lifestyle change may be difficult to adopt. The five-step cycle combines information discussed throughout this book to provide a guide for behavior change coaching. The five-step cycle uses empathy, aligning motivation, building confidence, setting smart stage-based goals, and setting accountability. The cycle helps to move practitioners from the EXPERT Approach ™ to the COACH Approach™. This cycle of patient-clinician collaboration is critical to paving the path to healthy behavior change.[8]

15.2.13 HARNESS THE POWER OF SOCIAL CONNECTION THROUGH GROUP INTERVENTIONS

Group interventions usually involve interactions with 8–12 patients per session. Some are led by mental health and other professionals functioning as educational or support groups. Group lifestyle medicine interventions are led by a physicians or other healthcare professionals focusing on specific chronic diseases. These group healthcare interventions also called group consultation models are classified by access, chronic care, and both access and chronic care. Access types include cluster visits or drop-in group medical appointments. Chronic care consultation models include shared medical appointments (SMAs), cooperative healthcare clinics, group lifestyle medicine interventions, and group visits. Models including both access and chronic care include class methods and group clinics. The recent pandemic introduced virtual group consultations to patient care resulting in hybrid models joined in person by some and virtually by others. Research reveals that these types group interventions improve health outcomes, lower hemoglobin A1c, reduce emergency room visits and patient healthcare costs.[9,10,11] Factors found to improve outcomes include a good facilitator, a focus on the process of change, and peer support as discussed in Chapter 13. Group interventions create connections in five areas: participant with the self, participant with facilitator, participant with individual participants, and participant with the whole group.

Table 15.1 provides key takeaway points from each chapter.

For further study, readers can access the recommended book in Table 15.2. This table provides examples of further reading for those looking for more material on the topics presented here.

TABLE 15.1
Main Takeaway Points from Each Chapter in the Book

13 Keys to Behavior Change

1. The patient's agenda is the guide	The COACH approach uses the patient's agenda to guide behavior change
2. Work with the patient's stage of change	Working with the patient's stage of change is essential to behavior change coaching. The Transtheoretical Model of Behavior Change is used to identify the patient's readiness for change and provides stage matched interventions to guide the patient through the stages of change
3. Build self-efficacy and confidence	Practitioners approach building self-efficacy in patients by prescribing lifestyle prescriptions for obesity, healthy eating, physical activity, and medication adherence throughout the change process. Confidence building occurs through mastery experience, vicarious experience, verbal persuasion, and emotional arousal
4. Tap into the patient's motivation	Collaboration between the practitioner and patient is strengthened with motivational interviewing (MI). MI acknowledges the patient's expertise and transfers ownership for behavior change to the patient
5. Honor the patient's autonomy	Recognizing the importance of patient autonomy to motivation guides practitioners to support patient goals. Practitioners identify patient strengths to build confidence and competence
6. Appreciate the positive and what is working well	Appreciative inquiry empowers the patient to take the lead in goal setting and problem solving with a focus on what is working or what has worked well in the past
7. Co-create goals with the patient	Co-creation of goals acknowledges the patient's expertise and values and uses that knowledge to build and support motivation
8. Maintain motivation	As practitioners, your focus on maintaining motivation improves the coaching relationship and patient outcomes. When motivation wanes, this requires reflection on whether you have reverted back into fixing mode
9. Overcome obstacles	Action planning helps overcome obstacles in a way that honors the patient's expertise. Consistent check-ins with the patient allow for real-time problem solving and provide accountability
10. Identify and use the patient's strengths	Identifying and using patient strengths sets the patient up to self-regulate goal-oriented activities. Using an exercise prescription, patients can self-regulate by gradually increasing the intensity of their exercise regime
11. Set accountability	Set accountability – The practitioner–patient relationship engages accountability in goal setting and achievement. Psychological safety is important as the patient is guided toward mastery of self-regulation and competency. Behavior change accountability is enhanced as the patient shares, writes, and monitors goals
12. Enjoy the process and five-step cycle of collaboration for behavior change	The five-step cycle uses empathy, aligning motivation, building confidence, setting smart goals, and setting accountability to move practitioners from the EXPERT approach to the COACH approach. This cycle of provider–patient collaboration is critical to paving the path to healthy behavior change
13. Group interventions and social support	Use group interventions and social support to power behavior change

TABLE 15.2
Examples of Further Reading Options

Topic	Book
Appreciative inquiry	*The Power of Appreciative Inquiry: A Practical Guide to Positive Change.* Whitney, D., and Trosten-Bloom, A. Berrett-Koehler Publishers. 2010
Appreciative inquiry	*Appreciative Inquiry: Change at the Speed of Imagination.* Magruder Watkins, J., Mohr, B., and Kelly, R. A Willey Company. 2001
Behavior change	*The Power of Habit: Why We Do What We Do in Life and Business.* Duhigg, C. Random House. 2014
Behavior change	*Changing for Good.* Prochaska J., Norcross J., and DiClemente C. Avon Books, 1995. *Changing to Thrive.* Prochaska, J. O. and Prochaska, J. M. Hazelden Publishing. 2016.
Behavior change	*Tiny Habits: The Small Changes That Change Everything.* Fogg, B. J. Houghton Mifflin Harcourt. 2020
Behavior change	*Atomic Habits: An Easy & Proven Way to Build Good Habits & Break Bad Ones.* Penguin: Avery. James Clear.
Behavior change	*How We Change: (And Ten Reasons Why We Don't).* Ellenhorn, R. Little, Brown Book Group. 2020
Behavior change	*Switch: How to Change Things When Change Is Hard.* Heath, C., Heath, D. Broadway Books. 2010
Behavior change	*Nudge: The Final Edition: Improving Decisions about Money, Health, and the Environment.* Thaler, R., Sunstein, R. 2021
Behavior change	*The Handbook of Behavior Change.* Hagger, M., Cameron, L. Cambridge University Press. 2020
Behavior change	*Social Learning Theory.* Bandura, A. J. Prentice Hall. 1977
Behavior change	*Self-Efficacy.* Bandura, A. W.H. Freeman and Company. 1997
Behavior change	*Principles of Behaviour Modification.* Bandura, A. Holt, Rinehart, and Winston. 1969
Behavior change	*Self-Determination Theory: Basic Psychological Needs in Motivation, Development, and Wellness.* Ryan, R. M., & Deci, E. L. 2017
Behavior change	*Why We Do What We Do: The Dynamics of Personal Autonomy.* Deci, E., & Flaste, R. Putnam's Sons. 1995
Behavior change	*On Second Thought: How Ambivalence Shapes Your Life.* Miller, W. Guilford Press. 2021
Behavior change	*The Joy Choice: How to Finally Achieve Lasting Changes in Eating and Exercise.* Segar, M. Hagette Book Group. 2022.
Behavior change/ coaching	*The Professional's Guide to Health and Wellness Coaching. American Council on Exercise.* Editors: Matthews, Bryant, Skinner & Green. 2019.
Coaching	*Helping People Change: Coaching with Compassion for Lifelong Learning and Growth.* Boyatzis, R., Smith, M., Van Oosten, E. Harvard Business Review Press. 2019.
Coaching	*Masterful Health and Wellness Coaching: Deepening Your Craft.* Arloski, M. Whole Person Associates. 2021.
Coaching	*How to Be a Health Coach: An Integrative Wellness Approach.* 3rd Edition. Jordan, M. Global Medicine Enterprises, Incorporated. 2022.

(Continued)

TABLE 15.2 (*Continued*)
Examples of Further Reading Options

Topic	Book
Coaching	*Coaching Psychology Manual*: Second Edition. Moore, M. Wolters Kluwer. 2015.
Coaching	*Coaching for Health: Why It Works and How to Do It*. Maini, A., A. Rogers, J. McGraw-Hill Education. 2016.
Coaching	*Coaching Questions: A Coach's Guide to Powerful Asking Skills*. Stoltzfus, T. 2008.
Coaching	*Developing Coaching Skills: A Concise Introduction*. Sternad, D. Econcise Publishing. 2021
Coaching	*The HeART of Laser-Focused Coaching: A Revolutionary Approach to Masterful Coaching*. Franklin, M. Thomas Noble Books. 2019
Group visits	*Running Group Visits in Your Practice*. Noffsinger, E. Springer. 2009
Health equity	*Health Equity: A Solutions-Focused Approach*. 1st Edition. K. Bryant Smalley, Jacob Warren, M. Isabel Fernandez. Springer Publishing. 2021
Lifestyle medicine	*PAVING the Path to Wellness: The Guide to a Healthy Body, Peaceful Mind, and Joyful Heart*. Frates, B., Tollefson, and M., Commander A. Healthy Learning. 2022
Lifestyle medicine	*Lifestyle Medicine Handbook*. 2nd Edition. Frates, B., Bonnet, J., Joseph, R., & Peterson, J. Healthy Learning. 2021
Lifestyle medicine	*Lifestyle Medicine*. 3rd Edition. Rippe, J. M. CRC Press. 2019.
Lifestyle medicine	*The Blue Zones, Second Edition: 9 Lessons for Living Longer from the People Who've Lived the Longest*. Buettner, D. National Geographic. 2012.
Lifestyle medicine	*Undo It!: How Simple Lifestyle Changes Can Reverse Most Chronic Diseases*. Ornish, D., Ornish, A. Random House Publishing Group. 2022.
Motivational interviewing	*Motivational Interviewing: Helping People Change*. 3rd Edition. Miller, W. R., & Rollnick, S. Guilford Press. 2013.
Self-care	*Harvard Medical School Special Health Report. Self-Care: A Step-by-Step Wellness Plan for Body, Mind, and Spirit*. Harvard Health Publishing. Harvard Medical School.
Self-efficacy	*Bandura A. Self-Efficacy: The Exercise of Control*. WH Freeman, 1997.

Now complete these same questions that you answered when you started this book. Compare your answers. What's different? What concepts do you want to continue exploring?

15.3 QUESTIONS TO PONDER NOW THAT YOU COMPLETED THE BOOK

Behavior Change Theories I know now:

Behavior Change Strategies I know that work:

Behavior Change Strategies I know that do not work:

Questions that I still have about Behavior Change:

This ends your learning journey with the book. By buying this book, you have joined a community of learners and teachers who are passionate about helping people to adopt and sustain change leading them to healthier practices and patterns. Thank you for joining this important journey. We look forward to hearing about your experience with this book. Feel free to contact Beth Frates with suggestions or comments (www.bethfratesmd.com).

REFERENCES

1. Frates, B., Bonnet, J., Joseph, R., & Peterson, J. (2020). *Lifestyle Medicine Handbook: An Introduction to the Power of Healthy Habits.* Healthy Learning, Monterey, CA.
2. Frates, B., Plaven, B., Agarwal, N., Dalal, M., & Tollefsen, K. (2020). *Teen Lifestyle Medicine Handbook: The Power of Healthy Habits.* Healthy Learning, Monterey, CA.
3. Ryan, R. M., & Deci, E. L. (2017). *Self-Determination Theory: Basic Psychological Needs in Motivation, Development, and Wellness.* Guilford Publishing, New York.
4. Ntoumanis, N., Ng, J. Y. Y., Prestwich, A., Quested, E., Hancox, J. E., Thøgersen-Ntoumani, C., Deci, E. L., Ryan, R. M., Lonsdale, C., & Williams, G. C. (2021). A meta-analysis of self-determination theory-informed intervention studies in the health domain: Effects on motivation, health behavior, physical, and psychological health. *Health Psychology Review, 15*(2), 214–244. https://doi.org/10.1080/17437199.2020.1718529.
5 Michie, S., Richardson, M., Johnston, M., Abraham, C., Francis, J., Hardeman, W., Eccles, M. P., Cane, J., & Wood, C. E. (2013). The behavior change technique taxonomy (v1) of 93 hierarchically clustered techniques: Building an international consensus for the reporting of behavior change interventions. *Annals of Behavioral Medicine: A Publication of the Society of Behavioral Medicine, 46*(1), 81–95. https://doi.org/10.1007/s12160-013-9486-6.
6. Joseph, R. P., Ainsworth, B. E., Keller, C., & Dodgson, J. E. (2015). Barriers to physical activity among African American women: An integrative review of the literature. *Women & Health, 55*(6), 679–699. https://doi.org/10.1080/03630242.2015.1039184.
7. Kelly, S., Martin, S., Kuhn, I., Cowan, A., Brayne, C., & Lafortune, L. (2016). Barriers and facilitators to the uptake and maintenance of healthy behaviours by people at mid-life: A rapid systematic review. *PLOS ONE, 11*(1), e0145074. https://doi.org/10.1371/journal.pone.0145074.
8. Frates, E. P., Moore, M. A., Lopez, C. N., & McMahon, G. T. (2011). Coaching for behavior change in physiatry. *American Journal of Physical Medicine & Rehabilitation, 90*(12), 1074–1082. https://doi.org/10.1097/PHM.0b013e31822dea9a.
9. Jaber, R., Braksmajer, A., & Trilling, J. S. (2006). Group visits: A qualitative review of current research. *Journal of the American Board of Family Medicine: JABFM, 19*(3), 276–290. https://doi.org/10.3122/jabfm.19.3.276.
10. Moitra, E., Sperry, J. A., Mongold, D., et al. (2011). A group medical visit program for primary care patients with chronic pain. *Professional Psychology: Research and Practice, 42*(2), 153–159. https://doi.org/10.1037/a0022240.
11. Housden, L., Wong, S. T., & Dawes, M. (2013). Effectiveness of group medical visits for improving diabetes care: A systematic review and meta-analysis. *Canadian Medical Association Journal, 185*, E635–E644.

Index

Note: **Bold** page numbers refer to tables; *italic* page numbers refer to figures.

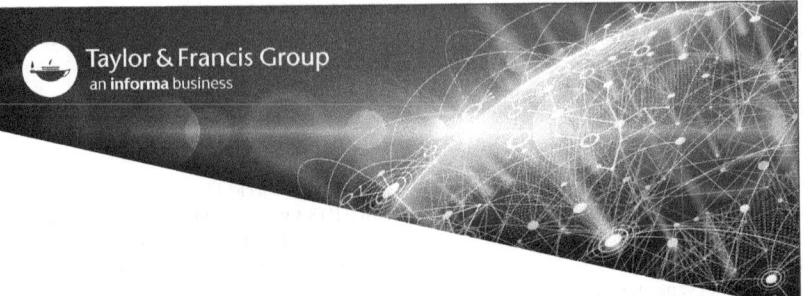
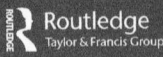
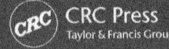